Surgical Anatomy
and Pathology
for Orthopaedic Surgeons

Surgical Anatomy and Pathology for Orthopaedic Surgeons

John V. Fowles, M.B., B.S. (Lond.), F.R.C.S.(C.)

Professeur Adjoint de Clinique
Département de Chirurgie
Université de Montréal, Montréal

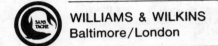

WILLIAMS & WILKINS
Baltimore/London

Library of Congress Cataloging in Publication Data

Fowles, John V.
  Surgical anatomy and pathology for orthopaedic surgeons.

  Bibliography: p.
  Includes index.
  1. Anatomy, Surgical and topographical. 2. Pathology. 3. Orthopaedic surgery. I. Title. [DNLM: 1. Musculoskeletal system—Anatomy and histology. 2. Orthopaedics. 3. Pathology, Surgical. WE 168 F789s]
  QM531.F74   617   82-7103
  ISBN 0-683-03317-4   AACR2

Composed and printed at the
Waverly Press, Inc.
Mt. Royal and Guilford Aves.
Baltimore, MD 21202, U.S.A.

To Deirdre,
    Because you were there during the difficult times.

Preface

This book on surgical anatomy and approaches and general surgical pathology is written mainly for orthopaedic and general surgical residents in their last two years of training. Practicing surgeons may also find the notes useful as an *aide mémoire*.

The book is not a textbook and should not be used as such. The reader will get the most out of it only if he already has a good working knowledge of the subject. A list of textbooks for further reading will be found at the end of this book.

The brief, lecture note style of writing, and the pocket format, will enable the resident to revise quickly the major points of these subjects while waiting for a bus or a friend, an attribute that may be particularly useful just before exams! The line drawings are easy to reproduce on paper or blackboard and may be colored in this book to facilitate differentiation of structures. The reader may also wish to annotate the text by adding or underlining facts that he considers important.

John V. Fowles

Acknowledgments

This book evolved over a period of several years of teaching in Montreal and with CARE-MEDICO in Tunisia and Afghanistan. The stimulus for the book came from the medical students, residents and surgeons themselves who were enthusiastic, quick to learn, and worked hard, often under very difficult circumstances. These men and women have earned my admiration and respect, and my gratitude for all that they have taught me.

I received a great deal of support from CARE doctors, volunteers and administrative staff alike, both abroad and at home, and I would like to thank them all for their help, understanding and patience. I would also like to thank Gerda Zaiane in Tunis, Belkise Shah in Kabul, and Carol-Ann Paul and Suzan Senechal in Montreal, for interpreting my handwriting and typing the various stages of the manuscript.

Finally, I am indebted to Frank Stansfield at the Royal College of Surgeons of England, and Alan W. Harrison at Toronto University, who showed me that anatomy and pathology could be fun.

Contents

PART I   **SURGICAL ANATOMY**

PART II   GENERAL SURGICAL PATHOLOGY

chapter 1

Posterior Triangle, Axilla and Brachial Plexus

Surgical Anatomy

POSTERIOR TRIANGLE OF THE NECK

Borders

- anterior border, the posterior edge of the sternocleidomastoid (SCM) muscle,
- posterior border, the anterior edge of trapezius and the
- inferior border (base), the middle third of the clavicle.
- the apex is posterior, the base is anterior.

Structures superficial to triangle

- skin, subcutaneous fat and platysma lie over the
- adipose tissue; this is crossed by supraclavicular sensory branches of the cervical plexus (C2, C3, C4);
- external jugular vein descends vertically in front of the SCM, then goes deep to pierce the cervical fascia, crosses the anterior corner of the triangle and drains into the subclavian vein.

Roof

- formed by cervical fascia (investing layer) which envelopes the SCM and trapezius muscles and is stretched between these muscles across the triangle.

Contents

- adipose tissue and lymph glands;

- omohyoid muscle runs across the anterior corner of the triangle, deep to clavicle and SCM, and is enveloped by septum from investing layer of cervical fascia;
- accessory nerve (cranial nerve XI and C1 to C5) from beneath SCM passes down and back to trapezius and supplies both muscles;
- supraclavicular nerves before they pierce the investing fascia;
- superficial transverse cervical artery from thyrocervical trunk passes between omohyoid and scalenus anterior, then posteriorly over scapular notch to supraspinatus and infraspinatus muscles;
- external jugular vein as it drains into subclavian vein.

Floor

- formed from above downwards by
  —levator scapulae
  —scalenus posterior
  —scalenus medius and
  —scalenus anterior;
- all three scalenes originate from cervical vertebrae; the latter two insert into the first rib, the posterior into the second rib;
- subclavian artery—lies on first rib, between anterior and middle scalenes, then becomes the axillary artery and crosses anterior corner of triangle to pass behind clavicle and into axilla;
- subclavian vein, below and in front of artery, crosses first rib in front of scalenus anterior, so that this muscle separates the vein from the artery. This vein is a continuation of axillary vein;
- trunks of brachial plexus, above and behind the artery;
- phrenic nerve lies on anterior surface of scalenus anterior, crossing from lateral to medial as the nerve descends.
- these structures are stuck down on the muscular floor by the prevertebral fascia.

AXILLA

Boundaries

- shaped like a pyramid with four walls and a base.
  Anterior wall
  - two pectoral muscles and
  - clavipectoral fascia.
  Medial wall
  - serratus anterior.

Posterior wall, from above downwards

- subscapularis
- teres major and
- latissimus dorsi twisting beneath teres major. In this wall is the
- quadrilateral space of Velpeau, formed by
  —subscapularis above,
  —long head of triceps medially,
  —teres major below and
  —humerus laterally. This space provides an
  —exit for axillary nerve and posterior circumflex artery from the axilla.

Lateral wall

- humerus and
- coracobrachialis.

Base

- superficial and
- deep aponeurotic layers.

Contents

Axillary artery

- continuation of subclavian artery, enters apex of axilla, leaves it at lower border of teres major to become brachial artery;
- divided into three parts by pectoralis minor;
- surrounded by fascia, the axillary sheath, which also surrounds the brachial plexus in the axilla.
- major branches are
  —superior thoracic artery (from first part) to pectoral muscles;
  —acromiothoracic and lateral thoracic from second part, and
  —subscapular, anterior and posterior circumflex humeral arteries from third part. For more detail, see Chapter 2, "Pectoral Girdle and Shoulder."

Axillary vein

- lies medial to artery and brachial plexus and
- continues over first rib as subclavian vein.

Brachial plexus and branches

- see below and Figure 1.1.

Lymph nodes

- pectoral group lies on medial wall and drains

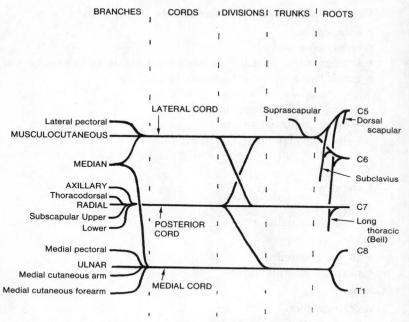

Figure 1.1. Diagram of brachial plexus.

—breast and
—upper, anterior trunk;
- scapular group on posteromedial wall of axilla, drains
  —tail of breast and
  —upper, posterior trunk;
- lateral group, medial to axillary vein, drains
  —upper limb;
- infraclavicular group, between pectoralis minor and deltoid, drains
  —upper part of breast;
- apical group, drains
  —all four groups mentioned above, and floor of axilla, and drains into
  —supraclavicular nodes in posterior triangle, thence into thoracic duct.

BRACHIAL PLEXUS (Fig. 1.1)

Roots

- anterior primary rami of C5, C6, C7, C8 and T1 lie between the scalenus anterior and medius muscles, beneath floor of posterior triangle.

Trunks

- at the lateral border of scalene muscles,
  - —C5 root joins C6 to form upper trunk,
  - —C7 continues as middle trunk,
  - —C8 joins T1 to form lower trunk.
- trunks lie in lower part of posterior triangle.

Divisions

- behind the clavicle, each trunk divides into an
  - —anterior and a
  - —posterior division to supply
  - —flexor and extensor muscle compartments, respectively.

Cords

- lie in the axilla;
- lateral cord, lying lateral to axillary artery, is formed by union of anterior divisions of upper and middle trunks;
- medial cord, lying medial to axillary artery, is formed from anterior division of lower trunk;
- posterior cord, lying posterior to axillary artery, is formed from union of all three posterior divisions.
- the cords
  - —approach first part of axillary artery (from lateral border of first rib to upper border of pectoralis minor),
  - —surround its second part (behind pectoralis minor) and
  - —give off their branches around the third part of the artery (from lower border of pectoralis minor to inferior border of teres major).

Branches

Branches from roots (3)

Dorsal scapular nerve (C5)

- goes posteriorly to supply rhomboids, and small branch to levator scapulae.

Nerve to subclavius (C5, C6)
- travels downward and forward to supply subclavius muscle.

Long thoracic nerve (C5, C6, C7)
- goes posteriorly to serratus anterior.

Branches from trunks (1)

- suprascapular nerve (C5, C6)
  - —arises from upper trunk (Erb's point) and
  - —goes posteriorly through suprascapular notch, beneath the fibrous band which bridges the notch; suprascapular artery goes over the bridge (Army over the bridge, Navy under it!). Nerve supplies supraspinatus,
  - —then turns around lateral end of scapular spine to infraspinatus.

Branches from divisions (0)

Branches from cords (13)

lateral cord (3)

Lateral pectoral nerve (C5, C6, C7)
- goes anteriorly to pectoralis major

Musculocutaneous (C5, C6, C7)
- to coracobrachialis, biceps, brachialis and to
- skin on lateral side of forearm.

Lateral head of median nerve (C5, C6, C7)

medial cord (5)

Medial pectoral nerve (C8, T1)
- goes anteriorly to pectoralis minor and pectoralis major.

Medial cutaneous nerve of arm (T1)
- to skin of distal half of medial side of arm.

Medial cutaneous nerve of forearm (C8, T1)

Ulnar nerve (C7, C8, T1)
- to flexor carpi ulnaris (C7), medial half of flexor digitorum profundus (C8) and intrinsics (T1).

Medial head of median nerve (C8, T1)
- crosses in front of third part of axillary artery to join lateral head of median nerve.

posterior cord (5)

Upper subscapular (C6)
- to subscapularis.

Thoracodorsal nerve (C6, C7, C8)
- to latissimus dorsi.

Lower subscapular (C6, C7)
- to teres major and subscapularis.

Axillary nerve (C5, C6)
- passes back, through quadrilateral space in posterior axillary wall, then laterally and anteriorly around surgical neck of humerus to supply
  —teres minor,
  —deltoid and
  —skin over deltoid.

Radial nerve (C5, C6, C7, C8, T1)
- leaves axilla by passing backwards through triangular space (teres major above, long head of triceps medially and humerus laterally) to wind posterolaterally around humeral shaft;
- in the axilla, radial nerve gives
  —motor branch to long head of triceps,
  —another to medial head of triceps (this branch accompanies ulnar nerve), and a
  —cutaneous branch, the posterior cutaneous nerve of the arm (contains all T1 fibers of radial nerve);
- ultimately supplies all extensor compartment muscles of arm and forearm.

Nerve root values of movements of upper limb
- shoulder
  C5—abduction and external rotation
  C6, C7, C8—adduction and internal rotation
- elbow
  C6, C7—flexion
  C7, C8—extension
- forearm rotation
  C6—supination
  C6—pronation
- wrist
  C6, C7—dorsiflexion
  C6, C7—palmar flexion
- fingers
  C7, C8—extension
  C7, C8—flexion
- hand intrinsics
  T1 (and C8 for thenar muscles)

- learn these, and you have a working knowledge of the root innervation of all upper limb muscles!

Injuries to the Plexus

- the plexus is stretched between two mobile segments, the cervical spine and the shoulder, and can be torn apart by violent injury to these segments.

UPPER PLEXUS INJURY

- C5, C6 and sometimes C7
- called Erb's paralysis;
- caused by traction due either to
  —birth trauma (breech) or
  —two-point landing (head and shoulder) from motorcycle.
- typical deformity (policeman's tip):
  —adduction and medial rotation of humerus (deltoid and lateral rotators paralyzed, C5)
  —extension of elbow (flexors paralyzed, C5, C6),
  —pronation of forearm (supinator paralyzed, C6) and
  —slight wrist flexion (wrist extensors paralyzed, C6, C7)
- if the following muscles are paralyzed:
  —serratus anterior,
  —levator scapulae and
  —rhomboids, then the lesion must involve the roots which are probably avulsed from the cord, and recovery is very unlikely;
- careful clinical examination is essential for a precise diagnosis;
- myelography may be helpful in establishing diagnosis and prognosis because traumatic meningoceles indicate root lesions;
- injury of the trunks has better prognosis than root injuries.

LOWER PLEXUS INJURY

- C8, T1 and sometimes C7
- Klumpke's paralysis;
- caused by traction during
  —birth injury (extended arms in breech),
  —fall onto outstretched arm or
  —arm pulled into machinery;

- paralysis involves
  —wrist and finger flexors (C6, C7, C8) and
  —all intrinsics of hand (C8, T1);
- if associated with Horner's syndrome
  —meiosis,
  —ptosis and
  —anhydrosis, then recovery is very unlikely because the roots are probably avulsed from the cord.

CORDS

- injuries usually caused by traction or penetrating injuries (gunshot, knife, road accident).

Lateral cord injury

- causes paralysis of:
  —biceps and brachialis (musculocutaneous nerve),
  —flexor carpi radialis and pronator teres (lateral head of median nerve);
- sensory loss of lateral side of forearm.

Posterior cord injury

- causes paralysis of:
  —internal rotation and abduction of humerus (axillary and subscapular nerves),
  —extension of elbow, wrist and metacarpophalangeal joints (radial nerve);
- sensory loss over shoulder, posterior part of arm and dorsum of first and second metacarpals and first web space.

Medial cord injury

- causes paralysis of:
  —flexors of the wrist (except flexor carpi radialis),
  —long flexors of fingers and
  —all intrinsic muscles of hand. Essentially, a combined median and ulnar nerve paralysis;
- sensory loss over:
  —front and medial side of arm,
  —medial side of forearm,
  —anterior surface of palm and fingers, and
  —posterior surface of palm and fingers except over first and second metacarpals and first web space.

Surgical Exploration

INDICATIONS

Open, penetrating wound

- an emergency if vascular injury is associated;
- primary (immediate) nerve repair is not recommended
  —wait until the wound is clean and closed.

Closed plexus injury

- repair of upper plexus gives better results than lower, but results are not good no matter where the injury.

COMPREHENSIVE SURGICAL APPROACH TO THE BRACHIAL PLEXUS

- this approach can be used in total or in part, depending on where the injury lies, and the approach is extensile (can be lengthened proximally or distally). Transverse incisions are not recommended because they cannot be lengthened.

Position of the patient

- on the back, a flat cushion between the shoulders,
- head turned to the opposite side with
- the arm free.

Skin incision (Fig. 1.2)

- starts 4 inches above clavicle, at anterior border of sternocleido-mastoid (SCM) muscle,
- goes laterally across the SCM muscle, parallel with the clavicle, then
- crosses the junction of middle and lateral thirds of the clavicle; the incision then
- follows the anterior border of the deltoid to the axilla and
- turns posteriorly for 2 inches, then distally.

Above the clavicle

- this is the posterior triangle.
- incise the subcutaneous tissue and platysma;
- ligate and divide the external jugular vein;
- cut the clavicular insertion of SCM;
- retract or cut omohyoid;
- ligate and cut the transverse cervical artery;
- retract the phrenic nerve medially, and
- cut, if necessary, the scalenus anterior.

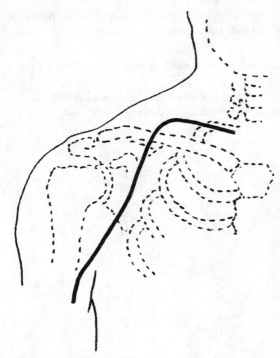

Figure 1.2. Comprehensive approach to the brachial plexus.

Below the clavicle
- the axilla.
- ligate and cut the cephalic vein;
- cut the pectoralis major tendon 1 cm from its insertion and retract it medially and distally;
- incise longitudinally the clavipectoral fascia;
- cut the pectoralis minor tendon;
- divide the clavicle in the middle with a Gigli saw and cut the tendon of subclavius;
- divisions of the plexus are visible behind clavicle,
- cords and branches visible in the axilla;
- retract
  —axillary vein laterally to see ulnar nerve,
  —axillary vein medially to see axillary artery,
  —axillary artery medially to see median nerve and

—axillary artery and vein, and the ulnar nerve laterally to see radial nerve (well posterior).

Closure

- plate on the clavicle, or threaded pins (not smooth pins because these migrate);
- resuture the muscles, platysma and skin, and apply
- Velpeau bandage, or spica, depending on the surgery.

chapter 2

Pectoral Girdle and Shoulder

Surgical Anatomy

JOINTS

- the pectoral girdle and shoulder have a complex of four joints.
  Scapulothoracic joint
  - the anterior surface of the scapula, embedded in muscles, slides on and around the muscle-covered posterolateral wall of the thorax.
  Acromioclavicular joint

  Articular surfaces
  - between the lateral end of the clavicle and the anteromedial part of the acromion.

  Ligaments
  - very strong;
  - acromioclavicular, blends with the superior part of the capsule;
  - coracoclavicular, in two separate parts
    —trapezoid from the stem of the coracoid process obliquely up and out to the anterolateral surface of the clavicle, and
    —conoid, short, thick and fan-shaped, from base of coracoid straight up to inferior surface of clavicle (conoid tubercle);
  - coracoacromial, forming an arch over the head of the humerus. Under this arch passes the tendon of supraspinatus.

  Movement
  - limited gliding
  Sternoclavicular joint

  Articular surfaces
  - medial end of clavicle articulates with the manubrium sterni and the first costal cartilage.

Ligaments

- anterior and posterior to manubrium;
- superior is very strong, blends with superior ligament of other side (interclavicular ligament);
- costoclavicular to first rib (strong).

Intra-articular disc (meniscus)

- attached above to the clavicle and below to first costal cartilage.

Relations

- sternohyoid and sternothyroid muscles immediately behind (posterior to) the joint;
- behind these muscles are the innominate vein and common carotid artery on left, bifurcation of innominate artery on right.

Movements

- gliding and rotation

Scapulohumeral joint

- this is a synovial ball and socket joint which is very shallow, is mobile, and has very little intrinsic stability.

Articular surfaces

- the glenoid cavity of the scapula looks upwards, laterally and 30° forwards. It is very shallow but is enlarged and deepened by the glenoid labrum, a fibrocartilaginous rim.
- the humeral head is one third of a sphere facing upwards, medially and 30° posteriorly;
- head/shaft angle is 130°;
- anatomical neck separates the head from the shaft, lies along the border of the articular cartilage, and forms an angle of 40° with the horizontal.

Stability of the joint

- depends on the capsule and ligaments (passive and weak) and muscles (active):

    Capsule
    - inserts around the edge of the glenoid labrum and around the superior part of the anatomical neck of the humerus; but
    - inferiorly the insertion lies nearer the surgical neck—the proximal humeral metaphysis is intracapsular here;
    - surgical neck lies horizontally at the level of the lesser tuberosity and the proximal growth plate.

Ligaments
- coracohumeral ligament
  —strongest of the ligaments;
- glenohumeral ligaments
  —these are three thickened bands in the front of the capsule,
  —superior (horizontal),
  —middle (oblique) and
  —inferior (horizontal) forming a Z.

Muscles
- short, stabilizing muscles arising from scapula; the tendons blend with the capsule, and form the rotator cuff:
  —subscapularis (anterior)
  —supraspinatus (superior)
  —infraspinatus (posterosuperior)
  —teres minor (posteroinferior).

Movements
- gliding and rotation.

MUSCLES

Muscles of pectoral girdle

Posterior group

Trapezius
- origin from skull (superior nuchal line), ligamentum nuchae (along tips of spines of cervical vertebrae), and all thoracic vertebral spines;
- inserted into lateral third of clavicle, acromion and spine of scapula above origin of deltoid;
- nerve supply is spinal accessory, C2, C3, C4;
- action is elevation of scapula and shoulder, and with serratus anterior it rotates the scapula.

Latissimus dorsi
- from spines of seventh to twelfth thoracic vertebrae, spines of all lumbar vertebrae, posterior part of iliac crest and inferior angle of scapula;
- runs laterally and twists around inferior border of teres major to form posterior wall of axilla, then
- inserts into floor of bicipital groove of humerus, between pectoralis major laterally and teres major medially (a lady between two majors);

- thoracodorsal nerve from posterior cord of brachial plexus, C6, C7, C8;
- adduction, internal (medial) rotation and extension of shoulder.

Levator scapulae
- from transverse processes of upper four cervical vertebrae;
- to upper quarter of medial border of scapula, above base of spine of scapula;
- special branches from cervical plexus, C3, C4, C5, and dorsal scapular nerve;
- pulls scapula medially and upwards, squares the shoulders.

Rhomboids
- from spines of C7 and T1 (minor) and T2 to T5 (major)
- to lower three quarters of medial border of scapula;
- dorsal scapular nerve, C5;
- action similar to levator scapulae.

Anterior group

Pectoralis major
- from medial half of clavicle, sternum and rectus abdominis aponeurosis;
- runs up and laterally, and tendon twists through 180° as it approaches humerus, so that lowest muscle fibers insert the highest; forms anterior wall of axilla;
- inserts into lateral lip of bicipital groove, covering long head of biceps;
- medial and lateral pectoral nerves, C6, C7, C8;
- adduction, flexion and internal (medial) rotation of arm.

Pectoralis minor
- from costochondral junction of third, fourth and fifth ribs;
- to medial border of coracoid;
- medial pectoral nerve, C8;
- depresses the shoulder, and with serratus anterior, it pulls scapula forwards around chest wall.

Serratus anterior
- from upper eight ribs anteriorly by interdigitations;
- to deep aspect of entire medial border of scapula;
- long thoracic nerve, C5, C6, C7;
- pulls scapula forwards and rotates it (push forward).

Muscles of shoulder joint

Subscapularis
- from entire surface of subscapular fossa of scapula;
- to lesser tuberosity of humerus;
- upper and lower subscapular nerves, C6, C7
- internal rotation of arm;
- bursa lies beneath this muscle and often communicates with synovial cavity of shoulder joint.

Supraspinatus
- from supraspinatus fossa of scapula;
- to superior facet on greater tuberosity of humerus;
- suprascapular nerve, C5;
- initiates abduction of shoulder.

Infraspinatus
- from infraspinous fossa;
- to middle facet of posterior surface of greater tuberosity;
- suprascapular nerve, C5;
- external (lateral) rotation of arm.

Teres minor
- from upper part of axillary border of scapula;
- to lowest facet of posterior surface of greater tuberosity;
- axillary nerve, C5;
- external rotation of arm.

Teres major
- from inferior angle of scapula;
- to medial lip of bicipital groove;
- lower subscapular nerve, C6, 7;
- internal rotation and adduction, and with teres minor, prevents upward movement of humeral head when shoulder is abducted.

Deltoid
- origin in three parts, from
  - —lateral third of clavicle,
  - —acromion (multipennate and very strong) and
  - —spine of scapula below insertion of trapezius;
- rounded shape of shoulder is due to deltoid over the humeral head;
- all three parts insert by common tendon into deltoid tuberosity on middle of lateral surface of humerus;

- axillary nerve, C5;
- action is threefold
  —central part abducts the arm after supraspinatus has started the movement;
  —anterior part flexes and
  —posterior part extends the arm, and both the anterior and posterior parts stabilize the humeral head in abduction;
- deltopectoral groove lies between deltoid and pectoralis major, and contains the cephalic vein.

ARTERIES AROUND THE SHOULDER

Subclavian branches

- thyrocervical trunk arises from first part of subclavian artery and divides into following branches:
  —transverse cervical divides into superficial branch to trapezius, deep branch to medial border of scapula and muscles;
  —suprascapular, with suprascapular nerve to supraspinous and infraspinous fossae and muscles, and
  —inferior thyroid.

Axillary branches

Second part of axillary artery:

Acromiothoracic (muscular)
- pierces clavipectoral fascia at upper border of pectoralis minor;
- four branches
  —acromial
  —deltoid
  —pectoral and
  —clavicular.

Lateral thoracic
- follows lower border of pectoralis minor;
- supplies pectoral muscles, serratus anterior and the breast.

Third part of axillary artery

Subscapular
- lies on posterior axillary wall, supplies
  —latissimus dorsi and
  —serratus anterior;
- circumflex scapular branch runs back through posterior wall to the

—subscapular and

—infraspinous fossae.

Posterior circumflex humeral

- accompanies axillary nerve posteriorly through the quadrilateral space,
- winds posteriorly then laterally around humerus 3 fingerbreadths below the acromion,
- supplies deltoid.

Anterior circumflex humeral

- small artery, runs around the front of surgical neck of humerus to supply muscles.

Arterial anastomoses

- around scapula and shoulder, branches from all these arteries anastomose with each other;
- this is an important anastomosis between branches of first part of subclavian and second and third parts of axillary arteries.

NERVES

- brachial plexus and its branches are in close association with the pectoral girdle and the shoulder joint;
- see Chapter 1.

MOVEMENTS OF SHOULDER

Normal range of motion

- arm at the side is starting position (zero)
- flexion: 180°
- extension: 30°
- abduction: 180°
- adduction: 30°
- external rotation: 80°
- internal rotation: 95° (the last 5° are important, for back scratching or zipping a zipper);
- circumduction—a combination of all the other movements.

Components of abduction

- first 60° of abduction is only in the scapulohumeral (SH) joint;
- the remaining 120° occurs equally in the SH and the scapulothoracic joints as the scapula slides forwards around the thorax and rotates upwards and laterally;
- during the last 90° of abduction, the humerus rotates 180° on its

axis to avoid impingement between the greater tuberosity and the acromion;

- clavicle rotates around its axis and is elevated 40°; this movement occurs mainly at the sternoclavicular joint.

Surgical Approaches

INDICATIONS

Anterior

- irreducible or recurrent anterior dislocation of the shoulder;
- anterior dislocation with fracture of the surgical neck;
- comminuted fracture of the humeral head and neck;
- soft tissue release and/or muscle transfer (Episcopo) for Erb's paralysis;
- arthroplasty;
- septic or TB arthritis, or osteomyelitis of proximal humerus.

Posterior

- irreducible or recurrent posterior dislocation of shoulder.

Acromioclavicular (AC)

- recent or old dislocation of the AC joint;
- internal derangement of the AC joint (meniscectomy).

APPROACHES

Anterior (Thompson-Henry) (Fig. 2.1)

- the major approach to the shoulder;
- this incision is extensile and can easily be lengthened distally and, with more difficulty, proximally.

Position

- patient supine (on back), cushion or sandbag behind the scapula, another beneath the buttock on affected side, the arm draped free; head turned away.

Skin incision

- starts at the acromioclavicular joint, continues
- medially just below and parallel to lateral third of clavicle, then at point just medial to tip of coracoid process the incision
- curves down and out to follow the deltopectoral groove to the point where the inferior border of deltoid crosses biceps.

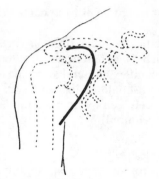

Figure 2.1. Anterior (Henry) approach.

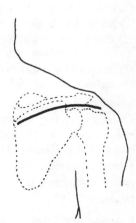

Figure 2.2. Posterior approach.

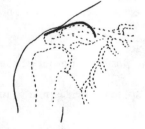

Figure 2.3. Robert's approach to the acromioclavicular joint.

Figures 2.1 to 2.3. Surgical approaches to the shoulder and acromioclavicular joints.

Dissection

- ligate and divide the cephalic vein and its tributaries;
- detach the anteromedial third of the deltoid by dividing it 1 cm from its clavicular origin;
- retract pectoralis major medially and deltoid laterally;
- for exposure of deep structures and the glenoid, drill a hole down the coracoid, then divide it with an osteotome and retract the attached muscles medially; or, divide pectoralis minor, cor-

acobrachialis and short head of biceps 1 cm from coracoid and retract them;
- incise subscapularis tendon vertically 2 cm from its insertion and likewise the capsule which is adherent to this tendon. Venous plexus and anterior circumflex humeral artery lie at the inferior border of the tendon and should be ligated first.
- joint and humeral head can be well seen by traction and lateral rotation of arm (good assistant required).

Closure
- screw coracoid or resuture muscles;
- with arm in internal (medial) rotation, overlap slightly and suture the subscapularis;
- then suture deep fascia and skin.

Posterior (Kocher) (Fig. 2.2)

Position
- patient semiprone (lying face down), cushion beneath chest and another beneath the pelvis on affected side, the arm draped free.

Incision
- starts lateral and just below the acromion,
- continues medially following the posterior border of the acromion, then
- parallel with and just below the spine of the scapula to its base.

Dissection
- detach posterior third of deltoid by dividing it 1 cm distal to its scapular origin;
- to avoid injury to the axillary nerve as it emerges from the quadrilateral space and enters the muscle, do not retract deltoid further distally than teres minor;
- to avoid injury to suprascapular nerve do not enter infraspinatus;
- expose the posterior joint capsule by retracting infraspinatus upward and teres minor downward, if necessary cutting these muscles 1 cm from their insertion into posterior surface of greater tuberosity.
- divide capsule vertically, parallel with and 1 cm lateral to the glenoid rim.

Closure
- resuture muscles with slight overlap, then
- fascia and skin.

Acromioclavicular (AC) approach (Roberts) (Fig. 2.3)

Position

- supine, cushion behind the shoulder, arm free, and patient's head turned to opposite side;
- surgeon sits at head of table.

Incision

- starts over lateral border of acromion, then
- medially over the AC joint and lateral quarter of the clavicle, then
- curves down for 1 inch.

Dissection

- expose capsule of AC joint and the coracoid by detaching the deltoid from the clavicle and anterior border of acromion, and gently retracting it distally (do not injure axillary nerve which adheres to its undersurface).

chapter 3

Arm and Elbow

Surgical Anatomy

HUMERUS

Important landmarks

Shape

- proximal end carries the head, anatomical and surgical necks, greater and lesser tuberosities, and is described in Chapter 2.
- shaft is triangular, apex anteriorly;
- distal third is flattened anteroposteriorly, and flares out medially and laterally into the epicondyles;
- distal epiphysis consists of
  —trochlea, shaped like an old-fashioned cotton reel, with a
  —lateral lip separating it from the hemispherical capitulum, and a
  —medial lip separating it from the large and prominent medial epicondyle (the funny bone!);
  —lateral epicondyle, on lateral side of capitulum, is small.
- nutrient foramen on anteromedial surface just below coracobrachialis insertion. Nutrient branch from brachial artery passes downward through cortex toward elbow.

Grooves

- spiral groove runs downwards and outwards around the posterior and lateral surfaces of the humerus;
  —separates origin of lateral head of triceps and deltoid insertion (above the groove) from the
  —medial head of triceps (below the groove);
  —radial nerve lies in the groove, in direct contact with bone.

- bicipital groove lies anteriorly on the proximal quarter of the shaft;
  —lesser trochanter lies medial to the upper end of this groove.

Muscle attachments

- proximal end, see Chapter 2.
- deltoid inserts into V-shaped tuberosity in the middle of the lateral surface;
- coracobrachialis inserts into medial surface opposite to and just below level of deltoid insertion;
- triceps by two heads from posterior surface;
- brachialis takes origin from distal half of anterior surface;
- extensor muscle origins along the lateral supracondylar ridge are, from above down,
  —brachioradialis;
  —extensor carpi radialis longus and
  —common extensor origin (extensor carpi radialis brevis, extensor digitorum communis, extensor carpi ulnaris and supinator);
- common flexor origin from front of medial epicondyle.

Ossification centers of proximal humerus

First appearance

- head at 1 year;
- greater tuberosity at 3 years, and
- lesser tuberosity at 5 years.

Fusion

- three secondary centers fuse together by the seventh year, and
- fuse with the shaft by the twentieth year.

Blood supply of a long bone

Periosteal supply

- periosteum contains mesh of small vessels and capillaries fed through attachments of surrounding muscles and sometimes by nearby arteries;
- supplies outer third of cortex through Volkmann's and Haversian canals.

Nutrient artery

- most long bones have only one nutrient artery. This

- pierces the cortex, divides into
  —ascending and descending branches in the medullary canal and forms
  —endosteal capillary network from which vessels radiate out through Volkmann's canals to connect with Haversian systems and supply
  —inner two thirds of cortex.
- either periosteal or nutrient system may take over supply of whole cortex if one or other system is damaged.
- direction of nutrient artery is usually away from the most active growth plate.

Metaphysis

- metaphyseal supply is by arterial and capillary loops from intramedullary and periosteal vessels as well as vessels which enter metaphysis from surrounding soft tissues.
- before end of growth these capillary loops reach the
  —growth plate, do not cross it and do not anastomose either, but
  —turn sharply back to empty into metaphyseal venous sinusoids. Relative
  —vascular stasis here may allow bacteria to proliferate and cause
  —osteomyelitis.
- after end of growth, metaphyseal and epiphyseal vessels anastomose freely across the closed growth plate.

Epiphysis

- supplied by
  —circumferential arterial ring. From this
- branches enter the epiphysis and then
- divide into smaller and smaller arcades ending in capillary loops beneath the articular cartilage and between the epiphyseal bone and resting layer on the growth plate. The
- growth plate derives nourishment by diffusion from these epiphyseal vessels.

Venous drainage

- venous drainage is into
  —intramedullary network of venous sinusoids which drain through

—periosteal, metaphyseal and epiphyseal veins and through the small vein accompanying the nutrient artery. The
* intramedullary venous sinusoids are large compared with arterial tree and constitute a
—high-volume low-pressure system.

ELBOW JOINT

Joint surfaces
* complex of three joints:

Humeroulnar
* hinge joint;
* trochlea of the humerus articulates with the trochlear notch of the olecranon (ulna);
* the trochlea is held in the jaws (coronoid and olecranon processes) of the proximal ulna like a nut in the jaws of a wrench;
* in flexion, some lateral movement is possible;
* in full extension the joint is locked, allowing no lateral movement.
* the olecranon and coronoid fossae of the humerus are intracapsular but extrasynovial;
* they receive the olecranon and coronoid processes of the ulna in extension and flexion, respectively.

Radiohumeral
* head of radius articulates with capitulum of humerus;
* capitulum is covered with articular cartilage anterosuperiorly, anteriorly and inferiorly but not posteriorly.
* head of radius is a short cylinder whose proximal surface is concave, to accommodate convex surface of capitulum, and is covered in articular cartilage;
* sides of cylindrical radial head articulate with annular ligament and ulna;
* radiohumeral joint allows rotation of the radius.

Proximal radioulnar
* circular side of the radial head articulates with the
—radial notch of the ulna (a facet continuous with the trochlear notch), and the
—inside of the annular ligament;
* annular ligament attaches to the anterior and posterior borders

of the radial notch of the ulna, and
- holds the radial head in place in all positions of the elbow.

Ossification centers

Distal humerus

First appearance
- *C*apitulum at 3 years (epiphysis, contributes to growth in length);
- *I*nternal epicondyle at 5 years (apophysis, no contribution to growth in length);
- *T*rochlea at 7 years (epiphysis) and
- *E*xternal epicondyle at 11 years (apophysis);
- remember the mnemonic
  —CITE 3, 5, 7, 11.

Fusion
- capitulum, internal (medial) epicondyle and trochlea fuse together at 14 years, and
- this fuses with the shaft at 16 to 17 years;
- lateral epicondyle fuses separately with the shaft at about 20 years.

Olecranon
- appears at 11 years (epiphysis), and
- fuses at 18 or sooner.

Radial head
- appears at 4 years and
- fuses at 18.

Capsule and ligaments

Capsule
- the three parts of the elbow joint have one common synovial cavity;
- the capsule inserts
  —above the coronoid and olecranon fossae,
  —around the articular margin of the trochlear notch (ulna),
  —into the annular ligament and is
  —continuous with radial and ulnar collateral ligaments;
- distal humeral metaphysis is partly intracapsular.

Medial collateral ligament
- from medial epicondyle, fans out in three bands to insert along medial border of trochlear notch and coronoid process;

- the ulnar nerve, after passing behind medial epicondyle and between heads of flexor carpi ulnaris, lies on the ligament.

Lateral collateral ligament

- from lateral epicondyle, fans out to blend with annular ligament, but
- posterior fibers pass over annular ligament and insert into lateral margin of ulna.

Annular ligament

- see above.

Movements

Flexion-extension

- flexion to approximately 135°;
- few degrees of hyperextension possible, especially in females;
- occurs at humeroulnar and radiohumeral joints.

Rotation

- 90° each of supination and pronation possible from point of midrotation which is 0°;
- rotation occurs at
  —proximal and distal radioulnar joints, the radial head rotating around its axis, the distal radius moving around the ulnar head; and at the
  —radiohumeral joint.

MUSCLES

- The anterior and posterior compartments of the arm are separated by medial and lateral intermuscular (IM) septa (see Figs. 3.1 to 3.4).

Anterior compartment

Biceps

- origin by
  —long head from supraglenoid tubercle, and
  —short head from coracoid process;
- long head is tendon,
  —lies within shoulder joint, surrounded by synovial sleeve (is extrasynovial), then
  —lies in bicipital groove of humerus,
  —on insertion of latissimus dorsi,
  —surrounded by synovial sleeve and
  —covered by transverse ligament.

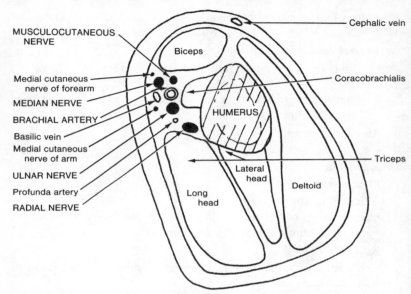

Figure 3.1. Transverse section through arm at junction of upper and middle thirds of humerus.

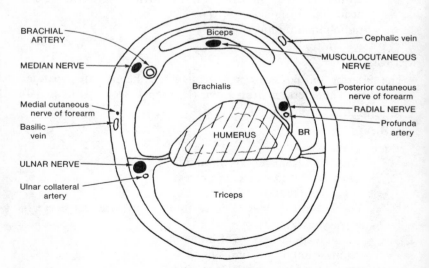

Figure 3.2. Transverse section through arm just below junction of middle and distal thirds of humerus.

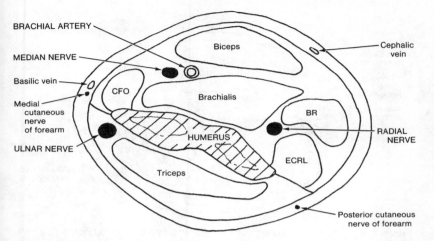

Figure 3.3. Transverse section of arm at level of humeral condyles. *CFO*, common flexor origin; *BR*, brachioradialis; *ECRL*, extensor carpi radialis longus.

- insertion by
  —tendon into back of bicipital tuberosity on medial side of proximal radial shaft, and by
  —bicipital aponeurosis into posterior (subcutaneous) border of ulna;
- nerve supply is musculocutaneous, C5, C6;
- action is
  —supination of forearm by radial insertion when elbow is flexed, and
  —flexion of elbow by both insertions. This muscle
  —puts in the cork screw,
  —pulls out the cork,
  —lifts the glass and
  —puts it down gently!

Coracobrachialis

- origin is tip of coracoid process and biceps muscle;
- inserted into medial surface of humeral shaft at its midpoint.
- musculocutaneous nerve, C7, which runs laterally and downward, between two parts of the coracobrachialis to supply it and reach the biceps and brachialis;
- weak adductor of the shoulder.

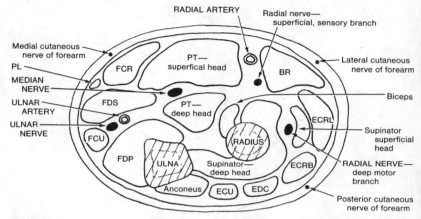

Figure 3.4. Transverse section of forearm at bicipital tuberosity of radius. *BR*, brachioradialis; *ECU*, extensor carpi ulnaris; *ECRB*, extensor carpi radialis brevis; *ECRL*, extensor carpi radialis longus; *EDC*, extensor digitorum communis; *FCR*, flexor carpi radialis; *FCU*, flexor carpi ulnaris; *FDP*, flexor digitorum profundus; *FDS*, flexor digitorum superficialis (sublimis); *PL*, palmaris longus; *PT*, pronator teres.

Brachialis

- origin from anterior surface of distal two thirds of humeral shaft, and from medial intermuscular septum;
- insertion into coronoid process of ulna;
- nerve supply is
  —musculocutaneous, C5, C6, and
  —radial nerve to lateral part which develops in extensor compartment in fetal limb.
- action is
  —elbow flexion and
  —controlled extension when putting an object down gently.

Posterior compartment

Triceps

- origin by
  —long head from infraglenoid tubercle,
  —lateral head from lateral tip of spiral groove, above deltoid insertion, and
  —medial head from medial side of spiral groove, lying deep to

other two heads, and separated from lateral head by radial nerve;

- inserts by common tendon into posterior surface of olecranon;
- nerve supply is radial nerve, C7, C8;
- extension of elbow.

Forearm muscles

Brachioradialis

- from upper two thirds of lateral supracondylar ridge of humerus,
- to styloid process of radius;
- radial nerve, C5, C6;
- flexion of elbow.

Extensor carpi radialis longus (ECRL)

- from distal third of supracondylar ridge of humerus,
- tendon passes beneath abductor pollicis longus (APL) and extensor pollicis brevis (EPB), and inserts
- into back of base of second metacarpal;
- radial nerve, C6, C7;
- extension and fixation of wrist and abduction of hand.

Superficial muscles of extensor compartment of forearm

- arise from common extensor origin (front of lateral epicondyle),
- pass distally over lateral side of elbow joint upon which they have little action (see Chapter 4).

Anconeus

- a superficial muscle of extensor compartment of forearm.
- origin from back of lateral epicondyle,
- fans out medially and distally to become triangular, covering radial head and
- inserts into lateral side of olecranon;
- radial nerve, C7, C8;
- slight abduction of ulna during pronation.

Supinator

- a deep muscle of posterior compartment of forearm.
- origin by
  —deep transverse fibers from supinator crest of ulna (just distal to radial notch), and by
  —superficial oblique fibers from back of lateral epicondyle, lateral collateral ligament and annular ligament;

- muscle
    - —passes laterally behind the radius,
    - —wraps itself anteriorly around the radius and
- inserts into the radial neck and shaft proximal to the oblique lines;
- posterior interosseous nerve (deep, motor branch of radial nerve), C6;
- supination of forearm, especially with elbow extended;
- importance in dissection is that the posterior interosseous nerve passes between the two heads of origin of the muscle to reach the forearm where the nerve supplies all the extensor muscles.

Superficial muscles of flexor compartment of forearm

- arise from common flexor origin (front of medial epicondyle), and
- pass distally in front of the medial side of the elbow joint, upon which they have little action (see Chapter 4).

BRACHIAL ARTERY

Main trunk

- continuation of the axillary artery;
- surface marking is a straight line drawn from the
    - —apex of the axilla to the
    - —center of the front of the elbow;
- artery lies on medial side of biceps, in front of long and medial heads of triceps, then on coracobrachialis, then brachialis;
- ulnar nerve is medial to the artery in upper arm. In lower arm the nerve passes to posterior compartment;
- median nerve is lateral to artery in upper arm, then crosses and becomes medial to it in lower arm;
- at the elbow, the artery is
    - —medial to the biceps tendon and passes
    - —beneath the bicipital aponeurosis.

Branches

- profunda brachii, travels posteriorly with radial nerve in radial groove, anatomoses with arteries around shoulder and elbow;
- nutrient, to nutrient foramen of humerus near coracobrachialis insertion;

- ulnar collateral, with ulnar nerve;
- supratrochlear, anterior and posterior branches, to elbow anastomosis;
- brachial artery divides into
  —two terminal branches,
  —radial and ulnar, at the
  —upper border of pronator teres, just distal to bend of elbow.

NERVES

Median

- from medial and lateral cords, C5, C6, C7, C8, and T1;

  Course in the arm

  - on lateral side of brachial artery in upper arm,
  - crosses in front of artery at level of coracobrachialis insertion,
  - continues on medial side of artery across front of elbow joint,
  - passes beneath bicipital aponeurosis,
  - enters forearm between the two heads of pronator teres.

  Branches in the arm

  - none.

Ulnar

- from medial cord, C7, C8 and T1;

  Course in the arm

  - on medial side of brachial artery in upper arm,
  - pierces medial intermuscular septum at level of coracobrachialis insertion and enters posterior compartment;
  - passes distally between the IM septum in front and the medial head of triceps behind, then
  - in the gutter between the medial epicondyle and the olecranon, under a fibrous roof. The nerve then
  - crosses medial to the medial collateral ligament of the elbow, and
  - enters the forearm between two heads of flexor carpi ulnaris.

  Branches in the arm

  - muscular to flexor carpi ulnaris, just above elbow joint.

Radial

- from posterior cord, C5, C6, C7, C8, and T_1.

Course in the arm

- winds posterolaterally and distally in spiral groove on humerus, lying directly on periosteum, then
- pierces lateral IM septum at level of coracobrachialis insertion and
- continues distally in front of the IM septum between brachio-radialis and brachialis, then
- in front of lateral epicondyle and the elbow joint, and
- into forearm under cover of brachioradialis.

Branches in the arm

- muscular, to medial and lateral heads of triceps, anconeus, brachioradialis, ECRL and lateral part of brachialis;
- lower lateral cutaneous nerve of arm;
- posterior cutaneous nerve of forearm;
- posterior interosseous nerve (deep motor branch), the major branch of the forearm,
    - leaves the radial nerve in front of lateral epicondyle,
    - crosses in front of radiohumeral joint, then
    - passes back beneath brachioradialis and between the two heads of supinator to reach the back of the forearm.

Musculocutaneous

- from lateral cord, C5, C6, C7.

Course

- perforates coracobrachialis,
- passes laterally between biceps and brachialis (behind) to become the
- lateral cutaneous nerve of forearm, lying anterior to the radial nerve at the elbow.

Branches in the arm

- muscular to coracobrachialis, brachialis and biceps.

Surgical Exploration of the Humerus

INDICATIONS FOR APPROACHES

Anterolateral

- osteotomy

- open reduction and internal fixation of recent fracture of humeral shaft
- tumor
- exploration of radial nerve in distal third of arm.

Lateral

- old fracture or pseudarthrosis
- osteomyelitis or TB of the shaft
- exploration of radial nerve in midarm
- open reduction and internal fixation of fracture of distal humeral metaphysis.

Posterior

- neurolysis, suture or graft of radial nerve in the groove;
- tendon transfer, second part of Episcopo (teres major and latissimus dorsi transferred posteriorly to posterolateral surface of humerus, to convert them from internal to external rotators), for Erb's paralysis.

Medial

- exploration of brachial artery, median or ulnar nerves in midarm.

SURGICAL APPROACHES

Anterolateral (Thompson-Henry) (Figs. 3.5, 3.9, and 3.10)

Position

- supine, cushion behind shoulder, arm free.

Incision

- starts in the deltopectoral groove halfway between the origin and insertion of deltoid,
- continues along anterior border of deltoid to its insertion, then
- down and slightly medially along lateral border of biceps to just above elbow joint.

Dissection

- retract deltoid laterally and biceps with cephalic vein medially;
- longitudinal incision through brachialis to reach the lateral surface of the humerus. Lateral part of cut brachialis protects radial nerve which supplies it. Brachial artery, musculocutaneous and median nerves are medial to incision.
- retract both parts of cut brachialis for clear view of humerus (biceps medially, brachioradialis laterally).

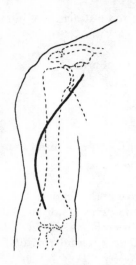

Figure 3.5. Anterolateral (Thompson-Henry).

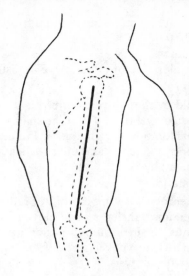

Figure 3.6. Lateral.

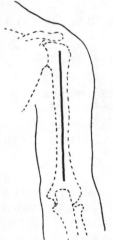

Figure 3.7. Posterior.

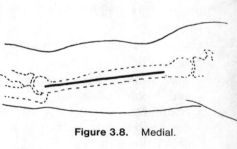

Figure 3.8. Medial.

Figures 3.5 to 3.8. Surgical approaches to humerus.

- this incision is extensile and can be easily lengthened proximally and distally;
- to approach the radial nerve in the distal third of the arm, the brachialis can be retracted medially (instead of cutting it), and the brachioradialis laterally.

Lateral (Figs. 3.6 and 3.10)

- to distal half of humerus and radial nerve.

    Position
    - prone, arm in slight abduction and external rotation, or
    - supine, abduction and internal rotation, arm free.

    Incision
    - from lateral epicondyle vertically to deltoid insertion.

    Dissection
    - identify radial nerve in distal part of incision, between brachialis (medially) and brachioradialis (laterally), and dissect it proximally. At proximal end of incision the radial nerve passes through the IM septum. Then
    - protect and gently retract the nerve; then
    - follow the intermuscular septum between triceps behind and brachioradialis in front, and you can reach the bone.

Posterior (Figs. 3.7, 3.9 and 3.10)

    Position
    - supine, the forearm across the chest, arm free; or
    - prone, the arm free in abduction.

    Incision
    - midline, from olecranon proximally.

    Dissection
    - retract long head of triceps medially and lateral head laterally to expose radial nerve in the radial groove;
    - dissect and protect the nerve.
    - can be enlarged proximally along posterior border of deltoid (protect axillary nerve entering deltoid), and distally by splitting longitudinally the triceps tendon and muscle (identify and protect the ulnar nerve).

Medial (Figs. 3.8, 3.9 and 3.10)

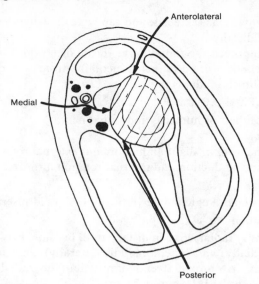

Figure 3.9. Similar section as in Figure 3.1, to show surgical approaches to humerus.

Position
- prone, arm in 90° abduction and internal rotation, arm free, or
- supine, arm abducted and externally rotated, arm free.

Incision
- line between medial epicondyle and center of axilla;
- make the incision in middle two thirds of this line (can be lengthened in both directions).

Dissection
- dissect behind or in front of basilic vein;
- incise deep fascia—ulnar nerve is immediately beneath this. Do not cut the nerve!
- in front of the ulnar nerve are the brachial artery and median nerve;
- expose the humerus and insertion of coracobrachialis, retract the brachial artery and median nerve forwards and the ulnar nerve posteriorly.
- if the incision is extended proximally, beware of the radial nerve passing from the axilla to the radial groove in the humerus.

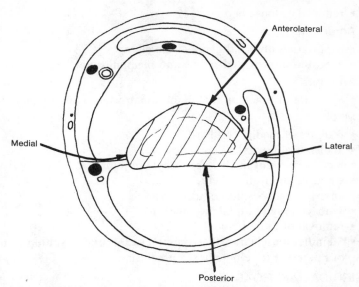

Figure 3.10. Similar section as in Figure 3.2, to show surgical approaches to humerus.

Surgical Exploration of the Elbow

INDICATIONS FOR APPROACHES

Posterior

- T fracture of distal humerus
- irreducible supracondylar fracture
- arthroplasty of elbow
- fusion of elbow
- untreated dislocation of elbow.

Posterolateral

- excision of radial head
- reduction of radial head (child)
- septic arthritis—drainage.

Lateral

- fractured radial head
- reduction of fracture of lateral condyle
- excision of fracture of capitulum
- synovectomy (with medial approach)

- removal of loose bodies

Anterolateral

- exploration of radial nerve at the elbow
- exposure of proximal radius and bicipital tuberosity.

Anterior

- exposure of brachial, radial and ulnar arteries and median nerve.

Medial

- fracture of medial condyle
- avulsion of medial epicondyle
- incarceration of medial epicondyle in joint
- exploration of ulnar nerve
- anterior transposition of ulnar nerve
- synovectomy (with lateral incision)
- removal of loose bodies
- Steindler muscle transfer (common flexor origin to anterior surface of humerus) for elbow flexor paralysis.

SURGICAL APPROACHES

- use a tourniquet when possible.

Posterior (Campbell) (Figs. 3.11, 3.17 and 3.18)

Position

- patient lying on the other side, arm free and 90° flexion at the shoulder, the elbow in 90° flexion, the arm supported on two cushions;
- or supine, with cushion beneath shoulder, the arm free across the chest.

Incision

- midline, starts 8 cm above olecranon, follows lateral border of olecranon and then the subcutaneous border (posterior) of the ulna for 8 cm.

Dissection

- find and protect ulnar nerve behind medial epicondyle, then
- the triceps is either
  —incised longitudinally to the olecranon, and both halves retracted laterally with the periosteum of the ulna, or
  —dissection is continued on both sides of triceps which can then be retracted first one way, then the other;

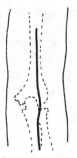

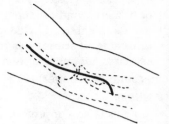

Figure 3.11. Posterior (Campbell).

Figure 3.12. Posterolateral (Kocher).

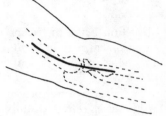

Figure 3.13. Lateral.

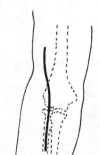

Figure 3.14. Anterolateral (Henry).

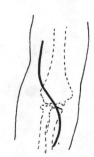

Figure 3.15. Anterior.

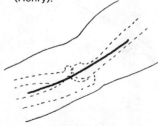

Figure 3.16. Medial.

Figures 3.11 to 3.16. Surgical approaches to elbow joint.

- expose subperiosteally the distal metaphysis and condylar region of humerus, and proximal end of ulna;
- expose radial head by dissecting and retracting anconeus.
- in closing, if triceps has not been divided horizontally, active exercises are possible soon after surgery.

Posterolateral (Kocher) (Figs. 3.12, 3.17 and 3.18)

Position

- same as lateral approach.

Incision

- as for lateral approach, but distal 3 cm are curved posteriorly and medially to subcutaneous border of ulna.

Dissection

- dissection between triceps posteriorly and brachioradialis and extensor carpi radialis longus anteriorly in arm, and between anconeus (medially) and extensor carpi ulnaris (laterally) in forearm.
- reflect muscles anteriorly and posteriorly from lateral epicondyle of humerus; retract distally the proximal fibers of supinator;

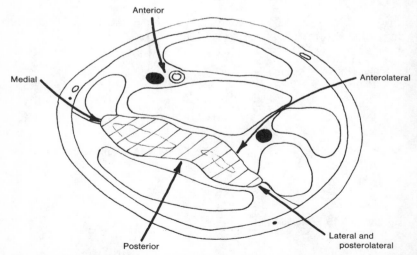

Figure 3.17. Similar section as in Figure 3.3, to show surgical approaches to elbow and proximal forearm.

- divide capsule longitudinally to expose lateral condyle and radial head and neck.

Lateral (Figs. 3.13, 3.17 and 3.18).

Position

- supine, arm free and supported on side table, cushion under shoulder.

Incision

- starts 8 cm above elbow and
- follows lateral supracondylar ridge to lateral epicondyle, then
- continues distally for 5 cm over lateral side of forearm.

Dissection

- dissection in arm between triceps (lateral head) and brachioradialis (in front); and in forearm between long wrist extensors (ECRL and extensor carpi radialis brevis (ECRB)) in front and the superficial extensor group behind (from common extensor origin);
- to expose the lateral epicondyle, the long extensor muscles are dissected off subperiosteally;
- radial head exposed by opening capsule between anconeus and common extensor attachment.
- the incision is extensile proximally in straight aline to deltoid insertion, but
- distal part of incision, in forearm, approaches deep motor branch of radial nerve which crosses radius from front to back 2 to 5 cm distal to radial head, and then enters supinator muscle. The nerve must not be injured. If in doubt, find it and protect it.

Anterolateral (Henry) (Figs. 3.14, 3.17 and 3.18)

Position

- supine, shoulder 90° abduction and external rotation, forearm in supination, arm free.

Incision

- start 5 to 8 cm above elbow joint, at lateral border of biceps;
- follow biceps tendon distally, then
- continue along medial border of brachioradialis.

Dissection

- retract biceps and brachialis medially, brachioradialis laterally;
- identify and retract laterally the radial nerve;

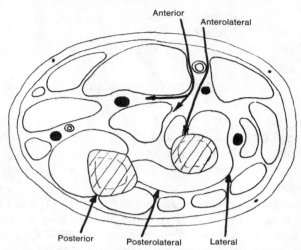

Figure 3.18. Similar section as in Figure 3.4, to show surgical approaches to elbow and proximal forearm.

- incise longitudinally the joint capsule to expose capitulum and radial head;
- to expose proximal radial shaft, reflect carefully the supinator and retract it laterally (will protect deep motor branch of radial nerve);
- in closing, it is essential to repair annular ligament (if this was cut or detached), unless the radial head and neck have been excised.

Anterior (Figs. 3.15, 3.17 and 3.18)

Position

- supine, arm in 90° abduction and external rotation, forearm supinated, arm free.

Incision

- S-shaped incision over middle of anterior surface of elbow.

Dissection

- dissect medially, incising bicipital aponeurosis and retracting biceps laterally to expose median nerve, brachial artery and its branches.

Medial (Figs. 3.16 and 3.17)

Position

- supine, cushion behind shoulder;
- arm free and, in abduction and external rotation, supported on a side table.

Incision

- start 5 cm proximal to medial epicondyle, cross just posterior to epicondyle and
- continue distally 5 cm in straight line.

Dissection

- identify and protect the ulnar nerve as it passes behind medial epicondyle and crosses the medial collateral ligament;
- separate, if necessary, the two heads of flexor carpi ulnaris to follow the ulnar nerve distally. Do not cut blindly in the vicinity of a nerve or vessel—always see the points of the scissors or knife;
- dissect and retract triceps posteriorly and brachialis anteriorly.
- expose medial side of elbow joint by incising capsule longitudinally. Greater exposure is gained by osteotomy of medial epicondyle. This should be reattached afterwards.

chapter 4

Forearm, Wrist and Carpals

Surgical Anatomy

BONES

Radius

- anterior surface is flat, bounded laterally by
  - —anterior oblique line in proximal third, and by
  - —anterior border distally.
- posterior surface is bounded laterally by posterior oblique line;
- lateral surface has rough area in middle for pronator teres (PT) insertion.
- medial border, attachment of interosseous membrane (IOM).
- bicipital tubercle lies medially at proximal confluence of oblique lines;
- styloid process is at distal extremity of lateral surface;
- Lister's tubercle, middle of posterior surface of distal epiphysis.
- shaft is gently bowed, convex laterally, to allow rotation of radius over ulna in pronation of forearm.
- nutrient foramen in proximal half of anterior surface for branch of anterior interosseous artery, directed towards elbow.

Ulna

- anterior surface separated from medial surface by anterior border;
- distal quarter of anterior border becomes pronator crest for pronator quadratus (PQ);
- posterior surface separated from medial surface by posterior border which is subcutaneous in its entire length.
- interosseous border, attachment of IOM;
- supinator crest is proximal quarter of interosseous border;
- styloid process is continuation of posterior border distally on head.

- nutrient foramen in proximal end of anterior surface for branch of anterior interosseous artery,
  - —directed towards elbow because
  - —long-bone growth is greater at the proximal end of humerus and distal radius and ulna than around the elbow;
  - —"to the elbow I go, from the knee I flee!"

Proximal carpal row
- from radial to ulnar side:
- scaphoid has tubercle anteriorly;
  - —blood supply from radial artery into center of dorsum, and from superficial palmar arch into anterolateral surface distally and distal pole (tubercle);
  - —proximal pole liable to avascular necrosis with fracture of waist or proximal third.
- lunate, with
  - —blood supply into anterior and posterior poles. But in one third of the population, only one of the two arteries is present.
- triquetrum;
- pisiform, a sesamoid bone in tendon of flexor carpi ulnaris (FCU), articulates only with triquetrum. You can feel it anteriorly in your own hand.

Distal carpal row
- from radial to ulnar side:
- trapezium, has groove anteriorly for tendon of flexor carpi radialis (FCR). Groove is bounded on radial side by ridge;
- trapezoid;
- capitate, largest carpal;
- hamate, has hook anteromedially; you can feel this.

Ossification centers
- distal radius, 2 years of age
- ulnar head, 4
- capitate, appears at 1 year of age,
- hamate, 2
- triquetrum, 3 (TRI = three; use this as mnemonic),
- lunate, 4
- scaphoid, 5
- trapezium, 6

- trapezoid, 7
- pisiform, 10 to 12 (the only sesamoid among the carpals is also the only bone that does not fit the orderly progression).

Remember that

—TRIquetrum is 3, and that

—appearance of centers follows an orderly progression around the carpals, in a circle.

JOINTS

Distal radioulnar joint

- synovial joint between the lateral two thirds of the lateral side of ulnar head and the medial side of the distal radial epiphysis.

Wrist joint

Joint surfaces

- distal radius has gently curved articular surface which is angled
  —15° toward the ulnar side and
  —15° toward the palm;
- triangular fibrocartilage covers distal surface of ulnar head, and is
  —attached to ulnar styloid medially and
  —medial border of distal radial epiphysis laterally;
- scaphoid articulates with radius;
- lunate articulates with radius and triangular fibrocartilage proximally, scaphoid laterally and triquetrum medially;
- triquetrum articulates with triangular fibrocartilage proximally.

Ligaments

- lateral collateral ligament, from radial styloid to scaphoid;
- medial collateral ligament, from ulnar styloid (which lies 1 cm proximal to radial styloid) to triquetrum.

Intercarpal joint

- between proximal and distal rows of carpals;
- scaphoid articulates distally with trapezium, trapezoid and capitate;
- lunate articulates distally with capitate and hamate;
- triquetrum articulates distally with hamate;
- capsule and intercarpal ligaments stabilize these articulations;
- pisohamate and pisometacarpal ligaments, from pisiform to

—hook of hamate, and to

—base of the fifth metacarpal, are continuation of FCU.

Carpometacarpal (CMC)

- trapezium has a saddle-shaped surface and articulates with first (thumb) and second metacarpals (MCs);
- trapezoid with second MC;
- capitate with second and third MCs, and
- hamate with fourth and fifth MCs.

Movements

- distal radioulnar joint
  —radius rotates 150° around ulnar head in pronation and supination.
- wrist
  —flexion 80°, extension 70°
  —ulnar deviation 30°, radial deviation 20°
  —circumduction, combination of all four other movements.
- intercarpal joints
  —limited gliding.
- carpometacarpal (CMC) joints
  —first CMC joint allows flexion, extension, abduction, adduction and circumduction. Opposition possible because of saddle-shaped joint surfaces.

MUSCLES

Anterior compartment

- separated from posterior compartment by radius, ulna and interosseous membrane (Figs. 3.4 and 4.1),
- enclosed by strong fascial envelope.
- superficial group arises, in part at least, from common flexor origin (CFO) on front of medial epicondyle;
- with palm of opposite hand on medial epicondyle, the thumb and four fingers represent the five superficial flexors in the following order, from lateral to medial:

  Pronator teres (PT)

  - origin by two heads, from
    —CFO (humeral head) and
    —medial side of coronoid process (ulnar head);
  - inserts into center of lateral surface of radial shaft;

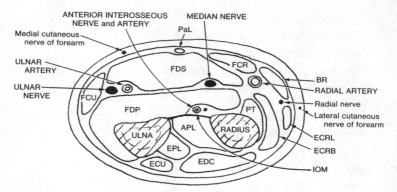

Figure 4.1. Transverse section of the midforearm. *APL*, abductor pollicis longus; *BR*, brachioradialis; *ECRB*, extensor carpi radialis brevis; *ECRL*, extensor carpi radialis longus; *ECU*, extensor carpi ulnaris; *EDC*, extensor digitorum communis; *EPL*, extensor pollicis longus; *FCR*, flexor carpi radialis; *FCU*, flexor carpi ulnaris; *FDP*, flexor digitorum profundus; *FDS*, flexor digitorum superficialis (sublimis); *IOM*, interosseous membrane; *PaL*, palmaris longus; *PT*, pronator teres.

- nerve is median, C6, C7;
- action is pronation of forearm.

Flexor carpi radialis (FCR)

- origin from CFO, forearm fascia and intermuscular septum;
- tendon lies in its own canal in transverse carpal ligament (flexor retinaculum of wrist), in groove on anterior surface of trapezium, and
- inserts into base, second MC;
- median nerve, C6, C7;
- acion is wrist flexion and abduction.

Palmaris longus (PL)

- absent in 30%;
- origin from CFO;
- inserts into central part of transverse carpal ligament and into palmar aponeurosis;
- median nerve, C6, C7;
- flexes wrist.

Flexor digitorum superficialis (sublimis) (FDS)

- origin by three heads

—CFO (humeral head) and medial collateral ligament,

—medial side of coronoid (ulnar head), and

—anterior oblique line of radius (radial head).

- in carpal tunnel, middle and ring finger tendons lie anterior to index and little finger tendons;
- tendons split over proximal phalanges (PPs) to allow flexor digitorum profundus (FDP) to pass through, then
- insert into sides of middle phalanx of four medial digits (not the thumb);
- median nerve, C7, C8, T1;
- flexes middle phalanx of finger, then proximal phalanx.

Flexor carpi ulnaris (FCU)

- origin by two heads from
  —CFO (humeral head) and
  —medial side of olecranon and proximal two thirds of posterior border of ulna (ulnar head);
- inserts into
  —pisiform, and thence by ligaments into
  —base fifth MC and hamate;
- ulnar nerve, C8, T1;
- flexes and adducts hand.
- deep group consists of following three muscles:

Flexor digitorum profundus (FDP)

- origin from front of ulnar shaft, olecranon, adjacent IOM and posterior border of ulna;
- tendons lie deep to FDS in carpal tunnel, pass through split in FDS tendons opposite PPs, and
- insert into base of palmar surface of distal phalanges of four fingers (not the thumb).
- nerve supply is C8, T1
  —ulnar to medial two tendons, and
  —median (anterior interosseous) to lateral two tendons;
- flexes distal phalanges.

Flexor pollicis longus (FPL)

- from front of radial shaft and adjacent IOM;
- inserts into base of palmar surface of DP of thumb;
- median nerve (anterior interosseous) C8, T1;
- flexes distal phalanx (DP).

Pronator quadratus (PQ)

- from pronator ridge on front of distal ulnar shaft
- to distal quarter of anterior surface and lateral border of radius;
- median nerve (anterior interosseous), C8, T1;
- pronates forearm.

Posterior compartment

- common extensor origin (CEO) is anterior surface of lateral epicondyle.
- superficial group has following seven muscles:

Brachioradialis (BR)

- see Chapter 3.

Extensor carpi radialis longus (ECRL)

- see Chapter 3.

Extensor carpi radialis brevis (ECRB)

- origin from CEO;
- tendon passes beneath abductor pollicis longus (APL) and extensor pollicis brevis (EPB) to
- insert into dorsum of base of third MC;
- deep radial nerve, C6, C7, supplies the muscle before the nerve enters supinator muscle;
- wrist extensor.

Extensor digitorum communis (EDC)

- from CEO and adjacent fascia;
- four tendons
  —connected to each other on back of hand by oblique bands; form
  —flat hoods over PPs of the fingers,
  —receive insertions of interossei and lumbricals; then each extensor hood
  —divides into three slips:
  —central slip inserts into dorsum of base of middle phalanx, the
  —two lateral slips insert into dorsum of base of DP;
- deep radial nerve, C6, C7, C8;
- extension of metacarpophalangeal (MP) joints.

Extensor digiti minimi (EDM)

- from CEO

- to DP little finger;
- tendon lies on ulnar side of EDC tendon;
- deep radial nerve, C6, C7, C8;
- extends little finger.

Extensor carpi ulnaris (ECU)

- from CEO and posterior border of ulna
- to base, fifth MC;
- deep radial nerve, C6, C7, C8;
- extends wrist and adducts hand.

Anconeus

- see Chapter 3.

- deep group comprises following five muscles:

Supinator

- see Chapter 3.

Abductor pollicis longus (APL)

- from posterior surface of ulnar shaft below anconeus insertion, the IOM and middle third of posterior surface of radial shaft;
- tendon crosses ECRL and ECRB tendons, forms anterior border of anatomical snuffbox, and
- inserts into radial side of base of first MC;
- deep radial nerve, C6, C7;
- abducts thumb.

Extensor pollicis brevis (EPB)

- from back of radial shaft and adjacent IOM distal to APL origin;
- tendon follows same direction as APL tendon,
- inserts into base of PP of thumb;
- deep radial nerve, C6, C7;
- extends PP thumb.

Extensor pollicis longus (EPL)

- from back of ulnar shaft and adjacent IOM below APL origin;
- tendon passes distally,
  - —turns around ulnar side of Lister's tubercle,
  - —forms posterior border of anatomical snuffbox,
  - —crosses tendons of ECRL and ECRB,
- inserts into base DP thumb;
- deep radial nerve, C6, C7, C8;

- extension of DP thumb.

Extensor indicis (EI)

- from back of ulna and adjacent IOM below EPL;
- inserts into ulnar side of EDC tendon to index at level of second MC head;
- deep radial nerve, C6, C7, C8;
- extends second MP joint.

Tendons at wrist (Fig. 4.2)

At level of distal radial and ulnar epiphyses, beneath the extensor retinaculum, from radial (lateral) to ulnar (medial) side:

- APL and EPB, in common fibrous tunnel and sharing synovial sheath, lie in groove on lateral side of radius;
- ECRL and ECRB, in common fibrous and synovial sheath, lie in groove on lateral side of posterior surface of radius. Synovial sheath separates distally into Y shape, one limb for each tendon;
- EPL, in separate fibrous synovial sheath, passes on medial side of Lister's tubercle and bends towards thumb;
- EDC and EI, in common fibrous and synovial sheath, on medial side of posterior surface of radius;
- EDM, separate synovial sheath, lies between radius and ulna;
- ECU, individual fibrous and synovial sheath in groove on back of ulna just lateral to ulnar styloid.
- these fibrous sheaths form the extensor retinaculum. Radial nerve crosses radial side of retinaculum.

Anatomical snuffbox

- triangular, base proximally;
- APL and EPB tendons anteriorly,
- EPL tendon posteriorly,
- radial styloid proximally and
- scaphoid and trapezoid in floor;
- radial artery crosses floor and
- superficial radial nerve crosses superficially.

ARTERIES

Radial

- terminal branch from brachial artery at the flexor crease of elbow;
- passes laterally to brachioradialis and, lying beneath this muscle,

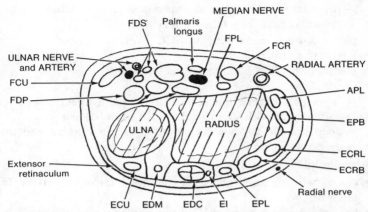

Figure 4.2. Transverse section through distal radial metaphysis to show tendons and extensor compartments. Abbreviations are the same as for Figure 4.1. Others: *EDM*, extensor digiti minimi; *EI*, extensor indicis; *EPB*, extensor pollicis brevis; *FPL*, flexor pollicis longus.

medial to sensory (superficial) branch of radial nerve, runs to wrist (felt as radial pulse), then

- turns backwards, crosses floor of anatomical snuffbox (beneath tendons of APL, EPB and EPL) to
- reach space between bases of first and second MCs. Artery
- passes forwards through this space, between two heads of first dorsal interosseous muscle to reach
- deep layer of palm and form deep palmar arterial arch with deep branch of ulnar artery.
- branches in forearm are muscular, and to anastomosis around elbow; superficial palmar branch leaves radial artery above wrist, crosses transverse carpal ligament, supplies thenar muscles, then forms superficial palmar arch with superficial palmar branch of ulnar artery.

Ulnar

- terminal branch of brachial, runs medially beneath all the superficial flexors to lie between FCU and FDS, lateral to ulnar nerve. Just below elbow gives off
  —common interosseous and

—two recurrent branches to anastomosis around elbow, and
—muscular branches. Ulnar artery then
- passes down forearm beneath FCU; at wrist, passes
- lateral to pisiform and
- medial to hook of hamate; at this level artery
- divides into
    —superficial branch, turns laterally in palm to form superficial palmar arch with superficial branch of radial artery, and
    —deep branch, follows deep branch of ulnar nerve and forms deep palmar arch.

Anterior interosseous
- one of two terminal branches of common interosseous artery (from ulnar artery);
- lies on anterior surface of IOM to wrist, has
- muscular branches and
- nutrient branches to radius and to
- ulnar and median nerves.

Posterior interosseous
- terminal branch of common interosseous just below elbow, turns
- backwards and passes between radius and ulna, proximal to IOM, to reach
- posterior compartment;
- lies between superficial and deep muscles as far as wrist;
- supplies muscles of posterior compartment.

NERVES
- all three major nerves enter forearm between heads of origin of muscles. General rules state that
- whenever a nerve
    —passes through a limb muscle or between its heads of origin, the nerve
    —supplies that muscle by a
    —branch which leaves the nerve proximal to the muscle; and
- when a nerve supplies a muscle, the nerve
    —receives sensory and proprioceptive fibers from the joint that the muscle crosses.
- nearly half of all fibers in a motor nerve are proprioceptive from muscles and joints.

Median

- enters forearm between heads of PT, then
- adheres to undersurface of FDS as far as distal third of forearm, then
- between FDS and FCR tendons and under PL tendon to carpal tunnel;
- supplies all anterior compartment
  —forearm muscles except FCU and medial half FDP, and sends
  —superficial palmar branch across (superficial to) transverse carpal ligament to skin of lateral two thirds of palm. Thus
  —palmar sensation not affected in carpal tunnel syndrome.

Ulnar

- crosses superficial to medial collateral ligament of elbow,
  —enters forearm between two heads of FCU, then
  —under that muscle, medial to ulnar artery, to wrist. In forearm
- supplies
  —FCU and medial half of FDP (to little and ring fingers), and sends
  —superficial palmar branch across (superficial to) transverse carpal ligament to skin of medial third of palm. Thus
  —palmar sensation is unaffected by nerve compression in canal of Guyon at wrist.
- at wrist passes through
  —canal of Guyon, lateral (radial) to pisiform, superficial to transverse carpal ligament, then curves around
  —ulnar side of hook of hamate beneath pisohamate ligament where it
- divides into
  —superficial terminal branch (sensation of little and medial side ring fingers) and
  —deep terminal branch (goes deep to hypothenar muscles and turns laterally across palmar interossei and long flexor tendons) to
  —all intrinsic muscles except opponens pollicis (OP), abductor pollicis brevis (APB), half flexor pollicis brevis (FPB) and lateral two lumbricals.

Radial

Deep radial nerve

- one of two terminal branches of radial nerve;
- leaves radial nerve in front of lateral epicondyle, passes
  —posterolaterally, beneath brachioradialis (BR), then
  —between two heads of supinator. At
  —exit from supinator breaks into fan of muscular branches.
- supplies all muscles of back of forearm except BR and ECRL, (these two are innervated by radial nerve above elbow; ECRB is innervated by deep radial nerve also above elbow).

Superficial radial

- the other terminal branch of radial nerve;
- lies beneath BR, on lateral side of radial artery; 5 cm above the wrist nerve
- passes posteriorly, beneath BR tendon, to back of wrist and hand, to
- skin of lateral three fourths of back of hand and fingers.

CARPAL TUNNEL

Boundaries

- anterior is the transverse carpal ligament, attached to
  —scaphoid tubercle and ridge of trapezium radially,
  —pisiform and hook of hamate medially. Its
  —proximal border lies at level of distal flexor crease of wrist (more distal than you think!), and it affords
  —origin to thenar and hypothenar muscles (Fig. 4.3).
- posterior are the carpal bones;
- medially are the pisiform and hook of hamate,
- laterally the scaphoid and trapezium.

Anterior relations

- superficial palmar branches of ulnar and median nerves cross the transverse carpal ligament;
- ulnar nerve and artery cross superomedial corner of ligament, just lateral to pisiform;
- PL tendon crosses in front of proximal border of ligament, then blends with ligament and palmar aponeurosis;
- APB and OP originate from ligament.

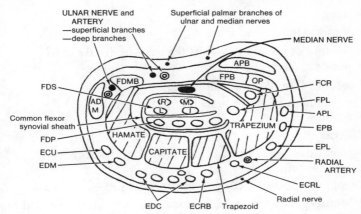

Figure 4.3. Transverse section through the distal carpal row. Abbreviations are the same as for Figures 4.1 and 4.2. Others: *ADM*, abductor digiti minimi; *APB*, abductor pollicis brevis; *FDMB*, flexor digiti minimi brevis; *FPB*, flexor pollicis brevis; *I*, index; *L*, little; *M*, middle; *OP*, opponens pollicis; *R*, ring.

Contents

- median nerve (soft, dull white, with blood vessel running longitudinally on its anterior surface, like most nerves) on radial side of FDS tendon to middle, and anterior to FDS tendon to index;
- four tendons of FDS (middle and ring fingers most superficial, index and little deeper);
- four tendons of FDP in one horizontal row. These tendons in a common synovial sheath with FDS;
- tendon of FPL is most lateral, in separate synovial sheath, and separated from tendon of FCR by septum from flexor retinaculum.
- tendon of FCR in separate synovial sheath and fibrous tunnel, lying in groove of trapezium.

Surgical Exploration of Forearm

INDICATIONS

Posterior, to ulna

- fracture or pseudarthrosis anywhere in the ulna
- osteomyelitis

- tumor.

Anterior (Henry), to radius

- fracture or pseudarthrosis of the shaft or distal radius
- tumor of shaft.

Posterior (Thompson), to radius

- exploration of motor branch of radial nerve.
- fracture of shaft.

Lateral

- fracture or pseudarthrosis radial shaft or distal end
- osteomyelitis.

Combined posterior (Boyd), to proximal radius and ulna

- Monteggia lesion (fractured ulna and dislocation of radial head)
- repair of annular ligament
- resection of proximal radioulnar synostosis.

SURGICAL APPROACHES

Posterior, to ulna (Figs. 4.4 and 4.9)

Position

- supine, the elbow flexed, forearm across the chest, arm free.

Incision

- along the posterior subcutaneous border from end to end, or along any part of this incision.

Dissection

- subperiosteal, reflecting FCU forwards and medially and ECU forwards and laterally;
- in distal third, identify and protect
  —dorsal cutaneous branch of ulnar nerve which
  —crosses medial surface and posterior border of ulna 4 cm above the ulnar head to reach the back of the wrist and hand.

Anterior (Henry), to radius (Figs. 4.5 and 4.9)

- whole length of radius can be exposed;
- any part of this approach can be used;
- incision is extensile.

Position

- supine, arm abducted 90°, forearm in supination, arm free.

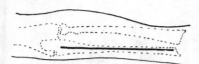

Figure 4.4.   Posterior approach to ulna.

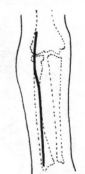

Figure 4.5.   Henry's anterior approach to radius.

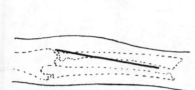

Figure 4.6.   Thompson posterior approach to radius.

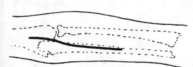

Figure 4.8.   Boyd posterior approach to proximal radius and ulna.

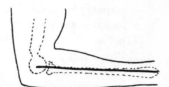

Figure 4.7.   Lateral approach to radius.

Figures 4.4 to 4.8.   Surgical approaches to forearm.

Incision

- starts lateral and proximal to biceps tendon, follows medial border of brachioradialis (BR) to wrist.

Dissection

- incise deep fascia; identify and tie recurrent radial vessels;
- retract BR, ECRL and ECRB, with elbow flexed;
- strip supinator muscle subperiosteally from radius and reflect it laterally (muscle protects deep motor branch of radial nerve);
- incise periosteum on radius as far as insertion of pronator teres (PT), to expose proximal radius;

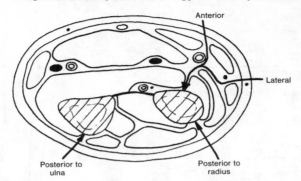

Figure 4.9. Similar section as in Figure 4.1, to show surgical approaches to forearm.

- distal to PT, dissect between BR laterally and FCR and radial vessels medially;
- protect sensory branch of radial nerve beneath BR;
- incise periosteum on radius lateral to attachments of FPL and pronator quadratus (PQ), and reflect these muscles medially. Pronation of forearm facilitates this; to
- expose midradius,
  —mobilize PT or
  —dissect it subperiosteally or
  —cut it near its radial insertion.

Posterior (Thompson), to radius (Figs. 4.6 and 4.9)

- for proximal and middle thirds of radial shaft.

  Position

  - supine, shoulder in 90° abduction, elbow flexed 90°, forearm in pronation, arm free.

  Incision

  - along the line between center of dorsum of wrist and lateral humeral epicondyle. Cut along proximal two thirds of this line.

  Dissection

  - between EDC (retract to ulnar side) and ECRB (to radial side) as far as elbow;
  - reflect APL off radius, and dissect the supinator subperiosteally off the radius, protecting the deep motor branch of the radial nerve (in the muscle);

• detach EDC from its origin (lateral humeral epicondyle) for better exposure of supinator and proximal radius.

Lateral (Figs. 4.7 and 4.9)

Position

• supine, shoulder abducted and internally rotated, elbow flexed 90°, supinated, arm free.

Incision

• cut on the line joining radial styloid with lateral humeral epicondyle;
• center the incision on the fracture.

Dissection

• between BR and radial vessels and sensory branch of radial nerve (retract anteriorly) and ECRB and ECRL (retract posteriorly). Start distally and work proximally;
• reflect subperiosteally the supinator, PT and PQ from anterior surface of radius, according to exposure required;
• do not remove more periosteum from radius than is necessary.

Combined posterior (Boyd), to proximal radius and ulna (Figs. 4.8 and 4.9)

Position

• patient on the side,
• shoulder flexion 90° and internal rotation 90°,
• elbow flexion 90°,
• forearm supinated,
• surgeon seated in front of the arm which is resting on pillows or a padded arm rest.

Incision

• starts 3 cm above the elbow at lateral border of triceps tendon,
• continues distally along lateral border of triceps, then
• lateral border of olecranon, finally along the subcutaneous (posterior) border of ulna to junction of proximal and middle thirds of ulna.

Dissection

• incise periosteum along posterior border of ulna and lateral edge of olecranon;
• detach subperiosteally anconeus, ECU and supinator from the

ulna and retract them together toward the lateral side, peeling supinator gently from around the radius;

- this exposes proximal third of ulna, proximal quarter of radius, posterior capsule of elbow joint and proximal quarter of IOM;
- deep branch of motor nerve is protected by the supinator.

Surgical Exploration of Wrist and Carpals

INDICATIONS

Posterior

- radiocarpal or radiometacarpal fusion
- synovectomy of wrist and intercarpal joints.

Lateral

- radial styloidectomy
- pseudarthrosis of scaphoid
- wrist fusion.

Anterior

- reduction of dislocated lunate
- scapholunate fusion
- synovectomy of wrist and intercarpal joints.

Medial

- excision of ulna head and neck (Darrach)
- excision of triangular fibrocartilage.

SURGICAL APPROACHES

Posterior (Fig. 4.10)

Position

- supine, shoulder abducted, elbow extended, forearm pronated, arm free.

Incision

- S-shaped incision with horizontal (transverse) limb of incision centered over and parallel with wrist joint.

Dissection

- define fibrous sheaths of extensor tendons and divide extensor retinaculum longitudinally on medial or lateral side or centrally, depending on exposure required. Do not damage tendons!

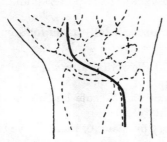

Figure 4.10. Posterior approach.

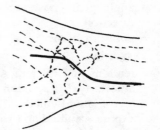

Figure 4.11. Lateral approach.

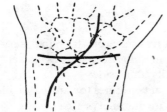

Figure 4.12. Anterior approaches.

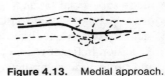

Figure 4.13. Medial approach.

Figures 4.10 to 4.13. Surgical approaches to wrist and carpus.

- retract tendons medially and laterally to expose capsule, and incise this.

Lateral (Fig. 4.11).

Position

- as above, but forearm in neutral rotation.

Incision

- 8 cm long, bayonet-shaped;
- starts over anterolateral border of distal radial metaphysis, continues
- distally to radial styloid, then

- angles gently posteriorly to cross snuffbox in posterior and distal direction. At
- posterior border of snuffbox it turns distally again for 2 cm

Dissection

- tendons of EPB and APL and the radial artery are retracted anteriorly, EPL tendon posteriorly;
- incise lateral collateral ligament and capsule longitudinally to expose scaphoid and wrist joint;
- protect radial artery and sensory branches of radial nerve to the thumb.

Anterior (Fig. 4.12)

Position

- as above, but forearm in supination.

Incision

- transverse, parallel with distal flexor crease; or
- longitudinal gently curved, following (but not in) skin creases where possible.

Dissection

- incise superficial fascia, identify and protect median nerve (beneath palmaris longus (PL) tendon when this is present) and incise flexor retinaculum on its ulnar side;
- if incision in flexor retinaculum continues toward palm, identify and protect motor branch of median nerve first;
- retract median nerve, PL and FPL laterally and FDS and FDP tendons medially;
- incise joint capsule to expose distal radius, lunate and scaphoid.

Medial (Fig. 4.13)

Position

- as above, but forearm pronated.

Incision

- longitudinal, gently curved, centered over ulnar styloid. Do not cut dorsal cutaneous branch of ulnar nerve.

Dissection

- incise capsule and medial collateral ligament longitudinally to
- expose triquetrum, styloid and head of ulna, and triangular fibrocartilage.

chapter 5
Hand

Surgical Anatomy

Note: The oral examiner's hands are very accessible, so learn the hand well!

OSTEOLOGY AND JOINTS

Five metacarpals (MCs)

- numbered from lateral (thumb, first) to medial (little, fifth);
- first lies
  —anterior to the other four, and is
  —rotated medially 90°. It
  —articulates separately with carpus (saddle joint of trapezius) and is
  —very mobile;
- medial four MCs articulate with
  —carpus and with each other at their bases. These joints have
  —capsules and strong ligaments, and
  —very little mobility. Second MC is least mobile, fifth is most mobile.
- third has a dorsal styloid process at its base;
- deep transverse metacarpal ligament binds together the medial four MCs at their heads;
- heads are wider anteriorly than posteriorly.

Metacarpophalangeal (MP) joints

- capsule is
  —thick and strong anteriorly (forms fibrocartilaginous volar plate) but
  —thin posteriorly. Thus
  —hyperextension is limited,

—flexion permitted.
- collateral ligaments attached to
  —posterior parts of MC heads, and are
  —lax in extension of MP joints, allowing abduction and adduction. But in
  —flexion these ligaments are stretched and tightened over broader anterior part of MC head, and MP joints are
  —locked (no lateral movement). So,
  —immobilize MP joints in flexion to avoid shortening of ligaments and stiffness.

Phalanges and interphalangeal (IP) joints

- base of proximal phalanx has a tubercle on each side for attachment of interosseous muscle.
- IP joints have capsules and collateral ligaments. No lateral movement is possible.

Secondary ossification centers:

- one for heads of the four medial MCs, and one for the base of every phalanx and for the first MC (which behaves like a phalanx in this respect).

MUSCLES

Extrinsic (see Chapter 4)

Flexor digitorum sublimis (FDS)

- tendon divides over proximal phalanx (PP) to let flexor digitorum profundus (FDP) tendon through;
- inserts into palmar surface of base of middle phalanx;
- flexes MP and proximal interphalangeal (PIP) joints.
- test for its function by holding other fingers in extension (to immobilize FDP) and asking patient to flex MP and PIP joints.

Flexor digitorum profundus (FDP)

- passes through FDS tendon in front of PP;
- inserts into palmar surface of base distal phalanx (DP);
- flexes MP, PIP and distal interphalangeal (DIP) joints (the only flexor of DIP).
- test for function by immobilizing MP and PIP joints in extension and asking patient to flex DIP joint.

Flexor pollicis longus (FPL)

- inserts into palmar surface, base of DP thumb.

- test for function by asking patient to flex IP joint of thumb.

Synovial and fibrous flexor sheaths (Fig. 5.1)

- common synovial sheath for FDS and FDP tendons under transverse carpal ligament with
  —extension into palm as far as distal border of thenar eminence; but
  —sheath for little finger tendons is continuous from wrist to tip of finger.
- separate synovial sheaths surround flexor tendons along
  —whole length of index, middle and ring fingers but
  —do not extend proximally into palm. Therefore
  —flexor tendons to index, middle and ring fingers have
  —no sheaths in distal two thirds of palm.
- FPL and flexor carpi radialis have separate sheaths.

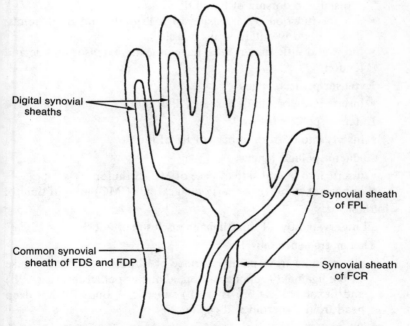

Digital synovial sheaths

Synovial sheath of FPL

Common synovial sheath of FDS and FDP

Synovial sheath of FCR

Figure 5.1. Diagram of palmar aspect of hand to show synovial flexor sheaths. *FCR*, flexor carpi radialis; *FDP*, flexor digitorum profundus; *FDS*, flexor digitorum superficialis (sublimis); *FPL*, flexor pollicis longus.

- fibrous tunnels along all the fingers
  —enclose the flexor tendons and synovial sheaths and
  —prevent bowstringing of the tendons during finger flexion. These sheaths are
  —strong over proximal and middle phalanges,
  —weak opposite IP joints.
- pyogenic tenosynovitis is caused by
  —direct innoculation (dirty knife) or
  —spread of pulp space infection.

Extensor digitorum communis (EDC)

- extensor hood over back of PP, a flat expansion of EDC tendon;
- tendon then splits into three slips
  —central slip inserts into dorsum of base of middle phalanx (boutonnière deformity results when this is ruptured),
  —two lateral slips continue on each side of central slip and distally to dorsum of base DP.
- test for function by extension of MP joints (not of IP joints; these extend by interosseous muscles).
- index and little fingers each have an extra extensor muscle and tendon.

Extensor pollicis longus

- inserts into dorsum of base of DP of thumb.

Extensor pollicis brevis

- inserts into dorsum of base of PP of thumb.

Abductor pollicis longus

- inserts into lateral side of base of MC of thumb;
- important stabilizer of carpometacarpal (CMC) joint of thumb.

Intrinsic

- all innervated by T1, but thenar muscles mainly C8.

  Thenar eminence muscles

- all originate from palmar surface of trapezium and transverse carpal ligament (opponens deep, abductor pollicis brevis (APB) and flexor pollicis brevis (FPB) superficial, but FPB has deep head from trapezoid and capitate);
- APB
  —inserts into lateral side of base of PP and extensor hood of thumb;

—mainly responsible for opposition;
- FPB
  —inserts through lateral sesamoid bone into lateral side of base of PP of thumb;
- opponens pollicis (OP)
  —inserts into whole length of anterolateral side of thumb MC;
- supplied by median nerve, except deep head FPB by ulnar nerve;
- action is opposition of thumb, brings pulp of thumb opposite to, and in contact with, pulp of other four fingers. This makes you different from monkeys!
- opposition entails the following movements of the thumb:
  —flexion at CMC joint,
  —medial rotation at CMC joint and
  —abduction at MP joint.

Adductor pollicis (ulnar nerve)

- origin from bases of second and third MCs (oblique head) and front of shaft of third MC (transverse head);
- inserts into medial side of base of PP of thumb through medial sesamoid.
- when adductor pollicis is paralysed, patient uses FPL to compensate when adducting the thumb, and the IP joint flexes. This is Froment's sign.

Hypothenar eminence (ulnar nerve)

- forms medial (ulnar) border of hollow of palm;
- surgically important only when atrophied, as a sign of ulnar nerve lesion.

Lumbricals (brown and slender, like earthworms—Latin)

- lateral two lumbricals are unipennate,
  —originate from FDP tendons of index and middle;
  —innervated by median nerve;
- medial two are bipennate,
  —originate from adjacent sides of FDP tendons of middle, ring and little fingers;
  —ulnar nerve.
- each lumbrical
  —passes to lateral (radial) side of its finger, anterior to deep transverse metacarpal ligament, and

—inserts into radial side of extensor hood of corresponding finger distal to insertion of interosseous muscle.
- action is to help
—flex MP and
—extend IP joints of fingers (no lumbrical to thumb).

Interossei
- ulnar nerve
  Palmar
  - three, all unipennate;
  - first originates from ulnar side of second MC shaft, passes on
    —ulnar side of MP joint of index,
    —inserts into ulnar side of extensor expansion of index, proximal to lumbrical, and
    —into tubercle on ulnar side of base of PP of index.
  - second and third from radial sides of shafts of fourth and fifth MCs, pass around
    —radial side of ring and little fingers,
    —insert into extensor expansion and
    —into tubercle on radial side of base of PP of ring and little fingers.
  - all interossei pass posterior to deep transverse metacarpal ligament.
  - individual action is adduct little, ring and index fingers toward middle finger, PAD (*P*almar *AD*duct).
  Dorsal
  - four, bipennate;
  - from adjacent sides of two MCs;
  - first and second pass
    —lateral to MP joints of index and middle fingers,
    —insert into extensor expansion and tubercle on radial side of base of PP of index and middle fingers;
  - third and fourth pass
    —medial to MP joints of middle and ring fingers,
    —insert into medial side of extensor expansion and base of PP of these two fingers.
  - individual action is abduction of index, middle and ring fingers, DAB (*D*orsal *AB*duct).

Combined actions of interossei

- flex MP joints of index, middle, ring and little fingers through insertion into base of PP;
- all extend IP joints by insertion into extensor expansions (hoods) of these four fingers.
- interossei and lumbricals (all small, weak muscles) act in concert with extensor digitorum communis (EDC) (large, strong muscle), the
  —EDC supplying the power, the
  —intrinsics redirecting this power as necessary (servomotor mechanism).
- with ulnar nerve lesion at wrist, patient is
  —unable to flex MP joints
  —nor to extend IP joints. Results in
  —ulnar clawhand (hyperextension of MP joints, flexion of IP joints),
  —least marked in middle and index fingers because lumbricals to these two fingers are supplied by median nerve and can compensate.
- first dorsal interosseous stabilizes PP of index at MP joint and prevents ulnar deviation of index during pinch (between pulp of thumb and index).

VESSELS

Superficial palmar arterial arch

- continuation of ulnar artery in palm;
- crosses palm between
  —flexor tendons posteriorly and
  —palmar aponeurosis anteriorly, at level of proximal transverse palmar skin crease.
- supplies digital branches to fingers; digital branches lie
  —superficial to digital nerves in palm,
  —cross the nerves in the web space and lie
  —posterior to digital nerves in fingers.
- other branches to muscles, bones and joints, skin.

Deep palmar arterial arch

- termination of radial artery and deep branch of ulnar artery;
- lies across base of MCs, level with distal border of thenar eminence

with thumb in abduction, between interossei posteriorly and flexor tendons anteriorly;
- anastomoses with digital branches of superficial arch. Other branches to surrounding structures.

Venous drainage
- drains mainly to dorsum of hand, thence by superficial veins to elbow where cephalic (lateral) and basilic (medial) veins form.

NERVES

Median nerve
- passes through carpal tunnel;
- motor branch recurves around distal edge of transverse carpal ligament to supply thenar muscles;
- median nerve continues into palm to supply
  —lateral two lumbricals, and
  —sensation to front and sides of lateral three and a half fingers.

Ulnar nerve
- superficial to carpal tunnel in the canal of Guyon;
- deep motor branch
  —turns around ulnar side of hook of hamate,
  —through opponens digiti minimi to
  —accompany deep ulnar arterial arch across the palm;
- supplies all the intrinsics except lateral two lumbricals, APB, superficial head of FPB, and OP, which are supplied by median;
- superficial branch
  —supplies sensation to medial one and a half fingers, and communicates with median nerve.

Radial nerve
- supplies skin over dorsum of hand (except over fifth MC) and radial three and a half digits
  —but autonomous area only covers base of index, thumb and first web space.

Digital neurovascular bundle
- each finger and thumb has two major neurovascular bundles which run along anterolateral and anteromedial borders of digit, the nerve anterior to the artery (you feel the prick before you see the blood!);
- incisions in the fingers must avoid these structures.

MIDPALMAR AND THENAR SPACES

- these are potential spaces that lie deep to flexor tendons, in close contact with flexor tendon sheaths (Fig. 5.2).

  Midpalmar space

  - bounded posteriorly by
    —third, fourth and fifth MCs,
  - anteriorly by
    —flexor tendons of middle, ring and little fingers;
  - separated from thenar space by vertical septum which runs backward from palmar aponeurosis to third MC.

  Thenar space

  - between
    —adductor pollicis posteriorly and
    —flexor tendons anteriorly, medial to thenar muscles.

  Infections

  - infections of these spaces usually caused by
    —purulent tenosynovitis of long flexor tendon sheath rupturing into the space, or by
    —extension from a web-space infection.
  - both pyogenic tenosynovitis and palmar-space infections are
    —surgical emergencies, and must be
    —widely drained, in the

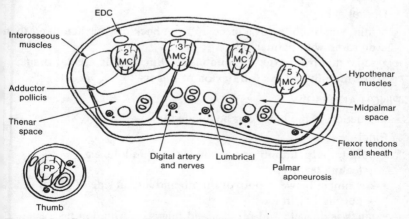

Figure 5.2. Transverse section of the hand through the midpalm. *EDC*, extensor digitorum communis; *MC*, metacarpal; *PP*, proximal phalanx.

—operating room, under
—general anesthesia, with
—full aseptic technique, by
—competent surgeon. These problems are
- NOT for the inexperienced doctor in the emergency room with local anesthesia.

PALMAR APONEUROSIS

- this is the deep fascia of the palm;
- continuous proximally with transverse carpal ligament and palmaris longus tendon;
- distally by digital slips it blends with fibrous flexor sheaths in the fingers.
- central part is thick, but
- parts over thenar and hypothenar eminences are thin.
- Dupuytren's contracture is a disease of this aponeurosis (Dupuytren was Chief Surgeon at Hôtel-Dieu Hospital, Paris).

SKIN

Palmar skin

- thick, tough, anchored to underlying fascia by fibrous bands and therefore relatively immobile and stable;
- covered in ridges and whorls which
- improve the grip.

Dorsal skin

- thin, very mobile; lift a piece up from back of your hand and then do same with palmar skin;
- separated from extensor tendons by thin, mobile areolar tissue;
- this mobility allows full flexion of fingers.

PINCH AND GRIP

- function of the hand can be divided into:

Pinch

- pulp to pulp, thumb opposes index and middle, e.g.,
  —feeling texture;
- key pinch, between pulp of thumb and lateral side of DP of index
  —putting key in lock;
- pinch is delicate and precise, and relays information because
  —skin over pulp is rich in sensory nerve endings.

Grip

- mainly by middle, ring and little fingers;
- strong, but little information about surface;
- grip is
  —strongest with wrist in extension,
  —weakest with wrist in flexion (force an assailant to drop a knife by very forcibly flexing his wrist!); thus
- wrist extensors contract synergistically with finger flexors to improve grip, e.g., holding a hammer.

Surgical Exploration

INDICATIONS

Proximal palmar

- carpal tunnel release
- exploration of median nerve at wrist and in proximal palm
- infection of midpalmar or thenar spaces
- tenosynovitis—pyogenic, TB, rheumatoid.

Distal palmar

- fasciectomy for Dupuytren's contracture (in combination with proximal palmar and anterior digital incisions as necessary)
- tendon suture, grafting (in combination with other incisions where necessary)
- trigger finger (stenosing tenovaginitis of flexor tendon sheaths)
- tenosynovitis
- open reduction of dislocation of MP joint of index finger.

Dorsum of hand

- repair of extensor tendons
- open reduction of MC fractures
- arthroplasty of MP joints.

Midlateral digital

- exploration of flexor tendons for repair or graft
- exploration of digital nerve for neuroma or repair
- release of contractures about IP joints (e.g., in rheumatoid)
- intra-articular fracture, open reduction
- fracture phalanx, open reduction
- drainage for tenosynovitis, osteomyelitis, septic arthritis.

Dorsal digital

- repair of extensor tendon rupture
- IP arthrodesis
- IP arthroplasty.

SURGICAL APPROACHES

General principles

- hand surgery deals with small anatomical structures, is time-consuming and tiring, and the surgical technique must be meticulous. So
- schedule the surgery early, when you are fresh;
- sit down, with your assistant, and
- place patient's hand on a side table;
- use a tourniquet.
- skin incisions should not be in creases, but close to them;
- incisions should be gently curved, not straight;
- incisions crossing flexor creases should curve obliquely across them, not cross them at right angles.
- incision must be long enough for easy exposure (wounds heal from side to side, not end to end!).
- two or more incisions may be used (as in fasciectomy for Dupuytren) but must not be too close together (to avoid skin necrosis).
- offset your incisions by making incision through fascia a little to one side of skin incision in order to avoid adherence to underlying structures, e.g., tendon, bone.

Technique

Proximal palm (Fig. 5.3)

Incisions

- incisions here are more longitudinal, and curve radially at their distal ends to parallel skin creases (look at your own hand).

Dissection

- incise fat down to deep palmar fascia and
- reflect skin and subcutaneous fat, as one flap, from the fascia (skin vessels run in the subcutaneous fat layer);
- identify and preserve motor branch of median nerve;
- incise deep fascia (resect part of it if necessary) to expose structures deep to it.

- superficial palmar arterial arch can be ligated and cut if deep dissection is necessary.

Distal palm (Fig. 5.3)

Incisions

- these should be nearly transverse (to parallel skin creases).

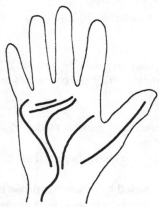

Figure 5.3. Palmar incisions.

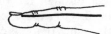

Figure 5.4. Transverse section of finger to show midlateral approach. *PP*, proximal phalanx.

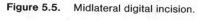

Figure 5.5. Midlateral digital incision.

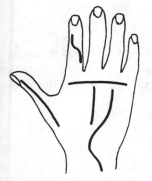

Figure 5.6. Dorsal incisions.

Figures 5.3 to 5.6. Surgical approaches in the hand.

Dissection
- deep palmar fascia is deficient between the MC heads, so do not cut too deeply too quickly!

Dorsum of hand (Fig. 5.6)

- longitudinal, to expose MCs or extensor tendons;
- transverse metacarpal, to expose MP joints.

Midlateral digital approach (fingers and thumb) (Figs. 5.4 and 5.5)

Incision
- longitudinal and straight,
- from MP joint to nail bed (or any part of this incision),
- just posterior to posterior extremity of IP flexor creases, along midlateral aspect of finger.

Dissection
- neurovascular bundle is anterior and can be retracted anteriorly or exposed by further dissection;
- dissect through fat anteriorly to expose flexor sheath, and incise this to expose tendons;
- phalanx and IP joints can be exposed by dissecting posteriorly;
- expose extensor hood and interossei tendons by developing dorsal flap.

Dorsal digital (Fig. 5.6)

Incision
- horizontal over back of joint; extend incision by proximal and distal longitudinal limbs on opposite sides to each other.

Dissection
- flaps developed to expose
  —extensor hood, central and lateral slips of extensor tendon (center the incision over PIP joint) and
  —distal insertion of extensor tendon (center over DIP joint).

chapter 6

Pelvis and Hip

Surgical Anatomy

PELVIS

Shape

- ring with two synovial joints (sacroiliac) posteriorly, and one fibrocartilaginous joint (symphysis pubis) in midline anteriorly;
- sacroiliac joints are oblique, can only be clearly seen in an oblique x-ray;
- joints held together with strong ligaments;
- each side of pelvis built from three bones—ilium, ischium and pubis, with sacrum posteriorly;
- pelvis supports the spinal column and rests on two legs.

Important features

Greater sciatic foramen

- apex is directly posterior to anterior inferior iliac spine (AIIS);
- divided into upper and lower parts by piriformis tendon;
- through upper part pass the
  —superior gluteal nerve and vessels;
- through lower part pass the
  —inferior gluteal nerve and vessels,
  —internal pudendal nerve and vessels,
  —sciatic nerve (already in lateral and medial divisions), and
  —nerves to obturator internus (OI) and quadratus femoris (QF).

Lesser sciatic foramen

- ischial spine and sacrospinous ligament divide
  —greater sciatic foramen (above) from
  —lesser sciatic foramen (below);

- OI passes through lesser foramen.

Pubic rami

- superior and inferior separated by obturator foramen which is medial and inferior to acetabulum.

Ischial tuberosity

- posterior, inferior and lateral to obturator foramen, below and behind acetabulum;
- on an anteroposterior x-ray of the pelvis, this is the most inferior part (you are sitting on two!).

Anterior superior iliac spine (ASIS)

- easily palpable, is excellent landmark;
- inguinal ligament runs from this medially and down to pubic tubercle;
- passing beneath ligament to reach thigh are
    —femoral nerve (laterally),
    —external iliac artery and vein and
    —femoral canal (medially—femoral hernia).

Anterior inferior iliac spine (AIIS)

- lies immediately above anterolateral angle of acetabulum and is
- good guide to acetabular rim during dissection.

Iliac crest

- palpable throughout its length;
- good cancellous bone for grafting lies in anterior quarter, and especially posterior quarter.

Posterior superior iliac spine (PSIS)

- palpable, lies immediately
- lateral to dimple (hollow in skin, obvious in children and women) which overlies sacroiliac joint.

Acetabulum

- lies between two strong bony columns
    —anterior (iliopubic) is superior pubic ramus and anteroinferior part of ilium,
    —posterior (ilioischiatic) is the posterior vertical part of ischium and posteroinferior part of ilium.

Inlet

- inlet of true pelvis is angled 45° anteriorly when standing so that

- top of sacrum is angled 45° too, and
- L5-S1 intervertebral disc is oblique;
- ASIS and symphysis pubis are in same coronal (vertical) plane.

HIP JOINT

- ball and socket joint, deep, inherently stable.

  Acetabulum (vinegar cup)

  - formed from the three pelvic bones—ilium, ischium and pubis;
  - develops from triradiate cartilage, centered in the acetabulum;
  - directed 45° (from coronal plane) laterally and downward (from vertical plane);
  - half a sphere, deepened by fibrocartilaginous labrum (similar in this respect to glenoid cavity of shoulder);
  - articular cartilage
    —shaped like a horseshoe inverted (upside down),
    —gap inferiorly is the acetabular notch
    —bridged by transverse acetabular ligament;
  - center of acetabulum inside the horseshoe is filled with fat and vessels;
  - ligament of femoral head (round ligament, ligamentum teres)
    —originates from transverse acetabular ligament,
    —crosses central fat pad and
    —inserts into notch on inferomedial part of femoral head;
    —arteries in ligament are from medial circumflex femoral and obturator arteries; enter ligament by passing beneath transverse acetabular ligament to supply small area of head in adult.

  Femoral head

  - three fifths of a near-perfect sphere, covered with articular cartilage except for insertion of round ligament (fovea capitis femoris);
  - directed upward 135° (neck-shaft angle), medially, and anteriorly 15° (anteversion);
  - growth plate of head lies across base of head and is convex toward the joint;
  - ossification center of head appears in first year after birth.
  - blood supply mainly by
    —retinacular vessels from medial and lateral circumflex femoral arteries which form anastomotic ring around base of neck; retinacular vessels
    —lie on surface of neck beneath synovial reflection and send

—branches into metaphysis and others into capital femoral epiphysis through small foramina at base of head; in the

—child these vessels reach epiphyseal ossific nucleus by passing through the cartilaginous anlage of the head and may be compressed here;

—major group in the adult is posteroinferior. At end of growth, epiphyseal and metaphyseal vessels anastomose so that head gains an intraosseous supply.

—arteries of the head (along round ligament) only supply small area around their entry point (fovea).

Capsule and ligaments

Capsule and synovium

- attached proximally to acetabular rim and transverse acetabular ligament,
- distally to middle of femoral neck posteriorly and intertrochanteric line anteriorly;
- most of femoral neck is intracapsular—important for spread of infection of femoral neck into hip joint.
- synovium is reflected along femoral neck to rim of head and has extension beneath transverse acetabular ligament to cover round ligament.

Ligaments

- these are strong;
- iliofemoral (Y-shaped ligament of Bigelow) from AIIS
  —lateral limb to upper part of intertrochanteric line,
  —medial limb spirals down to inferior part of intertrochanteric line. Tight in extension and medial rotation of femur;
- ischiofemoral, posterior, from back of acetabulum to capsule;
- pubofemoral, inferior.

Movements of hip

- normal values
  —neutral: 0°
  —flexion: 120° to 150°
  —hyperextension: 0° to 15°
  —abduction in extension or flexion: 45° to 60°
  —adduction: 20° to 30°
  —external rotation (in extension or flexion): 30° to 45°

—internal rotation (in extension or flexion): 60° to 90°

—circumduction: combination of other movements.

- measure hip movements with the
  —patient on his back on a
  —hard, flat surface, and the
  —pelvis locked by careful positioning of the opposite thigh, e.g., Thomas's test for hip flexion contracture.

Mechanical locking

- central axis of body when standing passes
  —through the body's center of gravity (just anterior to S2 vertebra)
  —behind the hip joints and
  —in front of the knees, therefore
- hips and knees are locked mechanically in extension, and do not require muscular contraction to maintain this posture. Thus it is possible to
- stand for long periods without fatigue.

FEMORAL NECK AND TROCHANTERIC REGION

Femoral neck

- mostly intracapsular;
- neck-shaft angle (angle between axes of neck and shaft) is normally 130° to 140° in adult. More than 140° is valgus of the head and neck, less than 130° is varus (coxa valga or vara);
- anteversion of the neck (anterior angulation of neck relative to coronal plane when the patella is facing forwards) is normally 40° in the infant. Stimulus of walking upright reduces this angle to 15° in the adult.

Trochanteric region

- lies between the greater and lesser trochanters;
- intertrochanteric line joins the two trochanters anteriorly,
- the intertrochanteric crest joins them posteriorly and has quadrate tubercle at its center;
- each trochanter has separate ossification center.

Bone structure

- in the femoral head, neck and trochanteric region the bone is cancellous, with two sets of trabeculae, both in the coronal plane;

- one set of trabeculae runs in an arc, convex proximally and laterally
  - from inferior part of head
  - to base of greater trochanter and into shaft;
  - this withstands tension (varus force);
- other set of trabeculae is nearly vertical and runs from superior part of head downwards and slightly laterally
  - to converge on calcar femoralis (strong thick cortex at inferior surface of neck) and into medial cortex of shaft. These trabeculae are aligned with trabeculae of ilium, above acetabulum, and
  - resist compression.

MUSCLES (Fig. 6.1)

Anterior iliac region

Psoas

- origin from
  - discs and adjacent areas of vertebral bodies between D12 and L5, from
  - fibrous arches stretching over segmental arteries running around vertebral bodies; and from
  - medial half of anterior surface of all lumbar transverse processes;
- descends
  - in front of iliacus (in iliac fossa), blends with this muscle, goes
  - beneath inguinal ligament, over pelvic brim and
  - forms part of floor of femoral triangle;
  - crosses anterior to hip joint capsule and turns posteriorly to
- insert into lesser trochanter. Bursa between tendon and femur;
- nerve supply is L2, L3 from lumbar plexus;
- action is
  - flexion (strongest when hip is already flexed more than 30°) and possibly
  - external rotation of hip. Iliopsoas is a
  - postural muscle.
- important facts:
  - muscle surrounded by thick sheath. This limits the psoas abscess of vertebral tuberculosis (Pott's disease);
  - lumbar plexus of nerves lies in muscle;

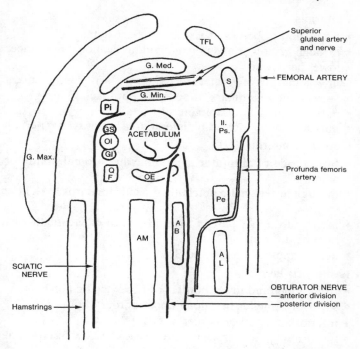

Figure 6.1. Diagram of sagittal section through the hip to show the important relations of the hip joint. *AB*, adductor brevis; *AL*, adductor longus; *AM*, adductor magnus; *G. Max.*, gluteus maximus; *G. Med.*, gluteus medius; *G. Min.*, gluteus minimus; *Gl*, gemellus inferior; *GS*, gemellus superior; *Il.*, iliacus; *OE*, obturator externus; *Ol*, obturator internus; *Pe*, pectineus; *Pi*, piriformis; *Ps.*, psoas; *QF*, quadratus femoris; *S*, sartorius; *TFL*, tensor fascia lata.

—tendon of iliopsoas lies beneath the muscle as it crosses pelvic brim.

Iliacus

- from most of medial surface of ilium (iliac fossa);
- blends with psoas, and has similar insertion and action;
- nerve supply is L2, L3 from femoral nerve.

Short lateral (external) rotators of thigh

- these are posterior, from above downwards:

Piriformis

- from front of bodies of S2, S3, S4, horizontally
- through greater sciatic notch, dividing the notch into upper and lower parts, and
- inserts into tip of greater trochanter by large round tendon
  —very good landmark in posterior approach to hip;
- nerve supply is S2, sometimes S1 and S3;
- muscle may be pierced by lateral division of sciatic nerve.

Obturator internus (OI)

- from inside of obturator membrane and around obturator foramen,
- through lesser sciatic notch, then bends forwards at right angles to
- insert into upper part of medial surface of greater trochanter, below piriformis;
- nerve supply is L5, S1 and S2.

Gemelli (twins)

- from upper and lower borders of lesser sciatic notch;
- superior gemellus lies along upper border of OI,
- inferior along lower border of OI;
- insert into greater trochanter above and below insertion of OI;
- nerve supply for
  —gemellus superior is L5, S1, S2 from nerve to OI, and for
  —gemellus inferior is L4, L5, S1 from nerve to quadratus femoris (QF).

Obturator externus (OE)

- from outer surface of obturator membrane and surrounding bone;
- to digital fossa at base of medial surface of greater trochanter;
- nerve supply is L2, L3, L4 posterior division of obturator nerve.

Quadratus femoris (QF)

- from lateral border of ischial tuberosity, flat, wide muscle running laterally below and parallel with OE;
- inserts into quadrate tubercle (middle of intertrochanteric crest);
- nerve supply is L4, L5, S1.

Glutei and tensor fascia lata (TFL)

Gluteus maximus
- origin from
  —lateral mass of sacrum,
  —posterosuperior area of ilium (above posterior gluteal line) and
  —back of sacrotuberous ligament;
- insertion has two parts
  —two thirds into fascia lata and iliotibial band,
  —one third into gluteal ridge (upper lateral margin of linea aspera of femur);
- nerve supply is inferior gluteal nerve, L5, S1 and S2;
- action is mainly
  —hip extension, but also
  —lateral rotation. This is a
  —postural muscle acting at hip and knee in standing;
- covers the hip joint, femoral neck, both sacral notches, short lateral rotators, sciatic nerve, and upper ends of hamstrings. Comes lower than the transverse gluteal fold (this is an extension crease of the hip joint).

Gluteus medius
- from outer surface ilium below crest and posterior gluteal line and above middle (anterior) gluteal line;
- inserts into upper and outer surface of greater trochanter;
- nerve supply is superior gluteal nerve, L4, L5, S1;
- action is abduction of thigh, or tilting up of opposite side of pelvis if leg is fixed (Trendelenburg test for weakness of gluteus medius). In walking, partly responsible for movement of the hips.

Gluteus minimus
- from outer surface of ilium between middle and inferior gluteal lines, lying beneath gluteus medius;
- inserts into front of greater trochanter;
- nerve supply is superior gluteal nerve, L4, L5, S1;
- action is abduction and medial rotation of thigh. Helps gluteus medius in walking.
- deep branch of gluteal artery and superior gluteal nerve run between the medius and minimus.

Tensor fascia lata (TFL)
- from outer surface of ilium below anterior third of crest;
- inserts into iliotibial tract, and through this into tubercle of Gerdy on anterolateral margin of lateral tibial condyle, with a slip to lateral femoral epicondyle;
- nerve supply is superior gluteal nerve, L4, L5, S1;
- action is complex. Assists in
  —abduction, flexion and internal rotation of thigh; assists in
  —extension of knee; muscle of
  —posture, stabilizing pelvis on femoral head and femoral condyles on tibia when standing with hips and knees flexed and in walking.
- fixed contracture of this muscle (as in polio) creates following deformities;
  Pelvis
  —forward tilt around coronal (lateral) axis and
  —upward tilt of opposite side of pelvis (pelvic obliquity) with
  —consequent lumbar lordoscoliosis.
  Hip
  —abduction, internal rotation and
  —flexion.
  Knee
  —flexion (because in slight flexion of knee, insertion of iliotibial tract is posterior to axis of flexion of knee, and flexes it further),
  —valgus of tibia and
  —external rotation of tibia.

Hamstring muscles
- all originate from ischial tuberosity (except short head of biceps femoris), extend the hip and flex the knee.

Semimembranosus
- from upper, lateral area of back of ischial tuberosity;
- for insertion, see Chapter 7.
- the nerve supply is medial division of sciatic nerve, L4, L5, S1.

Semitendinosus (ST)
- from inferomedial area of ischial tuberosity with long head of biceps; lies

- superficial to semimembranosus;
- inserts by long, round tendon (easily palpable) into
  —medial side of proximal tibial shaft
  —behind insertion of sartorius (S), and
  —behind and below insertion of gracilis (G) (*S*ay *G*race before *T*ea). These three tendons at their insertion form the
  —pes anserinus (goose's foot).
- nerve supply is by medial division of sciatic nerve, L4, L5.

Biceps femoris

- the only hamstring on lateral side of knee;
- long head from ischial tuberosity,
- short head from distal part of linea aspera and lateral supracondylar ridge;
- long head crosses semimembranosus and passes laterally and downwards, in back of thigh superficial to sciatic nerve, to join short head;
- inserts by tendon (easily palpable and has common peroneal nerve medial to it) into head of fibula anterior to styloid process of fibula;
- nerve supply of long head, L4, L5, S1, by medial division of sciatic nerve; short head, L5, S1, by lateral division of sciatic nerve.

Rectus femoris and sartorius

Rectus femoris

- the only member of quadriceps group which crosses the hip joint;
- origin by two heads
  —straight head from AIIS,
  —reflected head from superior margin of acetabulum (good guide to this acetabular margin) and from front of hip joint capsule;
- inserted by large tendon into superior pole of patella and with the three vasti, via the patella tendon, into tibial tubercle;
- nerve supply is from femoral nerve, L2, L3, L4;
- action is
  —hip flexion and
  —knee extension.

Sartorius

- from ASIS;
- inserts in front of gracilis and semitendinosus into medial side of proximal tibial shaft (crosses thigh from lateral to medial, anterior to quadriceps group);
- nerve supply from femoral nerve, L2, L3;
- action is
  —flexion, abduction and lateral rotation of thigh and
  —flexion of the knee;
  —both movements simultaneously and bilaterally result in squatting position of the tailor, hence the name sartorius;
- covers Hunter's canal and femoral artery in midthird of thigh.

Adductors

- these muscles adduct the thighs (custodes virginitatis).

Adductor magnus

- origin from inferior pubic and ischial rami and ischial tuberosity;
- insertion
  —part from rami inserts by flat sheet of muscle into linea aspera and medial supracondylar ridge;
  —part from ischial tuberosity inserts by tendon (easily palpable) into adductor tubercle (on middle of proximal border of medial femoral condyle);
  —gap in insertion of the two parts affords passage of femoral vessels to popliteal fossa;
  —perforating arteries pass through three or four holes in insertion of flat sheet;
- nerve supply:
  —L2, L3 by posterior division of obturator nerve
  —but ischial head L4, L5 by sciatic nerve.

Adductor brevis

- from outer surface of inferior pubic ramus, above and medial to magnus;
- runs laterally, in front of magnus, and inserts into upper part of linea aspera;
- nerve supply from both divisions of obturator nerve, L2, L3, L4;
- muscle separates the two divisions of obturator nerve.

Adductor longus

- longer, thinner, more oblique and anterior to brevis;

- origin from front of body of pubis;
- inserts into whole length of linea aspera;
- nerve supply is L2, L3, L4 anterior division of obturator nerve;
- action, as well as adduction of thigh, rotates it medially;
- separates femoral artery (in front of muscle) from profunda artery (behind).

Pectineus

- above and in same plane as adductor longus;
- from pectineal line (superior border) of pubis
- inserts into femoral shaft below lesser trochanter and anterior to adductor brevis;
- nerve supply is L2, L3 by femoral nerve; sometimes accessory obturator nerve too;
- action is adduction and medial rotation of thigh;
- forms floor of femoral triangle with adductor longus and iliopsoas.

Gracilis

- from inferior margin of pubis and inferior pubic ramus; runs vertically down medial side of thigh and
- inserts into proximal part of medial surface of tibia, behind sartorius, above and in front of semitendinosus;
- nerve supply is from anterior division of obturator nerve, L2, L3, L4;
- adducts thigh, flexes knee.

ARTERIES

Femoral artery

- continuation of external iliac. In
- upper third of thigh, anterior to hip joint, lies in femoral triangle between vein (medially) and nerve (laterally);
- can be palpated just below midpoint of line between ASIS and pubic symphysis;
- major branch is profunda, leaves posterior part of artery 2 to 5 cm below inguinal ligament, passes down, behind adductor longus, to lower third of thigh. Branches of profunda include
  —medial and lateral femoral circumflex arteries, to anastomoses around the proximal end of femur, and branch to ligament of femoral head, and

—three or four perforating branches to musculature of posterior and lateral thigh.

Gluteal arteries

Superior gluteal artery

- largest branch of internal iliac;
- leaves pelvis through greater sciatic foramen above piriformis,
- supplies gluteal muscles, ilium, and anastomoses around hip.

Inferior gluteal

- branch of internal iliac;
- leaves pelvis through greater sciatic foramen, below piriformis, goes to
- gluteal muscles and lateral rotators, sciatic nerve, and anastomoses around hip.

Obturator artery

- from internal iliac artery;
- leaves pelvis by groove in upper part of obturator foramen, gives off
- medial and lateral branches which supply
  —adductors, hamstrings and obturator muscles, a branch along
  —ligamentum teres to femoral head;
  —other branches anastomose with medial circumflex and inferior gluteal arteries.

NERVES

Lumbar plexus (Fig. 6.2)

- formed in psoas from anterior primary rami of D12 to L4, and gives following major branches

Psoas

- segmental, L2, L3.

Iliohypogastric, L1

- to skin over buttock and lower abdomen.

Ilioinguinal, L1

- skin over inside of upper thigh and genitalia.

Genitofemoral, L1, L2

- genitalia and front of upper thigh.

Lateral cutaneous nerve of thigh, L2, L3

- passes under inguinal ligament just medial to ASIS (meralgia paraesthetica due to compression here).

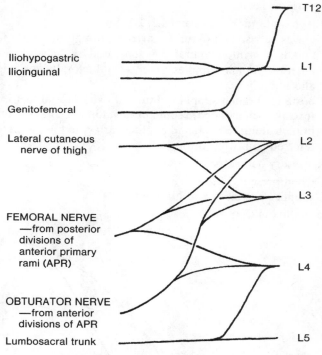

Figure 6.2. Diagram of lumbar plexus.

Femoral

- from dorsal divisions of L2, L3, L4;
- leaves psoas at its lateral border, descends in pelvis between psoas and iliacus, lying lateral to external iliac vessels,
- passes under inguinal ligament to femoral triangle;
- divides into branches to supply pectineus, sartorius and all four quadriceps muscles, also
- intermediate and medial cutaneous branches, and saphenous nerve (accompanies femoral artery to midthigh, then crosses posteromedial side of knee and accompanies great saphenous vein to anterior border of medial malleolus).
- lateral circumflex artery runs outwards between branches of the femoral nerve; branches to quadriceps and saphenous nerve are deep, the rest superficial to artery.

Obturator nerve

- from anterior divisions of L2, L3, L4;
- leaves pelvis, with obturator artery, through obturator foramen, and divides into two branches separated by the adductor brevis;
- anterior branch supplies gracilis, adductor longus and brevis and hip joint;
- posterior branch supplies obturator externus, adductor magnus (except ischial head), sometimes adductor brevis, and sends branch along femoral and popliteal artery to knee joint (explains referred pain from hip).

Accessory obturator

- when present, L3, L4;
- supplies pectineus and hip joint.

Sacral plexus (Fig. 6.3)

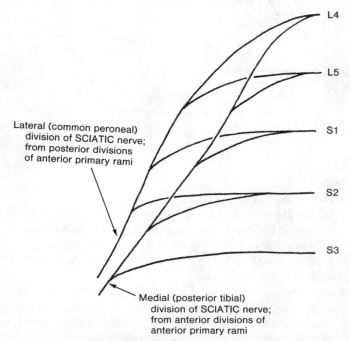

L4

L5

S1

S2

S3

Lateral (common peroneal)
division of SCIATIC nerve;
from posterior divisions
of anterior primary rami

Medial (posterior tibial)
division of SCIATIC nerve;
from anterior divisions of
anterior primary rami

Figure 6.3. Diagram of sacral plexus to show constitution of sciatic nerve. Other branches of plexus are not shown.

- formed on piriformis from anterior rami of L4, L5 (lumbosacral trunk) and S1, S2, S3;
- lies behind internal iliac artery, rectum and pelvic fascia;
- divides into anterior and posterior divisions

Branches:

Muscular
- to piriformis (S1, S2), obturator internus and gamellus superior (L5, S1, S2), quadratus femoris and gamellus inferior (L4, L5, S1).

Superior (L4, L5, S1) and inferior gluteal (L5, S1, S2) nerves.

Posterior cutaneous nerve of thigh (S2, S3) and perforating cutaneous (S2, S3).

Sciatic (L4, L5, S1, S2, S3)
- leaves pelvis posteriorly through greater sciatic foramen, beneath piriformis tendon at junction of upper and middle thirds of line drawn between posterior inferior iliac spine and ischial tuberosity;
- passes laterally and obliquely downwards on ischium, then on obturator internus and gamelli. Here it is behind the hip joint and easily injured in posterior dislocation of the hip;
- then passes vertically down on (superficial to) quadratus femoris. Here it lies midway between ischial tuberosity (medially) and greater trochanter (laterally). IM injection into upper, outer quadrant of buttock is safe;
- in its entire course in the buttock, the nerve is covered by gluteus maximus;
- enters thigh deep to hamstrings, lying on (superficial to) adductor magnus;
- branches of the trunk to all hamstrings from medial component (except short head of biceps from lateral component), and to ischial (medial) part of adductor magnus.

Hypogastric and pelvic plexuses

- autonomic nervous system.
- hypogastric plexus lies in front of lumbar and first sacral vertebrae (sacral promontory), between the two common iliac arteries, and is a sympathetic plexus; the
- two pelvic plexuses are derived from the hypogastric plexus. These

pelvic plexuses lie on each side of the rectum, prostate and bladder in the male and the rectum, cervix and bladder in the female and

- receive parasympathetic nerves from S2, S3, S4. The hypogastric and pelvic plexuses control involuntary rectal and bladder sphincters in both sexes, erection of penis and ejaculation of semen in the male;
- damage to the hypogastric plexus, during anterior fusion of L5 to S1 disc space, may cause impotence (failure of erection) or infertility (failure to ejaculate semen) in the male.

Surgical Exploration

INDICATIONS

Iliofemoral

- cup arthroplasty
- intra-articular fusion with or without graft
- drainage of hip
- anterior dislocation of hip
- pelvic osteotomy
- acetabuloplasty
- soft-tissue release of hip contracture
- arthrodesis

Ilioinguinal

- fracture of anterior column of acetabulum
- transverse fracture of acetabulum
- fracture of both acetabular columns
- sacroiliac arthrotomy (posterior part of incision)

Anterolateral

- total hip replacement
- open reduction and internal fixation of subcapital or transcervical fractures

Posterolateral

- open reduction of subcapital or transcervical fracture
- arthrodesis
- arthroplasty—cup, total

Posterior

- femoral replacement arthroplasty (Moore, Thompson)

- intra-articular fusion with or without graft
- comminuted, irreducible or unstable subcapital fracture
- arthroplasty
- irreducible posterior dislocation
- posterior fracture dislocation
- fracture of posterior acetabular lip
- fracture of posterior column of acetabulum
- septic arthritis of hip—drainage
- osteomyelitis of femoral neck
- excision of head and neck (Girdlestone)

In general

- anterior incisions bleed more than posterior incisions;
- posterior incisions are best for osteomyelitis of the neck or septic arthritis because gravity aids drainage (always work with nature, not against her); but beware sciatic nerve!

SURGICAL APPROACHES

Iliofemoral (Smith-Petersen) (Fig. 6.4)

Position

- supine, leg free.

Incision

- starts 1 cm below the center of the iliac crest,
- runs forward parallel with and below the crest to the ASIS, then
- down front of thigh, parallel with lateral border of sartorius for 15 cm.

Dissection

- TFL dissected off crest and retracted laterally, together with gluteus medius and minimus, to capsule of hip joint;
- sartorius and rectus femoris retracted medially (protect femoral nerve and vessels);
- reflected head of rectus is landmark for edge of acetabular roof and is detached and retracted;
- T incision in capsule, the bar of the T close to acetabular margin, the stem along axis of femoral neck;
- hip can be dislocated anteriorly (hyperextension, adduction and external rotation of femur) after cutting ligament of the head (ligamentum teres).

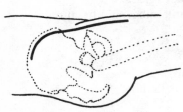

Figure 6.4.   Iliofemoral (Smith-Peterson).

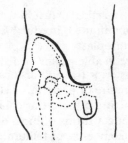

Figure 6.5.   Ilioinguinal (Judet and Letournel) approach to pelvis.

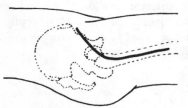

Figure 6.6.   Anterolateral (Watson-Jones).

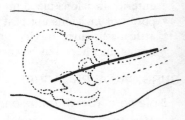

Figure 6.7.   Posterolateral (Gibson).

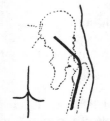

Figure 6.8.   Posterior (Osborne).

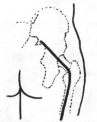

Figure 6.9.   Posterior (Moore).

Figures 6.4. to 6.9.   Surgical approaches to the pelvis and hip joint.

Ilioinguinal (Judet and Letournel) (Fig. 6.5)
- for almost all the inside of the bony pelvis.
  Position
  - supine.
  Incision
  - along anterior two thirds of iliac crest, then

- medially from ASIS, slightly curving up to a point 1 or 2 cm above the symphysis pubis.

Dissection
- dissect the abdominal muscles from the entire length of sacro-iliac crest, from ASIS to PSIS;
- incise aponeurosis of external oblique just above the inguinal ligament and above the superficial inguinal ring from ASIS to the midline;
- incise the inguinal origins of internal oblique and transversus abdominis to expose iliopsoas fascia;
- retract iliopsoas and femoral nerve gently;
- retract the spermatic cord (or cut the round ligament in female)
- divide the conjoined tendon (internal oblique and transversus abdominis, forming posterior wall of inguinal canal) just above its insertion to expose the cave of Retzius (the retropubic space);
- free by blunt dissection the femoral vessels and retract.
- this approach affords the following exposures:
- by retracting iliopsoas and femoral nerve medially
  —whole of iliac crest
  —whole of medial surface of ilium
  —sacroiliac joint
  —posterior and lateral part of pelvic inlet;
- by retracting femoral vessels and spermatic cord medially or laterally
  —whole of superior pubic and anterior part of ilium from ASIS to symphysis pubis (anterior column of acetabulum)
  —roof of acetabulum
  —anterior part of pelvic inlet;
- by retracting vessels medially and psoas laterally
  —quadrilateral (pelvic) surface of ilium forming
  —medial wall of acetabulum,
  —greater sciatic notch
  —posterior column of the acetabulum (ilioischiatic column).

Closure
- suture of muscles layer by layer with accurate apposition;
- drain.

Anterolateral (Watson-Jones) (Fig. 6.6)
- reasonably bloodless.

Position

- supine, with sandbag beneath the buttock of same side, leg free.

Incision

- 1 inch below ASIS, down and back to greater trochanter, then
- straight down thigh, in axis of femur, for 15 cm.

Dissection

- fascia lata incised in line of distal incision;
- interval between gluteus medius and TFL incised (bloodless plane);
- retract TFL anteriorly, clear space in front of femoral neck and head to expose anterior capsule;
- incise capsule longitudinally;
- dissect origin of vastus lateralis subperiosteally to expose base of greater trochanter and proximal femoral shaft;
- for wider exposure, divide anterior fibers of gluteus medius from greater trochanter.

Posterolateral (Gibson, Kocher and Langenbeck) (Fig. 6.7)

Position

- on the side, lower leg flexed at hip and knee;
- kidney rests or pillows in front and behind trunk to stablize patient,
- leg free.

Incision

- start 6 cm anterior to PSIS, below iliac crest,
- continue distally and slightly anteriorly to posterosuperior pole of greater trochanter, then for
- 12 cm down anterior border of greater trochanter and femur.

Dissection

- incise longitudinally the fascia lata in distal part of incision;
- extend incision of deep fascia proximally along anterior border of gluteus maximus, palpating the sulcus here with the hip in abduction;
- retract muscles anteriorly and posteriorly to expose greater trochanter and short lateral rotators of hip behind the femoral neck;
- identify tendon of piriformis (the most proximal of the lateral rotators, lies at superior margin of femoral neck) and interval between it and gluteus medius; then partially

- divide gluteus medius and minimus muscles 1 cm from insertion into greater trochanter and retract forwards;
- anterior and superior joint capsule is now seen;
- incise capsule longitudinally along superior surface and transversely at medial (acetabulum) and lateral (trochanter) ends;
- dislocate hip anteriorly (flexion, abduction and external rotation).

Closure

- closure of anterior capsule to prevent redislocation.

Posterior (Osborne) (Fig. 6.8)

Position

- on the side, with kidney rests back and front, and the lower leg flexed at the hip and knee.

Incision

- start just lateral and distal to PSIS;
- continue down and lateral (parallel with fibers of gluteus maximus) as far as posterosuperior angle of greater trochanter, then
- straight down along posterior border of greater trochanter for 10 cm.

Dissection

- split gluteus maximus in the line of its fibers, parallel with skin incision;
- divide insertion of gluteus maximus into fascia lata along length of distal limb of incision;
- rotate the thigh internally;
- identify piriformis tendon, divide this, gemelli, obturator internus (and quadratus femoris if larger exposure required) 1 cm from their insertions into trochanter;
- retract these short lateral rotators medially—they protect the sciatic nerve which lies superficial to them under gluteus maximus; if in doubt, identify and retract the nerve gently;
- femoral neck, posterior capsule and posterior lip of acetabulum are exposed;
- incise posterior capsule in T;
- dislocate hip posteriorly by flexion, adduction and internal rotation.

Posterior (Moore) (Fig. 6.9)

- good for fracture of posterior acetabular lip.

Position

- identical to Osborne approach.

Incision

- starts 10 cm distal to PSIS; continues
- down and laterally, parallel with gluteus maximus fibers, to greater trochanter; then
- follows posterolateral border of greater trochanter and femoral shaft for 10 cm.

Dissection

- split gluteus maximus in line with its fibers;
- divide proximal part of gluteus maximus insertion into linea aspera. Retract the muscle proximally and distally;
- identify and protect sciatic nerve;
- divide short lateral rotators near their insertion and retract medially;
- incise posterior capsule in T or H;
- femoral neck, hip joint and posterior wall of acetabulum are exposed.

chapter 7
Thigh and Knee

Surgical Anatomy

FEMORAL SHAFT

Shape

- femur is the longest, largest bone in the body;
- slightly bowed, convex anteriorly and laterally;
- mechanical axis of femur, from center of head to center of knee jont, is about 6° medial to anatomical axis (down center of shaft);
- nutrient arteries from perforating branches of profunda enter cortex along proximal half of linea aspera directed away from knee.

Muscle origins

- gives origin to muscles in upper two thirds of anterior and lateral surfaces and whole linea aspera;
- anterior surface of distal third separated from muscles by supra-patellar bursa (part of knee joint synovium) to facilitate gliding of quadriceps in flexion and extension of knee;
- linea aspera (Fig. 7.1) is a
  —raised ridge in central three fifths of posterior femoral surface;
  —medial lip of linea aspera continuous proximally with spiral line and intertrochanteric line, distally with medial supracondylar line;
  —provides origin for (medial to lateral) vastus medialis (whole length of the linea aspera), adductor brevis (upper half) and adductor longus (lower half), adductor magnus (whole length), gluteus maximus (upper half) and biceps short head (lower half), lastly the vastus lateralis (upper half).

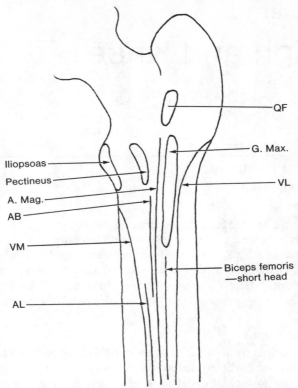

Figure 7.1. Diagram of proximal end of linea aspera to show muscle insertions. Not drawn to scale. *AB*, adductor brevis; *AL*, adductor longus; *A. Mag.*, adductor magnus; *G. Max.*, gluteus maximus; *QF*, quadratus femoris; *VL*, vastus lateralis; *VM*, vastus medialis.

KNEE and PATELLOFEMORAL JOINTS

Osseous structure

Femur

- two eccentrically curved condyles with long axis in anteroposterior direction;
- anterior part is oval, posterior part is semicircular;
- articular surface of medial condyle longer than lateral;
- lateral condyle lies in sagittal (anteroposterior (AP)) plane,

medial condyle angled 22° anterolaterally;
- condyles separated by intercondylar notch posteriorly;
- anteriorly condyles meet in midline and form patellar groove for articulation with patella;
- lateral wall (on lateral condyle) of patellar groove is larger and more prominent than medial wall.

Tibia

- two condyles, lateral shorter than medial in anteroposterior axis, each supporting a flat, oval, articular surface partly covered with a meniscus;
- intercondylar area lies between the condyles, with two tubercles, medial and lateral, in the middle;
- order of insertion of structures in intercondylar area, from anterior to posterior;
  —anterior horn *M*edial meniscus
  —*A*nterior cruciate ligament
  —anterior horn *L*ateral meniscus (MAL)
  —tubercles
  —posterior horn *L*ateral meniscus
  —posterior horn *M*edial meniscus
  —*P*osterior cruciate ligament (LMP)
- tibial tuberosity is anterior, at junction of proximal tibial epiphysis and metaphysis, and is not articular.

Patella (Latin—small pan)

- sesamoid bone in tendon of quadriceps muscle;
- triangular, base proximal;
- posterior surface covered with articular cartilage in proximal three quarters, divided by rounded ridge into lateral (larger) and medial articular facets;
- quadriceps inserted into base (proximal pole) of patella and into sides by retinacular (flat, tendinous) fibers;
- patellar tendon, thick and strong,
  —from apex (distal pole of patella),
  —inserts into tibial tuberosity;
- blood supply from circumferential plexus fed by all genicular arteries, with principal supply entering through distal pole. In transverse fracture, proximal fragment may be avascular.

Extra-articular structures

Capsule

- attached to femoral condyles and superior border of intercondylar notch posteriorly (femur);
- anteriorly to margins of patella (but is perforated superiorly by suprapatellar pouch) and to patellar tendon;
- inferiorly, to the periphery of the menisci and the upper margins of tibial condyles (meniscotibial portions called the coronary ligaments).
- capsule has several thickenings (see below).
- synovium
  —lines the capsule and retropatellar fat pad,
  —covers the cruciates and supplies them with blood vessels, and
  —forms the suprapatellar bursa lying between quadriceps tendon and distal femur, allowing tendon to glide on femur during flexion and extension of knee.

Anterior aspect of knee

- capsule
- patellar tendon, thick and strong;
- quadriceps expansions from vastus lateralis and medialis form the retinacula to sides of patella and patellar tendon, with expansions to tibial condyles anteriorly, medially and laterally, and
- reinforce the capsule in these areas.

Medial aspect of knee

Tibial (medial) collateral ligament

- strong, flat band;
- origin from medial epicondyle and condyle of femur;
- deep fibers (also called medial capsular ligament) insert into medial meniscus and edge of medial tibial condyle;
- superficial fibers down and forwards to tibial shaft 10 cm distal to condyle, beneath tendons of pes anserinus (sartorius, gracilis, semitendinosus) and separated from these by bursae. Ligament
- glides backwards and forwards over femoral condyle in flexion and extension;
- stabilizes knee against valgus stress (superficial part) and rotation (deep part).

Posterior oblique ligament
- thickening in posteromedial capsule, blending with deep part of tibial collateral ligament in front and with oblique popliteal ligament behind;
- resists rotary stress of the knee.

Pes anserinus
- tendons of sartorius (S) (in front) and gracilis (G) and semi-tendinosus (ST) (behind) (*S*ay *G*race before *T*ea!)
- insert into medial side of proximal tibial shaft;
- protect knee against rotary and valgus stress.

Posterior aspect

Semimembranosus ramifications
- direct insertion into posteromedial corner of medial tibial condyle;
- indirect insertions through four expansions, all originating from direct insertion;
  - oblique popliteal ligament (of Winslow) upwards and laterally to lateral femoral condyle near origin of lateral head of gastrocnemius, reinforces posterior capsule centrally;
  - expansion into posterior horn of medial meniscus and adjacent capsule;
  - long expansion forwards, in groove along margin of medial tibial plateau just below articular surface; inserts into tibia beneath tibial collateral ligament;
  - distal expansion to posteromedial part of proximal tibial metaphysis, and to fascia covering popliteus.
- semimembranous
  - internally rotates tibia and
  - tightens capsule posteriorly and posteromedially, thus helping stabilize knee against rotary stress; also
  - pulls posterior rim of medial meniscus backwards during flexion.

Posterior oblique ligament
- blends with oblique popliteal ligament (see above) and reinforces posteromedial capsule.

Arcuate complex
- consists of
  - posterior capsule, lateral part of

—oblique popliteal ligament,
—short fibular collateral ligament and expansions from
—popliteus muscle origin and
—biceps femoris tendon.
- reinforces posterolateral capsule and
- stabilizes knee against rotary and varus stress.

Meniscofemoral ligaments
- from posterior horn of lateral meniscus, two small ligaments pass upward and medially, and lie
  —anterior (Humphrey) and
  —posterior (Wrisberg) to posterior cruciate ligament;
- insert into medial femoral condyle just anterior and posterior to insertion of posterior cruciate. These ligaments help
- stabilize knee through meniscal attachment to capsule and arcuate complex.

Lateral aspect

Fibular (lateral) collateral ligament
- round,
- from lateral epicondyle of femur
- down and back to head of fibula anterior to styloid, beneath biceps tendon;
- no capsular attachments;
- separated from lateral meniscus by popliteus tendon.
- provides stability against varus stress, especially with knee extended.

Short fibular collateral ligament
- lies posteromedial and parallel with fibular collateral ligament;
- may contain a sesamoid bone (fabellar);
- reinforces posterolateral corner of capsule.

Iliotibial tract
- longitudinal thickening in fascia lata;
- inserts into
  —lateral femoral epicondyle, then passes between lateral border of patella and biceps tendon to insert into
  —lateral tibial tubercle (Gerdy's tubercle);
- moves back and forth over femoral condyle in flexion and extension,

  • stabilizes knee against varus stress.
  Biceps and popliteus tendons
  • see below for anatomy.
  • both enhance lateral stability against varus and rotary stress.

Intra-articular structures

Menisci

• fibrocartilage, triangular in cross section with the base toward periphery of tibial condyles;
• superior surface of each is concave;
• medial is shaped like a large, open C; the lateral, a small closed C;
• attached peripherally to the tibia by joint capsule, (coronary ligament) except where popliteus tendon intervenes laterally;
• medial meniscus also attached to deep fibers of tibial collateral ligament medially and to semimembranous posteriorly;
• lateral meniscus attached to popliteus fibers posteriorly;
• anterior and posterior horn of each meniscus attached firmly to intercondylar area of tibia, and
• both anterior horns connected to each other by transverse ligament.
• menisci are avascular, and have no nerves.
• functions may include
  —deepening of tibial articular surface to stabilize femoral condyles,
  —guidance of femoral condyles in flexion and extension,
  —shock absorbers in weight-bearing, and
  —distribution of synovial fluid within the joint.
• menisci move back and forth (lateral more mobile than medial) during movements of knee.

Cruciates

• both cruciates are intracapsular but extrasynovial;
• anterior cruciate ligament
  —from medial part of anterior intercondylar fossa of tibia,
  —upward, backward and laterally to posterior part of medial surface of lateral femoral condyle, in intercondylar notch;
  —small, anteromedial portion is tight in all knee positions, while
  —large posterolateral part is taut only in extension.

- posterior cruciate
  - —from posterior part of posterior intercondylar area of tibia,
  - —upward and medially to posterior part of lateral surface of medial femoral condyle, crossing the anterior cruciate;
  - —bulk (anterior portion) is tight in flexion, loose in extension;
  - —smaller posterior part is loose in flexion, tight in extension.
- cruciates prevent
  - —anteroposterior (sagittal) displacement of tibia on femur (maximum normal displacement is about 5 mm);
- cruciates
  - —wind around each other and tighten in internal rotation of tibia on femur, thus limiting internal rotation;
  - —unwind in external rotation, thus permitting greater AP displacement and external rotation in this position.

MUSCLES (Fig. 7.2)

Adductors

- adduct the hip (see Chapter 6).

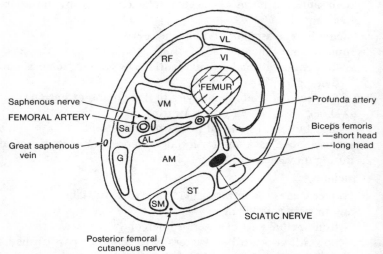

Figure 7.2. Transverse section through midthigh. *AL*, adductor longus; *AM*, adductor magnus; *G*, gastrocnemius; *RF*, rectus femoris; *Sa*, sartorius; *SM*, semimembranosus; *ST*, semitendinosus; *VI*, vastus intermedius; *VL*, vastus lateralis; *VM*, vastus medialis.

Extensors (of the knee)

- quadriceps group, consists of four muscles, all with similar
  —nerve supply, femoral, mainly L4 but also L2 and L3, and with similar
  —action, extension of the knee.

Rectus femoris

- fusiform, bipennate, superficial to vasti;
- origin from anterior inferior iliac spine (AIIS) and superior acetabular lip by two heads;
- insertion into superior pole of patella by outer layer of trilaminar quadriceps tendon.

Vastus lateralis

- origin from proximal half of lateral lip of linea aspera by aponeurosis, muscular fibers obliquely run down and medially;
- inserts into
  —side of quadriceps tendon, forming middle layer with vastus medialis,
  —retinacular (tendinous) fibers into side of patella and patellar tendon, and
  —expansion to anterior part of lateral tibial condyle.

Vastus medialis

- origin from spiral line, medial lip linea aspera, and medial supracondylar ridge, down and forward;
- inserts into
  —medial side of quadriceps tendon, blends with vastus lateralis,
  —lower muscle fibers horizontally to medial side of patella (prevent lateral dislocation),
  —retinacular fibers to medial side of patellar tendon and
  —expansion to anterior margin of medial tibial condyle.

Vastus intermedius

- lies beneath other three quadriceps muscles;
- origin from upper two thirds of front and lateral surface of femur;
- inserts into posterior edge of proximal pole of patella via deep layer of quadriceps tendon.

Flexors (of the knee)

- hamstrings, sartorius and gracilis—see Chapter 6.

Gastrocnemius

- origin by two heads from posterior surface of distal femur, one above lateral condyle, the other above medial condyle
- two heads
  —descend over back of femoral condyles, and
  —converge to blend with each other in midcalf,
  —forming inferolateral and inferomedial borders of popliteal space. In
  —midcalf, muscle fibers replaced by aponeurosis which then
  —unites with tendon of soleus to become the
  —Achilles tendon (named because it was the only vulnerable part of the body of Achilles, the Greek mythological hero who fought at Troy about 3,500 years ago);
- insertion by Achilles tendon into back of calcaneum;
- nerve supply is posterior tibial, S1, S2;
- action is flexion of knee and plantar flexion of foot.

Plantaris

- small muscle with long tendon;
- origin from distal part of lateral supracondylar ridge of femur;
- downwards on soleus, beneath gastrocnemius,
- inserts into Achilles tendon;
- nerve supply and
- action similar to gastrocnemius.

Popliteus

- origin by three tendinous heads:
  —main tendon from lateral surface of lateral femoral condyle, just distal to insertion of fibular collateral ligament; runs down and back, separating lateral meniscus from capsule and fibular collateral ligament (bursa here); muscle's
  —fibula head passes upward and medially to join the main tendon and form the arcuate ligament; third head is
  —medial, from posterior capsule and posterior horn of lateral meniscus, runs down and laterally to join other two heads;
- three conjoined heads pass down and medially to muscle belly which lies obliquely on posterior surface of proximal tibial metaphysis and shaft; muscle
- inserts into back of tibia above oblique soleal line;
- nerve supply is posterior tibial, L4, L5, S1;

- action is to rotate femur laterally on tibia (or tibia medially on femur), and thus unlock knee and
  - —enable flexors to flex the knee (does not flex the knee itself); also
  - —prevents lateral meniscus being crushed between condyles during flexion, and
  - —provides rotary and sagittal stability to knee.

Popliteal space (fossa)

- lies behind the distal femur, knee jont and proximal tibia;
- shaped like a diamond;
- bounded by
  - —biceps tendon above and laterally,
  - —semitendinosus and semimembranosus tendons above and medially, and
  - —both heads of gastrocnemius inferiorly;
- roof is fascia lata;
- floor is (from above downwards)
  - —femur
  - —oblique popliteal ligament
  - —tibia
  - —popliteus;
- contents are (from superficial to deep)
  - —short (small) saphenous vein and posterior femoral cutaneous nerve,
  - —tibial and common peroneal nerves,
  - —popliteal vein and tributaries and
  - —popliteal artery and its genicular branches,
  - —all buried in fat containing lymph nodes.

Fascia lata

- the deep fascia completely surrounding the thigh with intermuscular (IM) septa between major muscle groups (extensors, adductors and flexors).
- attached proximally to iliac crest, inguinal ligament, ischiopubic ramus and sacrum;
- attached below to tibial condyles and sides of patella and patella ligament (blends with retinacula of quadriceps).
- iliotibial tract is longitudinal, thickened band in lateral part of fascia lata, receives insertions of tensor fascia lata (TFL) and two

thirds of gluteus maximus, and inserts into lateral epicondyle of femur and tubercle on anterolateral aspect of lateral tibial condyle.

VESSELS

Femoral artery

- continuation of external iliac artery.
- in upper third of thigh, lies in
  —femoral triangle. Borders of triangle are
  —sartorius laterally,
  —medial margin of adductor longus medially and
  —inguinal ligament above;
  —floor is iliopsoas laterally and pectineus and adductor longus medially.
- in the triangle, the artery lies between femoral vein (medial) and femoral nerve (lateral to artery).
- in middle third of thigh lies in subsartorial canal of Hunter (John Hunter, eighteenth century English surgeon, anatomist and researcher);
  —laterally and anteriorly to canal is vastus medialis,
  —behind is adductor longus above and magnus below,
  —roof is fascia and sartorius muscle with saphenous nerve (from femoral) and femoral vein.
- at junction of middle and lower thirds, artery goes posteriorly through opening in adductor magnus and becomes popliteal artery.
- surface marking, with thigh in abduction and external rotation, is
  —proximal two thirds of line joining
  —adductor tubercle of medial femoral condyle to
  —midpoint of line between ASIS and symphysis pubis.
- for branches, see Chapter 6.

Popliteal artery

- from opening in adductor magnus (junction middle and lower thirds of thigh) where it is continuation of femoral artery,
- runs down and slightly laterally, lying deep in popliteal space on femur, then capsule, then popliteus. It is
- crossed superficially, from lateral to medial, by poplital vein and, superficial to that, by tibial nerve.
- at lower border of popliteus muscle, artery divides into anterior and posterior tibial arteries.

- branches around the knee (easily cut during surgery, and bleed a lot)
  - —superior medial genicular runs medially above femoral condyle, beneath semimembranosus and adductor magnus;
  - —superior lateral genicular runs laterally above lateral femoral condyle, under biceps;
  - —inferior medial genicular runs medially around medial tibial condyle, beneath medial head of gastrocnemius and medial ligament;
  - —inferior lateral genicular runs laterally along periphery of lateral meniscus, under lateral head of gastrocnemius, popliteus tendon and lateral ligament.
- all the branches form rich anastomosis around the knee joint.

Popliteal vein

- formed at lower border of popliteus muscle by anterior and posterior tibial veins;
- runs up and medially, between artery (deep) and medial popliteal nerve (superficial), to opening in adductor magnus where it becomes femoral vein;
- tributary is short (small) saphenous vein lateral to posterior cutaneous nerve of calf between two heads of gastrocnemius.

NERVES

Femoral

- see Chapter 6.

Sciatic

- origin described in Chapter 6.
- enters thigh deep to hamstrings and is crossed in midthigh by long head of biceps femoris;
- branches to all hamstrings and ischial part of adductor magnus.
- in distal thigh enters poplital space as tibial and peroneal nerves (division occurs at varying level between sacral plexus and lower thigh).

Tibial nerve

- L4, L5, S1, S2, S3
- enters popliteal space at apex, superficial to both femoral vessels,
- runs straight down middle of popliteal space to inferior angle, enters the posterior compartment of the leg between two heads

of the gastrocnemius, then deep to soleus to lie on deep posterior compartment muscles.
- branches
  —muscular, to gastrocnemius, plantaris and popliteus;
  —posterior cutaneous nerve of calf (sural nerve) runs down between two heads of the gastrocnemius and superficial to this muscle, then with short saphenous vein around back of lateral malleolus to supply skin over lateral margin of foot and little toe. Receives communicating branches from superficial and deep peroneal nerves.

Common peroneal
- L4, L5, S1, S2
- runs down and laterally, beneath and medial to biceps tendon;
- leaves popliteal space by passing down and laterally, superficial to lateral head of gastrocnemius, to fibula;
- winds forward around fibula neck (below fibula head) and divides into superficial peroneal (musculocutaneous) and deep peroneal (anterior tibial) nerves;
- branches of common peroneal nerve are
  —lateral cutaneous nerve of calf and
  —sural communicating.

Obturator nerve
- posterior branch receives an articular branch from the knee; this branch ascends alongside the popliteal artery, and
- may explain pain referred from hip to knee.

Saphenous nerve
- from femoral nerve;
- runs with femoral artery to lower end of subsartorial canal of Hunter, then
- medially beneath sartorius to join long (great) saphenous vein as far as foot, posterior to medial ligament of knee, anterior to medial malleolus;
- supplies skin over front of knee (usually cut by medial parapatellar incision and resultant hypoesthesia may be bothersome), anterior and medial surface of leg, medial side of foot and great toe.

MOVEMENTS AT KNEE

Patellofemoral joint

- the patella glides up and down in the patellar groove between the femoral condyles; this sesamoid bone
- improves the mechanical advantage (lever arm) of the quadriceps mechanism, and thereby increases by 30% the power of the quadriceps in extending the knee jont.

Knee joint

- during first 20° to 30° of flexion the femoral condyles rock and glide on the tibial condyles; the remainder of flexion is pure gliding, the menisci and ligaments guiding the femoral condyles; the menisci themselves move back and forth on the tibial condyles;
- vertical axis of rotation of knee passes near center of the joint;
- during the last 15° of extension, the femur rotates medially on the tibia, and this movement locks the knee in extension (standing is thus possible without muscular contraction). This rotation is partly due to the articular surface of medial femoral condyle being longer than the lateral;
- weight of body (center of gravity) passes anterior to locked knee and prevents accidental unlocking;
- before the extended knee can be flexed, it must be unlocked, (lateral rotation of femur on tibia). This is done by contraction of popliteus muscle.
- lateral movement of the tibia on femur is zero with knee in full extension, and a few degrees with the knee flexed 10° (posterolateral and posteromedial parts of capsule are relaxed). Compare both knees.
- anteroposterior movement of tibia on femur is limited to a few degrees in flexion, zero in extension (compare both knees);
- stability of the knee depends on capsule, ligaments and muscles (especially quadriceps).

Surgical Exploration of the Femur

INDICATIONS FOR APPROACHES

Posterolateral

- all shaft fractures—open reduction and IM nail or plate
- subtrochanteric fracture

- supracondylar fracture—nail plate, in combination with medial (Henry) approach when necessary
- exploration of common peroneal nerve
- osteomyelitis
- supracondylar or femoral osteotomy
- epiphyseodesis

Lateral (trochanteric region)

- closed reduction and nail plate for subcapital, transcervical and intertrochanteric fractures
- open reduction and nail plate of intertrochanteric fracture

Medial, subsartorial canal

- exploration and repair of femoral vessels in canal

Medial (Henry), posterior surface distal femur

- supracondylar fracture
- supracondylar osteotomy
- epiphyseodesis

Posterior (Bosworth)

- exploration of sciatic nerve in thigh
- tumor of posterior femoral shaft

SURGICAL APPROACHES

Posterolateral (Figs. 7.3 and 7.7)

- to entire length of femur.
- any part of this incision may be used.

  Position
  - on the side, kidney rests front and back, lower leg flexed at hip and knee. Leg free.

  Incision
  - from base of greater trochanter to middle of lateral femoral condyle, straight.

  Dissection
  - incise fascia lata along anterior border of iliotibial tract,
  - dissect vastus lateralis off lateral intermuscular septum and retract muscle forwards;
  - follow lateral IM septum to linea aspera, identify, ligate and divide perforating vessels (branches of profunda femoris),
  - divide periosteum and reflect vastus intermedius anteriorly with periosteum as far as necessary.

- in supracondylar region, incise the fascia lata transversely and do not enter suprapatellar pouch.
- incision can be extended distally across knee joint to fibula head and neck, for exploration of common peroneal nerve.

Lateral (Figs. 7.3 and 7.7)

- to trochanteric region and proximal shaft.

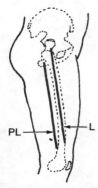

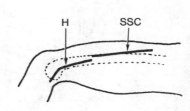

Figure 7.4. Henry's medial approach (*H*) and medial approach for subsartorial canal (*SSC*).

Figure 7.3. Posterolateral (*PL*) and lateral (*L*) approaches.

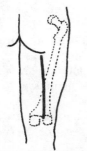

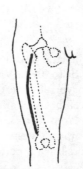

Figure 7.5. Posterior approach.

Figure 7.6. Anterolateral approach.

Figures 7.3 to 7.6. Surgical approaches to femoral shaft.

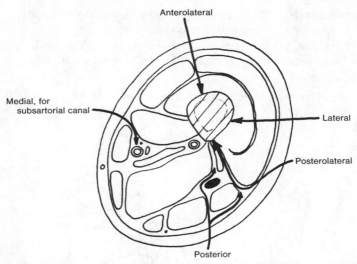

Figure 7.7. Section similar to Figure 7.2, to show surgical approaches to femoral shaft.

Position

- on the side, lower leg flexed, kidney rests back and front. Leg free.

Incision

- start 5 cm proximal and anterior to greater trochanter,
- incise as far as trochanter, then
- vertically and distally, parallel with femoral shaft, for 10 to 15 cm.

Dissection

- incise fascia lata distally, and split it with scissors proximally just posterior to TFL. Vastus lateralis is now exposed;
- divide transversely the origin of vastus lateralis from inferior ridge of greater trochanter, then divide this muscle longitudinally 1 cm from its origin on linea aspera.
- ligate perforating vessels before cutting them (otherwise they retract across linea aspera, and hemorrhage cannot be controlled easily).
- incise periosteum and retract vastus lateralis and intermedius anteriorly to expose lateral and anterolateral surfaces of femur.

- base of femoral neck can be exposed anteriorly by further subperiosteal dissection of vastus lateralis and intermedius and by incision of anterolateral part of hip joint capsule and its insertion on intertrochanteric line.
- this approach can be transformed into Watson-Jones anterolateral approach to hip joint, or continued distally as far as knee, as necessary.

Medial (Figs. 7.4 and 7.7)

- for vessels in subsartorial canal.

  Position

  - supine, thigh in abduction and external rotation.

  Incision

  - follows anterior border of middle third of sartorius, anterior to adductor magnus.

  Dissection

  - retract sartorius posteriorly with long (great) saphenous vein;
  - incise fascia to expose femoral vessels.

Medial (Henry) (Fig. 7.4).

- for posterior surface femur in popliteal space.

  Position

  - supine, leg abducted and in external rotation.

  Incision

  - start 15 cm proximal to adductor tubercle, and
  - cut parallel to adductor magnus tendon to the tubercle, then
  - 5 cm beyond it and a little posteriorly.

  Dissection

  - dissect along anterior border of sartorius and retract this posteriorly (do not enter synovium of knee);
  - this exposes adductor tendon. Retract this and vastus medialis anteriorly to expose posterior surface of femur, femoral vessels and posterior tibial nerve;
  - retract neurovascular bundle posteriorly

Posterior (Bosworth) (Figs. 7.5 and 7.7)

- beware of injury to sciatic nerve by rough handling!

  Position

  - prone.

Incision

• vertical, midline, from gluteal fold to apex of popliteal space.

Dissection

• incise deep fascia.
• to expose proximal part of shaft, dissect between long head of biceps and vastus lateralis, and retract biceps medially;
• for middle of shaft, retract vastus medialis origin medially and vastus lateralis laterally;
• for distal part of shaft, dissect between biceps and semitendinosus, and retract biceps laterally with sciatic nerve.
• for whole of shaft, divide long head of biceps distally, and retract it medially with sciatic nerve. Do NOT retract biceps laterally, or you may damage sciatic nerve.
• when linea aspera has been exposed, expose the femur by subperiosteal dissection (beware of perforating vessels).

Anterior (Figs. 7.6 and 7.7)

• these are all muscle-splitting approaches, are bloody,
• likely to cause limitation of movement of the knee, and are
• not advised.

Surgical Exploration of the Knee

INDICATIONS FOR APPROACHES

Anteromedial

• synovectomy
• patellectomy
• debridement of knee for osteoarthritis
• arthroplasty, partial or total replacement
• repair of ruptured anterior cruciate, or medial collateral ligament and capsule
• tendon transfers for medial rotary instability
• transposition of patella ligament
• osteochondral femoral fracture
• displaced or depressed intra-articular fracture of medial tibial condyle

Medial parapatellar

• arthrotomy (exploratory)

- medial meniscectomy
- IM nailing of tibial fracture
- removal of loose bodies
- septic arthritis (drainage)

Anterior transverse

- knee fusion
- reduction and internal fixation of fractured patella
- patellectomy for comminuted fracture

Anterolateral

- fracture of lateral tibial condyle
- fracture of lateral femoral condyle
- repair of lateral collateral ligament and capsule

Lateral transverse (Bruser)

- lateral meniscectomy

Posterolateral

- removal of loose bodies confined to this compartment
- drainage
- soft-tissue release and tendon lengthening

Posterior

- exploration of neurovascular bundle
- excision of Baker's cyst
- posterior capsulotomy
- repair of ruptured posterior cruciate ligament

Posteromedial

- removal of loose bodies
- drainage
- soft-tissue release and tendon lengthening

SURGICAL APPROACHES

Points to note:

- under anesthesia, BEFORE the incision, examine the knee again.
- this is articular surgery, and the knee is very susceptible to infection, with severe consequences.
- tourniquet for no longer than 90 minutes; then pack the wound, apply firm and even pressure, release the tourniquet for 10 minutes and examine the leg or toes to confirm that circulation has returned. Tourniquet may then be reapplied for 60 minutes.

- do not remove periosteum around the knee—will provoke periarticular calcification.
- use absorbable sutures in synovium, because nonabsorbable sutures may cause hydrarthrosis. Use nonabsorbable sutures in capsule and muscular aponeuroses.
- active quadriceps exercises (taught before surgery) should be started as soon as possible after surgery, unless contraindicated. Remember that without active physiotherapy, the success of your treatment will be jeopardized.

Anteromedial (Langenbeck) (Fig. 7.8)

Position

- supine, leg free.

Incision

- start 10 cm above patella at medial border of quadriceps tendon, then continue
- distally in a gentle curve around medial border of patella and gently back to midline just medial to tibial tubercle.
- if the curve around the patella is too sharp, the skin over the patella may slough.

Dissection

- incise fascia;
- incise between vastus medialis and quadriceps tendon, and capsule and synovium in same line;
- incise retinacular fibers, capsule and synovium 1 cm medial to patella, then continue incision to medial border of patellar tendon.
- retract patella laterally to expose anterior compartment and medial tibial condyle and metaphysis;
- exposure can be increased by lengthening incision proximally; or partially detaching patella tendon medially from tibial tuberosity and dislocating patella laterally, then flexing knee.

Medial parapatellar (Fig. 7.9)

- this is the distal half of the preceding approach and is used particularly for medial meniscectomy.
- to see clearly the posterior horn of medial meniscus, and to be sure not to leave part of this horn behind, make a
  —second vertical incision 8 cm long behind medial collateral ligament, through capsule and synovium. This gives

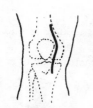

Figure 7.8. Anteromedial (Langenbeck).

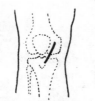

Figure 7.9. Medial parapatellar.

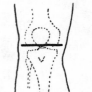

Figure 7.10. Anterior transverse.

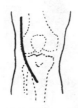

Figure 7.11. Anterolateral (Kocher).

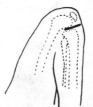

Figure 7.12. Lateral (Bruser).

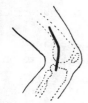

Figure 7.13. Postero-lateral.

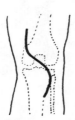

Figure 7.14. Posterior.

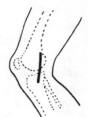

Figure 7.15. Posteromedial (Henderson).

Figures 7.8 to 7.15. Surgical approaches to the knee joint.

—clear view of posterior horn, its posterior peripheral attachment, and the tibial attachment of posterior cruciate ligament.

Anterior transverse (Fig. 7.10)

Position

• supine, leg free.

Incision

- transverse, from midpoint of medial surface of knee to midpoint of lateral surface of knee,
- centered either over patella (for patella fracture) or over knee joint (for fusion of knee joint).

Dissection

- centered over knee joint for fusion, incise fascia, patella tendon, retinacular and aponeurotic fibers of quadriceps, then incise in same transverse line the capsule and synovium. Retract patella proximally to expose anterior compartment of knee joint.

Anterolateral (Kocher) (Fig. 7.11)

- not the equal of anteromedial approach

Position

- supine, sandbag beneath buttock of same side. Leg free.

Incision

- start just lateral and 8 cm proximal to patella,
- continue distally 1 cm lateral to patella, then
- curve medially to 3 cm below tibial tuberosity (never cross the midline because an incision here is painful when the patient kneels).

Dissection

- incise retinacular and aponeurotic fibers in line of skin incision;
- incise capsule and synovium, and
- retract patella medially (it cannot be dislocated medially);
- lateral compartment of joint, lateral tibial condyle and proximal metaphysis of tibia are exposed;
- to expose lateral femoral condyle, extend incision proximally.

Lateral (Bruser) (Fig. 7.12)

Position

- supine, knee fully flexed, leg free.

Incision

- start incision at joint line just lateral to patellar tendon, and
- continue posteriorly along joint line as far as vertical axis of fibula.

Dissection

- split iliotibial tract in direction of its fibers;

- do not cut lateral collateral ligament which is relaxed and lies at posterior end of incision;
- retract iliotibial tract and identify inferior lateral genicular artery; protect it or ligate and divide it;
- incise synovium to expose lateral meniscus.

Posterolateral (Henderson) (Fig. 7.13)

Position

- supine, knee flexed, leg free.

Incision

- start in middle of lateral surface of thigh 10 cm above lateral femoral condyle;
- continue straight down thigh to posterolateral border of lateral condyle, then
- curve incision gently back to end just anterior to fibula head (thus avoid common peroneal nerve).

Dissection

- trace anterior surface of IM septum to linea aspera in proximal part of incision;
- expose lateral femoral condyle;
- identify femoral origin of lateral collateral ligament;
- retract posteriorly the popliteus tendon (lies between biceps femoris tendon and lateral collateral ligament) and incise longitudinally the capsule and synovium.

Posterior (Fig. 7.14)

- dangerous. Know your anatomy!
- the flexion crease at back of knee lies 2 to 3 cm proximal to line of knee joint.

Position

- prone.

Incision

- S-shaped. Proximal limb follows semitendinosus 5 cm to knee joint, then gentle curve laterally for 5 cm to lateral head of gastrocnemius, then
- curves distally 5 cm.

Dissection

- identify posterior cutaneous nerve of calf (sural nerve) lying

under fascia beneath two heads of gastrocnemius (small saphenous vein pierces lower part of popliteal fascia lateral to nerve and enters popliteal vein);
- trace this nerve proximally to origin from tibial nerve;
- tibial nerve is key to dissection of popliteal space;
- trace tibial nerve distally, find and protect branches to gastrocnemius (both heads) and soleus (accompanied by vessels);
- trace tibial nerve proximally to find common peroneal nerve;
- trace common peroneal nerve distally, beneath tendon of biceps;
- protect lateral cutaneous nerve of calf.
- expose popliteal artery and vein (deep to tibial nerve);
- identify and protect superior genicular vessels;
- retract popliteal vessels gently.
- open posteromedial compartment of joint between medial head of gastrocnemius and semimembranosus, retracting tendinous origin of medial head of gastrocnemius laterally (thus protecting popliteal vessels);
- open posterolateral compartment between lateral head of gastrocnemius and biceps tendon.

Posteromedial (Henderson) (Fig. 7.15)

Position

- supine, thigh abducted, knee flexed 25°. Leg free.

Incision

- start at adductor tubercle and descend parallel to medial collateral ligament, anterior to tendons of sartorius, gracilis, semitendinosus and semimembranosus.

Dissection

- incise capsule posterior to medial collateral ligament and enter posteromedial compartment of knee.

chapter 8

Leg and Ankle

Surgical Anatomy

TIBIA AND FIBULA

Tibial shaft

Surfaces

- medial (entirely subcutaneous) between anterior and medial borders. No muscle attachments;
- lateral, between anterior and interosseous (IO) borders. Proximal third covered with muscle;
- posterior, between interosseous and medial borders. Soleal line runs down and medially over upper part, and vertical line runs straight down center of proximal half of this surface. Proximal three fifths covered with muscle.
- nutrient artery, from posterior tibial artery, enters posterior surface just distal to soleal line, in direction away from knee joint: "to the elbow I go; from the knee I flee!"

Borders

- anterior (entirely subcutaneous);
- medial (subcutaneous);
- interosseous, has interosseous membrane (IOM) attached to most of its length.

Fibula shaft

- Latin—pin or brooch
- fibula is placed lateral and posterior to tibia.

Surfaces

- all surrounded by muscle;
- anterior between anterior and interosseous borders;

- lateral between anterior and posterior borders;
- posterior between interosseous and posterior borders. Upper two thirds of posterior surface is divided in two by vertical ridge called medial crest;
- nutrient artery from peroneal branch of posterior tibial enters posterior surface in distal direction.

Borders

- anterior,
- interosseous and
- posterior.

Tibiofibular joints

Superior tibiofibular joint

- posterolateral (fibula is more posterior than you think);
- synovial;
- between head of fibula and undersurface of lateral tibial condyle;
- supported by capsule and anterior and posterior ligaments.

Interosseous membrane

- deficient above (anterior tibial artery passes forwards into anterior compartment), and below (perforating peroneal artery).
- fibers directed down and out.

Inferior tibiofibular joint

- strong IO ligament 3 cm wide just above ankle, essential for stability of ankle;
- anterior and posterior inferior tibiofibular ligaments (latter comes below distal tibia posteriorly to deepen socket for talus)

ANKLE JOINT

Joint surfaces

Ankle mortice

- constructed from three surfaces;
- distal tibial articular surface forms the roof (takes five sixths of standing weight);
- medial malleolus, with comma-shaped articular surface is medial wall, and
- lateral malleolus (fibula) is the lateral wall. Tip of this lateral malleolus is 1½ cm more distal and posterior to medial malleo-

lus, and slopes obliquely laterally (takes one sixth of standing weight).

Talus
- body of talus fits into mortice;
- dome-shaped superior surface of body of talus is broader anteriorly than posteriorly (lateral stability greater in dorsiflexion than plantar flexion).
- medial articular facet is comma-shaped, matching that on medial malleolus, and
- lateral articular facet is triangular for lateral malleolus.

Capsule and ligaments

Capsule
- thin, attached round margins of articulating surfaces.

Medial collateral (deltoid) ligament
- from tip, anterior and posterior borders of medial malleolus;
- divides into deep and superficial parts
  —deep part to talus,
  —superficial part fans out in triangular shape to navicular tuberosity, plantar calcaneonavicular (spring) ligament, sustentaculum tali (of calcaneus) and posterior talus.

Lateral collateral ligament
- consists of three bands
  —anterior talofibular band to talar neck;
  —calcaneofibular ligament, downward and posteriorly to calcaneum just posterior to peroneal tubercle, and
  —posterior talofibular ligament, from pit (depression) on posteromedial surface of lateral malleolus passes horizontally to posterior talar tubercle.

Movements
- dorsiflexion (extension), 20°,
- plantar flexion (flexion), 50°.
- in plantar flexion, some abduction and adduction is possible (see above).

MUSCLES (Fig. 8.1)
- in the leg, these are surrounded by strong fascia which is attached to anterior tibial border, sweeps laterally, posteriorly and medially to

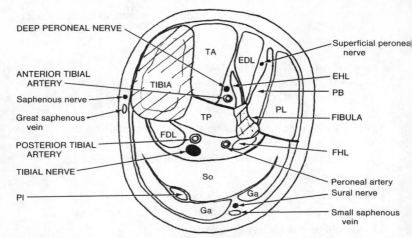

Figure 8.1. Transverse section through middle of leg. *EDL*, extensor digitorum longus; *EHL*, extensor hallucis longus; *FDL*, flexor digitorum longus; *FHL*, flexor hallucis longus; *Ga*, gastrocnemius; *PB*, peroneus brevis; *Pl*, plantaris, *PL*, peroneus longus; *So*, soleus; *TA*, tibialis anterior; *TP*, tibialis posterior.

surround all muscle groups, and reattaches to medial tibial border.
- muscles are in three groups:

Anterior group

- between tibia and fibula in front of IOM. All tendons easily visible and palpable around ankle and foot.
- all supplied by deep peroneal nerve, mainly L5.

Tibialis anterior (TA)

- origin from upper-two thirds lateral surface tibia and IOM,
- to medial and inferior surface of base of first metatarsal (MT) (of big toe) and medial cuneiform;
- separate tendon sheath (synovial) beneath both retinacula;
- nerve supply L4, L5;
- action is dorsiflexion of foot, and inversion with tibialis posterior (TP).

Extensor hallucis longus (EHL)

- from midthird anterior surface fibula and IOM;
- to dorsal surface of base of terminal phalanx of great toe
- separate sheath at ankle;

- nerve is L5, S1;
- action is extension of great toe (attempts to dorsiflex foot when tibialis anterior is paralyzed as in poliomyelitis and causes classic cockup deformity of great toe with depressed first MT).

Extensor digitorum longus (EDL)
- from proximal two thirds of anterior surface fibula and IOM;
- to dorsal aspect of base of middle and distal phalanges of all four lateral toes (similar to long extensor tendons of fingers);
- has common synovial sheath for all four tendons;
- nerve is L5, S1;
- action is extension of toes (and of foot when tibialis anterior is paralyzed).

Extensor retinacula
- in two parts across front of ankle joint;
- superior, from lateral (fibular) malleolus to tibia just above medial malleolus; pierced by tibialis anterior tendon, the others run beneath it;
- inferior, from lateral surface calcaneum; one band passes superomedially to medial malleolus, the other inferomedially to plantar aponeurosis; pierced by all extensor tendons.

Relations of tendons (Fig. 8.2).
- in front of ankle the order in which the structures cross the ankle joint, from medial to lateral side, is:
  —*T*ibialis anterior
  —extensor *H*allucis longus
  —*V*ena comitans (one of two companion veins of the artery)
  —anterior tibial *A*rtery
  —*V*ena comitans
  —deep peroneal *N*erve
  —extensor *D*igitorum longus
- *T*imothy *H*ath *V*exed *A*ll *V*ery *N*ervous *D*amsels.

Lateral group
- both supplied by superficial peroneal nerve, L5, S1.

  Peroneus longus
  - from proximal two-thirds lateral surface fibula;
  - tendon lies
    —posterior to peroneus brevis tendon in groove behind lateral malleolus, then

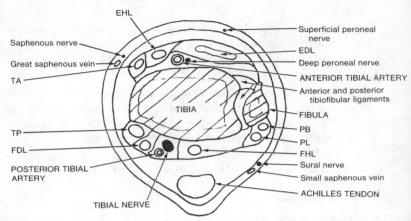

Figure 8.2. Transverse section through distal tibia and fibula just above ankle joint. Abbreviations are the same as for Figure 8.1.

—crosses lateral collateral ligament and ankle,
—turns through 90° around cuboid to run in groove beneath cuboid forwards and medially in sole of foot;
• inserts into lateral and inferior aspect base of first MT and medial cuneiform;
• action is
—eversion (and plantar flexion of foot with TP and triceps surae), and
—support of transverse arch of foot.

Peroneus brevis
• from lower two-thirds lateral surface fibula, anterior to peroneus longus;
• tendon lies
—anterior to peroneus longus behind lateral malleolus,
—passes above peroneal tubercle on lateral surface of calcaneum, and
• inserts into styloid process of base fifth MT (palpable);
• action is eversion of foot (and plantar flexion in concert with TP and triceps surae).

Peroneal retinacula and sheaths
• common fibrous tunnel (retinaculum) and synovial sheath for both tendons behind lateral malleolus;

- synovial sheath splits to follow the tendons individually on both side of peroneal tubercle.

Posterior group

- gastrocnemius, soleus and plantaris are superficial, the rest are deep.
- all supplied by tibial nerve, mainly S1.

Gastrocnemius (see Chapter 7)

- this muscle and the soleus form the triceps surae.

Soleus

- origin from
  - soleal line on posterior surface of tibia and middle third of medial border of tibia,
  - proximal quarter of posterior surface of fibula and
  - fibrous arch over popliteal vessels and tibial nerve;
- lies deep to gastrocnemius and
- inserts into deep aspect of tendocalcaneus and thereby into calcaneum;
- nerve is L5, S1, S2;
- action (in concert with gastrocnemius) is
  - plantar flexion of ankle (and of foot through plantar aponeurosis), and thus
  - push off.

Plantaris (see Chapter 7)

Popliteus (see Chapter 7)

Tibialis posterior (TP)

- from lateral half posterior surface tibia below soleal line, IOM and fibula;
- to tuberosity of navicular (palpate it), and by fibrous slips to all tarsals (except talus) and all MTs (except fifth);
- nerve is L4, L5;
- action
  - very strong invertor of foot; also
  - plantar flexion with peroneals and triceps surae, and
  - supports longitudinal arch of foot.

Flexor digitorum longus (FDL)

- from posterior surface tibia below soleal line;
- to four lateral toes, plantar surface of base of distal phalanges,

after splitting and passing through tendons of flexor digitorum brevis (similar to flexor digitorum profundus and flexor digitorum superficialis in hand);
- nerve is L5, S1, S2;
- action
  —flexes lateral four toes and
  —lifts heel off ground in walking, using heads of four lateral MTs as fulcrum.

Flexor hallucis longus (FHL)

- large, powerful, multipennate, with muscle fibers as far as the ankle joint;
- origin from lower three-quarters posterior surface fibula and IOM;
- tendon grooves back of talus and under surface of sustentaculum tali (a bony process on medial side of calcaneum which supports talus);
- inserts into plantar surface of base of distal phalanx great toe;
- nerve is L5, S1, S2;
- action is
  —flexion of great toe, and
  —lifts heel off ground in walking (heel off) by using ball of foot (head of first MT) as fulcrum; also
  —supports medial longitudinal arch of foot.

Relations of tendons (Fig. 8.2)

- behind the ankle the order in which structures cross the ankle joint, from medial to lateral side, is:
  —*T*ibialis posterior
  —flexor *D*igitorum longus
  —*V*ena comitans
  —posterior tibial *A*rtery
  —*V*ena comitans
  —tibial *N*erve
  —flexor *H*allucis longus
- *T*imothy *D*oth *V*ex *A*ll *V*ery *N*ervous *H*ousewives.

ARTERIES

- popliteal artery ends at lower border of popliteus muscle (in the popliteal space) where it divides into two terminal branches anterior and posterior tibial arteries.

Anterior tibial artery

- passes forward, between two heads of tibialis posterior and through proximal defect in IOM (between proximal tibial metaphysis and neck of fibula) to anterior tibial compartment;
- travels straight down leg, beneath TA, on anterior surface of IOM, to cross ankle midway between the two malleoli, beneath extensor retinacula,
- lying directly on tibial periosteum just above ankle where it becomes the dorsalis pedis artery.
- relations:
  - —in leg, TA is medial, EDL and EHL are lateral, but the EHL tendon crosses in front of the artery in the lower leg to lie medial to the artery at the ankle;
  - —deep peroneal nerve is lateral to the artery.
- branches:
  - —to anastomoses around the knee and ankle,
  - —to soleus, peroneus longus and muscles of anterior compartment of leg.

Posterior tibial artery

- passes down back of leg, between triceps surae (gastrocnemius and soleus) and deep muscles of posterior compartment;
- distally, lies between tendo achillis and medial border tibia (can be palpated here);
- behind ankle divides into two terminal branches
  - —medial and
  - —lateral plantar arteries.
- branches:
  - —peroneal, down medial border of fibula, gives nutrient branch to fibula;
  - —nutrient branch to tibia;
  - —muscular to posterior and lateral compartments of leg;
  - —calcaneal, arises near ankle and supplies skin and fat of heel (must not be damaged during talectomy or Syme's amputation);
  - —anastomotic to anterior compartment and around ankle joint.

NERVES

Common peroneal nerve

- from posterior (dorsal) divisions of L4, L5, S1, S2 nerve roots;
- leaves popliteal space beneath tendon of biceps femoris and

- runs around lateral aspect of neck of fibula to peroneus longus; before reaching this muscle the nerve divides into two branches:
  - —superficial peroneal nerve, supplies peroneal muscles and skin of lateral side of leg, dorsum of foot and all the toes; and the
  - —deep peroneal nerve, which lies on front of IOM, lateral to anterior tibial artery, and supplies muscles of anterior compartment, extensor digitorum brevis and dorsal skin between the first and second toes.

Tibial nerve

- leaves inferior angle of popliteal space,
- enters the leg between the two heads of gastrocnemius, beneath soleus,
- descends in leg, lateral to posterior tibial artery, lying on deep muscles beneath gastrocnemius; then lies medial to Achilles tendon in lower part of leg. Behind the ankle it divides into
- two terminal branches, the
  - —medial and
  - —lateral plantar nerves;
- branches from tibial nerve in the leg to
  - —muscles of the posterior compartment and
  - —skin over heel, and by the
  - —sural nerve (which receives anastomotic branch from common peroneal nerve) it supplies skin over posterior surface of leg and lateral side of foot.

Surgical Exploration of the Leg

INDICATIONS

Transverse medial
- high tibial osteotomy for genu valgum

Transverse lateral
- high tibial osteotomy for genu varum

Anterior
- osteomyelitis—drainage, saucerization
- open reduction and plating of fracture of tibia
- graft for pseudarthrosis
- derotation osteotomy of shaft
- removal of tibial cortex for use as graft

Posteromedial
- posterior graft of tibia

Posterolateral
- osteomyelitis of fibula
- removal of fibula shaft for use as graft
- osteotomy of fibula
- posterior tibiofibular graft

SURGICAL APPROACHES

Transverse medial (Fig. 8.3)
- for proximal tibial metaphysis, medial aspect (not extensile).

  Position
  - supine, thigh in abduction and external rotation,
  - leg free.

  Incision
  - transverse, from superomedial border of tibial tuberosity medially to posteromedial angle of tibia, parallel with and just below the medial condyle (do not cut long saphenous vein);
  - do not cross tibial tuberosity.

  Dissection
  - incise periosteum in line with skin incision, dissecting beneath (but not cutting) the patellar tendon and medial collateral ligament;
  - dissect subperiosteally the posterior surface of tibia.

Transverse lateral (Fig. 8.4)
- for proximal tibial metaphysis, lateral aspect (not extensile).

  Position
  - supine, with sandbag beneath buttock of same side.
  - leg free.

  Incision
  - from superolateral point of tibial tuberosity, laterally parallel with and just below tibial condyle, to or across head of fibula;
  - do not cross tibial tuberosity.

  Dissection
  - reflect origin of TA from lateral surface of tibia for 5 cm below condyle. Do not go further or you may injure anterior tibial artery;

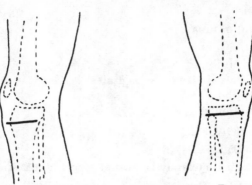

Figure 8.3. Transverse medial.   **Figure 8.4.** Transverse lateral.

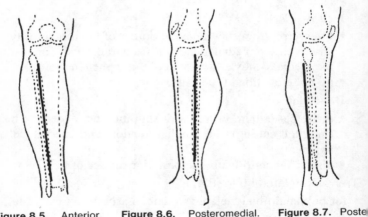

Figure 8.5. Anterior.   **Figure 8.6.** Posteromedial.   **Figure 8.7.** Poste
                                                                      lateral.

Figures 8.3 to 8.7.   Surgical approaches to the tibia and fibula.

- dissect proximal tibial metaphysis subperiosteally laterally, a
  medially beneath patellar tendon; proximal part of insertion
  this tendon can be detached from tibial tuberosity for grea
  exposure.
- if fibula head is to be excised, the common peroneal nerve m
  first be identified, freed and retracted gently;
- excision of fibula head and neck permits subperiosteal expos
  of posterior surface of tibia as far as the medial border.

Anterior (Figs. 8.5 and 8.8)

Position

- supine.

Incision

- longitudinal, immediately lateral to anterior border of tibia.

Dissection

- incise periosteum over tibia, and reflect periosteum medially (anterior surface) and periosteum and anterior compartment muscles laterally.

Posteromedial (Figs. 8.6 and 8.8)

Position

- supine, thigh in external rotation and abduction, knee flexed.

Incision

- longitudinal, along medial border of tibia (do not cut long saphenous vein).

Dissection

- reflect subperiosteally the posterior compartment muscles, and the periosteum from the medial surface.

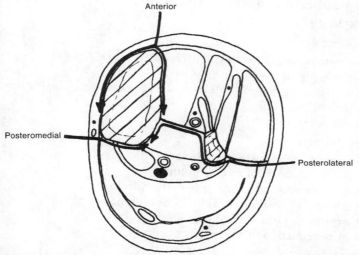

Figure 8.8. Section similar to Figure 8.1, to show surgical approaches to the tibia and fibula.

Posterolateral (Henry and Harmon) (Figs. 8.7 and 8.8)

Position

- prone, or on side, leg free.

Incision

- longitudinal, along posterior border of fibula, as long as necessary.

Dissection

- if proximal shaft or fibula head is to be exposed, identify an
protect common peroneal nerve first;
- dissect between soleus (behind) and peronei (in front) to fibula
- expose fibula subperiosteally;
- to expose posterior surface of IOM and lateral surface of tibia
    —dissect fibula subperiosteally to its IO border (beware pero
    neal artery); then
    —reflect posterior compartment muscles from IOM until th
    tibia is reached, and
    —expose subperiosteally the lateral surface of tibia (posterio
    tibial nerve and vessels are protected by deep muscles).

Surgical Exploration of the Ankle

INDICATIONS

Anterolateral

- comminuted, intra-articular fracture of distal tibia
- ankle fusion
- pantalar arthrodesis (ankle, subtalar, talonavicular and calcanec
cuboid joints)
- talectomy

Posterolateral

- ligamentoplasty (Watson-Jones) of lateral collateral ligament
ankle, or repair of recent rupture
- fracture of distal fibula or lateral malleolus
- fracture of posterolateral lip of distal tibial epiphysis
- exploration of peroneal tendons
- open reduction of fractured calcaneum.

Posterior

- inlay ankle fusion

- inlay subtalar fusion (Gallie)
- fracture posterior lip tibia
- tendo achillis repair, or lengthening and posterior capsulotomy of ankle.

Posteromedial

- fracture of medial malleolus and posterior lip of tibia
- rupture of medial collateral ligament
- posteromedial soft-tissue release for club foot
- exploration of posterior tibial neurovascular bundle

Anterior

- fracture of neck and talus.

SURGICAL APPROACHES

Anterolateral (Figs. 8.9 and 8.13)

Position

- supine, leg free, sandbag under buttock of same side.

Incision

- start 5 cm above ankle on anterolateral surface of leg, halfway between fibula and anterior tibial border;
- continue straight down and end at base of fourth MT.

Dissection

- incise fascia and extensor retinacula,
- detach origin (from calcaneus) of extensor digitorum brevis muscle and reflect distally,
- retract medially the extensor tendons, anterior tibial artery (dorsalis pedis) and deep peroneal nerve, and
- incise ankle joint capsule.
- for exposure of intertarsal joints
  —expose talonavicular joint (beneath extensor tendons) and calcaneocuboid joint and incise capsule transversely;
  —dissecting distally, expose joints between cuboid and fourth and fifth MTs, and between navicular and lateral cuneiform;
  —dissect through fat on lateral and inferior surfaces of talar neck to expose subtalar joint.

Posterolateral (Kocher) (Figs. 8.10 and 8.13)

Position

- supine, sandbag beneath same buttock, leg free.

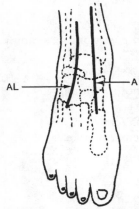

Figure 8.9. Anterolateral (AL) and anterior (*A*).

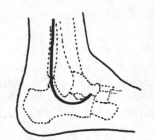

Figure 8.10. Posterolateral.

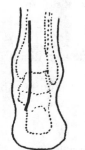

Figure 8.11. Posterior.

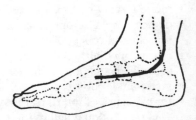

Figure 8.12. Posteromedial.

Figures 8.9 to 8.12. Surgical approaches to the ankle joint.

Incision

- start 5 to 10 cm proximal to tip of lateral malleolus, 1 cm behind posterior border of fibula,
- continue vertically down behind lateral malleolus and
- swing incision forward, 2 to 3 cm below tip of lateral malleolus, then upward and forward to head of talus.

Dissection

- incise fascia over peroneal tendons and retract them posteriorly;
- distal fibula can be exposed subperiosteally;
- lateral malleolus can be exposed by subperiosteal dissection, and the calcaneofibular ligament can be cut if necessary.
- expose the ankle joint by
  - osteotomy through distal fibula shaft,
  - dividing the IOM and anterior and posterior malleolar ligaments and turning lateral malleolus downwards, hinging it on lateral collateral ligament (technique of Gatellier and Chastang).
- expose subtalar joint and talar neck by reflecting distally the extensor digitorum brevis and fat pad in the sinus tarsi.
- fibula must be replaced and fixed with a transverse screw into tibia;
- repair tendon sheaths and retinacula.

Posterior (Figs. 8.11 and 8.13)

Position

- prone, leg free.

Incision

- longitudinal, halfway between Achilles tendon and back of medial malleolus;
- start 2 cm above ankle joint and end at calcaneum.

Dissection

- retract tendo achillis laterally;
- identify and retract medially the posterior tibial vessels and tibial nerve, with TP and FDL;
- retract FHL laterally (or medially);
- identify posterior capsule of ankle joint (do not confuse with subtalar joint) and incise transversely.

Posteromedial (hockey stick) (Figs. 8.12 and 8.13)

Position

- supine, sandbag beneath same buttock, leg free.

Incision

- start 6 or 8 cm above medial malleolus, just behind postero-medial border of tibia,

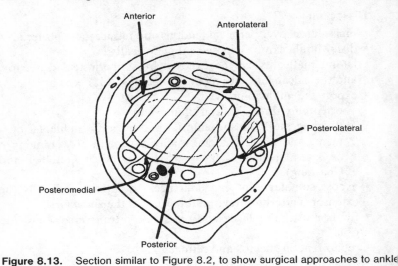

Figure 8.13. Section similar to Figure 8.2, to show surgical approaches to ankle joint.

- descend vertically behind medial malleolus, then swing forward below tip of malleolus;
- can be extended forward as far as head of first MT.

Dissection

- medial malleolus can be exposed subperiosteally (do not divide medial collateral ligament).
- fracture of posterior lip and medial malleolus can be exposed by
  - posterior retraction of posterior tibial vessels, tibial nerve, FHL, and
  - anterior retraction of TP and FDL, after incising their sheaths.
- dissection can be carried forward to first MT for soft-tissue release.

Anterior (Figs. 8.9 and 8.13)

Position

- supine, leg free.

Incision

- start lateral to anterior border of tibia, 8 cm above ankle joint and

- continue distally onto foot 5 cm distal to ankle joint;
- can be extended.

Dissection.

- dissect between TA (medially) and EHL (protect anterior tibial vessels and deep peroneal nerve) laterally;
- expose ankle joint and incise capsule;
- both malleoli are easily exposed.
- dorsal (superior) aspect of neck of talus and talonavicular joint can be exposed through distal part of incision.

chapter 9
Foot

Surgical Anatomy

OSTEOARTICULAR STRUCTURE

Topography
- hindfoot is
  —talus and
  —calcaneus (Fig. 9.1);
- midfoot is
  —remaining tarsals;
- forefoot is
  —metatarsals and phalanges;

Talus (astragalus)
- has no tendon or muscle attachments;
- body is dome-shaped, almost completely covered with articular cartilage, and articulates
  —superiorly with tibia and
  —inferiorly with calcaneus (two articular facets separated by sulcus tali).
- body carries
  —lateral, triangular facet, base proximally, sloping down and out articulates with lateral malleolus,
  —medial facet for medial malleolus, and
  —posterior tubercle (sometimes separate, the os trigonum) for attachment of posterior talofibular ligament. Medial to tubercle is
  —groove for flexor hallucis longus (FHL) tendon.
- head covered with articular cartilage, articulates
  —anteriorly with navicular bone and
  —inferiorly with plantar calcaneonavicular (spring) ligament

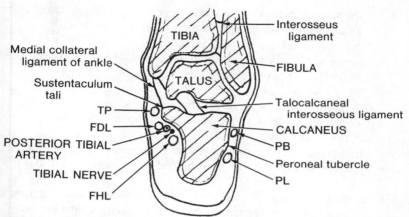

Figure 9.1. Coronal section through ankle joint and hindfoot. *FDL*, flexor digitorum longus; *FHL*, flexor hallucis longus; *PB*, peroneus brevis; *PL*, peroneus longus; *TP*, tibialis posterior.

which runs from distal border of sustentaculum tali (on calcaneus) to navicular tuberosity.
- neck has no articular cartilage.
- blood supply of talus is precarious. Main supply of head and body is through
  —superior surface of neck from anterior tibial artery and
  —inferior surface of neck by anastomosis of branches from posterior tibial artery and perforating branch of peroneal artery in the sinus tarsi. Fracture of neck may cause
- avascular necrosis of the body. Other
- branches from posterior tibial artery enter body
  —beneath medial collateral ligament and through
  —posterior tubercle.

Calcaneus (os calcis)

- cortex is thin, fragile, and
- interior is cancellous bone.
- superior surface anteriorly carries
  —two articular facets for talus, the anterior and posterior, separated by a groove, the
  —sulcus calcanei. This and the sulcus tali form a canal or tunnel,
  —the sinus tarsi. The anterior facet is on the superior surface of

—the sustentaculum tali, a bony process projecting medially from anteromedial corner of calcaneus. This process is

—grooved inferiorly by FHL tendon;

- superior surface is angled like a pitched roof in the sagittal (antheroposterior) plane, forming an angle of

—25° to 40°, called

—Böhler's angle. Decrease of angle may indicate a

—depressed fracture of the articular platform.

- anteriorly, calcaneus articulates with cuboid;
- anterior process is the prominent anterosuperior angle of calcaneus.
- posterior surface has large tuberosity for insertion of Achilles tendon.
- lateral surface has peroneal tubercle (trochlear process); peroneal tendons run on either side of it, brevis in front, longus behind.
- posteroinferiorly are

—two tubercles, medial and lateral, and a

—transverse ridge between them, for attachment of the

—superficial intrinsic muscles and the

—plantar aponeurosis.

Navicular (scaphoid)

- articulates with talar head proximally, three cuneiforms distally and cuboid laterally;
- tuberosity (on medial side, easily palpable) receives tibialis posterior tendon and spring ligament; may have separate ossification center.

Cuboid

- calcaneocuboid and talonavicular joints comprize the midtarsal joint of Chopart, and function as one unit;
- cuboid also articulates with fourth and fifth metatarsals (MTs) distally and with navicular and third cuneiform medially;
- inferior surface grooved by peroneus longus tendon which may have a sesamoid bone here.

Cuneiforms

- three bones;
- articulate proximally with the navicular and
- distally with the first, second and third MTs. The
- second cuneiform is more proximal than the other two, making a mortice for the base of the second MT, so that this MT is

—locked into the tarsals, and is therefore the

—key to fracture-dislocations of the tarsometatarsal joint, (the joint of Lisfranc, surgeon with Napoleon's Grande Armée).

Joints

Subtalar

- consists of
  - —two joints (anterior and posterior talocalcaneal) separated by sinus tarsi (a tunnel containing fat, interosseous ligament and an artery):
  - —posterior joint between talar body (concave facet) and calcaneus;
  - —anterior between talar (convex facet) and calcaneus, sustentaculum tali and plantar calcaneonavicular (spring) ligament, and is continuous with talonavicular joint.
- axis of rotation is directed forwards and slightly medially;
- movements are eversion and inversion of the foot, acting with midtarsal joint.

Other joints

- all synovial, and
- held together by capsules and very strong ligaments;
- little movement occurs at the intertarsal and tarsometatarsal joints, except subtalar and midtarsal.

Ossification centers

- radiographic appearance:
  - —calcaneus, talus and cuboid are present at birth;
  - —third (lateral) cuneiform, first year of age;
  - —first (medial) cuneiform, second year;
  - —second (intermediate) cuneiform and navicular, third year.

Tarsal angles

- on anteroposterior (AP) radiograph of foot, angle between longitudinal axes of
  - —talus (in line with first MT) and
  - —calcaneus (in line with fifth MT) is normally
  - —20° to 40°, open distally;
  - —varus foot reduces the angle (less than 20°),
  - —valgus foot increases it (more than 40°).
- on lateral radiograph, angle between

  —long axes of talus and calcaneus is between
  —30° and 50°, open posteriorly;
  —clubfoot reduces this angle (less than 30°),
  —congenital vertical talus increases it (more than 50°).
- longitudinal axis of foot follows second MT.

Arches

- plantar surface of foot is shaped like half a dome; both feet together form a
- complete, shallow dome.
- foot has three major weight-bearing areas,
  —head of first MT,
  —head of fifth MT and
  —posterior tubercles of calcaneus.
- medial longitudinal arch lies between calcaneal tubercles behind and head of first MT in front, and includes in its structure the
  —calcaneus, talus, navicular, three cuneiforms and the medial three MTs. Center of this arch is the
  —highest point of plantar vault.
- lateral longitudinal arch, from calcaneus to fifth MT, includes
  —calcaneus, cuboid and lateral two MTs.
- transverse arch is formed by
  —heads of all five MTs.
- apex of plantar vault is
  —toward posterior part of foot, beneath the tibia. Thus
  —weight of patient is spread forwards and backwards by these arches (like a stone arch in a Gothic cathedral);
- integrity of arches is maintained by
  —long tendons of extrinsic muscles passing forward in sole,
  —tibialis anterior,
  —intrinsic muscles of foot,
  —interosseous ligaments, and
  —plantar fascia.

MUSCLES

- extrinsic muscles are tendinous in the foot (see Chapter 8);
- intrinsic muscles have their origins and insertions within the foot.

  Dorsum

  - dorsum of foot has one intrinsic muscle only, the extensor digitorum brevis (EDB);

- from anterolateral part of superior surface of calcaneus, divides into
- four tendons; the
- most medial tendon inserts into dorsum of base of proximal phalanx (PP) great toe, the other
- three tendons insert into sides of extensor digitorum longus tendons to the second, third and fourth toes;
- nerve is deep peroneal, L5, S1;
- action is extension of PP of four medial toes.

Sole

- sole of foot has extrinsic tendons and intrinsic muscles in four layers.

First layer

- most superficial layer,
- contains three muscles:

Abductor hallucis

- from medial calcaneal tubercle and plantar aponeurosis
- to medial side of base of PP of great toe;
- nerve is medial plantar, S2, S3;
- abducts great toe.

Flexor digitorum brevis (FDB)

- from medial calcaneal tubercle and plantar aponeurosis; divides into
- four tendons, for the four lateral toes. Each tendon
- divides opposite PP to allow flexor digitorum longus (FDL) tendon to pass through (similar to flexor digitorum profundus and flexor digitorum superficialis in hand), then unites to
- insert into sides of middle phalanx;
- nerve is medial plantar, S2, S3;
- flexes proximal interphalangeal (PIP) joints of lateral four toes.

Abductor digiti minimi

- no surgical importance.

Plantar aponeurosis

- from posteroinferior border of calcaneus, passes
- forwards, superficial to all muscles, and
- divides into five slips which blend with flexor tendon sheaths in toes (similar to palmar aponeurosis in hand);

- central portion is thick and strong, medial and lateral parts are thin.

Second layer

Lumbricals
- origin from FDL tendons;
- inserted into extensor hoods of four lateral toes;
- nerve to medial lumbrical is medial plantar, to the other three is lateral plantar nerve, S2, S3;
- action is metacarpophalangeal (MP) flexion, PIP and distal interphangeal (DIP) extension.

Quadratus plantae (flexor accessorius)
- not important.

Note: long flexor tendons, FDL and FHL, pass through this layer.

Third layer

Flexor hallucis brevis (FHB)
- from inferomedial surface cuboid and third cuneiform;
- divides into two tendons; one
- inserts into medial side of PP (blends with abductor hallucis), the other
- inserts into lateral side of PP of great toe (blends with adductor hallucis); each tendon has a
- sesamoid at its insertion, with FHL tendon lying between them;
- nerve is medial plantar, S2, S3;
- flexes MP of great toe.

Adductor hallucis
- by two heads, oblique and transverse, from second, third and fourth MTs to
- insert into lateral side base of PP of great toe, with FHB;
- nerve is lateral plantar, S2, S3;
- adducts great toe.

Flexor digiti quinti minimi
- unimportant.

Note: lateral plantar artery and nerve cross the sole between the third and fourth layers.

Fourth layer

- interossei
  —three plantar and four dorsal. These are

—similar to hand, but
—central axis of foot is
—second toe, not third (as in hand);
—nerve is lateral plantar, S2, S3;
—dorsal abduct (DAB), plantar adduct (PAD).

ARTERIES

Dorsalis pedis artery

- continuation of anterior tibial artery in the foot,
- follows lateral border of tendon of extensor hallucis longus, then
- passes into the sole between bases of medial two MTs and inter-ossei (vulnerable here in tarsometatarsal fracture-dislocation) to anastomose with lateral plantar;
- branches to EDB, tarsi and joints, and the artery of sinus tarsi (anastomoses with branch from posterior tibial).

Lateral plantar artery

- terminal branch of posterior tibial, starts halfway between medial malleolus and heel,
- runs forward and laterally, between first and second layers of sole, then
- goes deep and runs medially, between third and fourth layers; forms plantar arch with dorsalis pedis.

Medial plantar artery

- terminal branch of posterior tibial; runs forward on medial side of foot, between first and second layers, then becomes more superficial.

NERVES

Deep peroneal nerve

- divides at ankle into
  —medial branch, accompanies dorsalis pedis, supplies skin of first web space; and
  —lateral branch, to EDB.

Lateral plantar nerve

- terminal branch of tibial, arises halfway between heel and medial malleolus;
- lies on medial side of lateral plantar artery, and accompanies this across sole;

- distribution corresponds to ulnar nerve, i.e., supplies all
  - —intrinsic muscles of sole (except abductor hallucis, FDB, FHB and first lumbrical) and supplies
  - —skin of lateral side of sole.

Medial plantar nerve

- terminal branch of tibial nerve;
- lies on lateral side of medial plantar artery, and accompanies it to forefoot;
- distribution corresponds to median nerve in hand, i.e., supplies
  - —abductor hallucis, FDB, FHB, first lumbrical and
  - —medial two thirds of skin of sole and medial 3½ toes.

Sural nerve

- branch of tibial with fibers from peroneal via sural communicating;
- accompanies short (small) saphenous vein forward beneath lateral malleolus to lateral border of foot and little toe.

Saphenous nerve

- branch from femoral nerve;
- travels with long (great) saphenous vein, forward beneath medial malleolus, to medial side of leg and foot (not toes).

Superficial peroneal nerve

- supplies skin of front of leg and dorsum of foot and toes except lateral border and first web space.

Nerve root values of movements of lower limb:

- hip
  - —flexion, L2, L3
  - —extension, L4, L5
- knee
  - —extension, L3, L4
  - —flexion, L5, S1
- ankle
  - —dorsiflexion, L4, L5
  - —plantarflexion, S1, S2
- subtalar
  - —inversion, L4
  - —eversion, L5, S1
- each joint is innervated by four segments except subtalar;
- the more distal the joint, the more distal the segment;

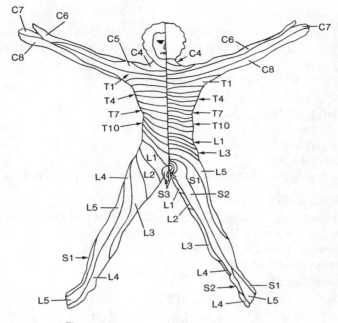

Figure 9.2.   Sensory dermatome pattern.

- learn these nerve root values by moving your own limb and chanting the appropriate numbers;
- remember, the price of final exam success is CONSTANT REPETITION!

Sensory dermatomes

- for both limbs and trunk, see Fig. 9.2.

Surgical Exploration

INDICATIONS

Anterolateral

- triple arthrodesis
- exploration, drainage or fusion of most tarsal joints.

Lateral (Ollier)

- Grice, extra-articular subtalar arthrodesis
- triple arthrodesis (subtalar, talonavicular and calcaneocuboid joints)
- septic arthritis of subtalar joint.

Others, for

- tendon transfers
- fractures and fracture-dislocations
- interphalangeal fusions
- hallux valgus
- osteomyelitis and septic arthritis of tarsals or tarsal joints.

SURGICAL APPROACHES

- cardinal rule is always protect vessels, nerves and tendons;
- the foot does not tolerate well too much surgery at one time;
- where people walk barefoot, the patient should be protected against tetanus before surgery.

Anterolateral

- see Chapter 8 (Figs. 8.9 and 8.13).
- all tarsals and tarsal joints can be reached through distal half of this incision except the joints between navicular and medial two cuneiforms.

Lateral (Ollier) (Fig. 9.3).

- for subtalar and midtarsal joints.

Position

- supine, sandbag beneath buttock of same side, leg free.

Incision

- start 2 to 3 cm below tip of lateral malleolus (at anterior border of peroneal tendons, in front of peroneal tubercle of calcaneus), and
- gently curve forward and upward to talonavicular joint.

Dissection

- cut extensor retinaculum and
- retract common extensor tendons medially;
- peroneal tendons lie at posterior end of wound—protect them!
- incise down to bone along superior, posterior and inferior margins of sinus tarsi,

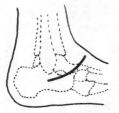

Figure 9.3. Lateral (Ollier's) approach to subtalar and midtarsal joints.

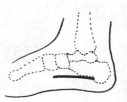

Figure 9.4. Steindler approach to plantar aponeurosis.

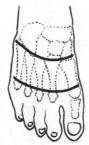

Figure 9.5. Transverse dorsal approaches to tarsals and metatarsals.

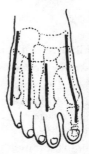

Figure 9.6. Longitudinal dorsal approaches to tarsals and metatarsals.

Figures 9.3 to 9.6. Surgical approaches to the foot.

- detach the fat pad from inside the sinus tarsi and
- reflect it and the EDB distally to expose sinus tarsi, subtalar joint (anterior part) and calcaneocuboid joint.
- talonavicular joint can be exposed by dissecting superiorly and medially beneath long extensor tendons and the neurovascular bundle.

Others (Figs. 9.4 to 9.6)

- in addition to these, other medial, lateral, dorsal, longitudinal and transverse approaches can be used to expose small, individual areas of tarsal and MT joints.

chapter 10

Spine and Spinal Cord

Surgical Anatomy

OSTEOLOGY

Typical cervical vertebra

- C3 to C7.

   Body
   - small, oval and concave superiorly in transverse (coronal) plane.

   Transverse process
   - attached to posterolateral area of body (by homologue of rib) and anterolateral area of pedicle (by true transverse process);
   - concave superiorly for nerve root which passes laterally behind vertebral artery;
   - contains foramen transversarium for the vertebral artery (lies in front of nerve root) and vein (in front of vertebral artery).

   Pedicles
   - project backwards and laterally and unite the posterior arch (lamina) with the body.

   Articular facets
   - placed at junction of pedicle and lamina;
   - angled 45°, superior facet looking up and back, inferior facet downwards and forwards. Flat and oval.

   Posterior arch
   - lamina is thin and weak;
   - spine is bifid and small except C7 which is long and not bifid.

   Vertebral canal
   - triangular and large.

Atlas

- first cervical vertebra.

  Body
  - atlas has no body. This is represented by the odontoid process and is part of axis (C2).

  Anterior arch
  - anterior arch unites the two lateral masses and has small articular facet on posterior surface for odontoid.

  Lateral masses and articular facets
- lateral masses carry
  - —large articular facets superiorly which
  - —articulate with occipital condyles and
  - —carry weight of head (hence the name atlas, after the Greek mythological hero who carried the world on his shoulders). Shape is
  - —concave and horizontal, and
  - —allows flexion and extension of head. Also
  - —small facets inferiorly articulate with axis and allow
  - —rotation.
- transverse ligament runs between the masses, behind anterior arch, attached to a tubercle on inside of each lateral mass.

  Transverse processes
- lie lateral to lateral masses;
- structurally similar to transverse processes of typical cervical vertebra,
- big and strong to provide muscles with leverage for rotation of the atlas (and thus the head) around the odontoid. Tips are palpable in front of mastoid process.
- vertebral artery passes
  - —up through foramen transversarium of atlas, immediately
  - —turns back, then
  - —medially around posterior part of lateral mass lying on posterior arch, then passes
  - —beneath the posterior atlantooccipital membrane into the vertebral canal, then
  - —up through foramen magnum into skull.

- first cervical nerve passes over posterior arch
  - —laterally, behind lateral mass, beneath the vertebral artery, then divides into
  - —anterior division which runs forward along lateral border of lateral mass, medial to vertebral artery, and
  - —posterior division which enters suboccipital triangle.

Posterior arch

- unites the two lateral masses posteriorly. Has
- groove on superior surface, behind lateral mass, for vertebral artery and first cervical nerve;
- has no spinous process but has a small posterior tubercle.

Axis

- second cervical vertebra.

Body

- this carries the odontoid superiorly.

Odontoid

- represents body of atlas;
- ossifies from three centers, and
- fuses with axis at 4 years.
- blood supply is by
  - —anterior and posterior branch from each vertebral artery,
  - —small branch from internal carotid, and branches along
  - —alar, apical and accessory ligaments. These
- nutrient arteries enter odontoid through foramina around
  - —base, along
  - —lateral and anterolateral surface and on
  - —apex. Avascular necrosis of odontoid is rare.

Articular facets

- superior facets lie
  - —posterolateral to odontoid at junction of body and transverse process and
  - —articulate with inferior facets of lateral masses of atlas (slope down and laterally);
- inferior facets lie
  - —posterior to transverse process, look downward and forward like typical cervical inferior facets, and
  - —articulate with third cervical vertebra.

Transverse process

- has foramen transversarium for the vertebral artery which passes upwards and outwards to reach foramen of atlas (which is more lateral than the others).
- nerve root passes out behind the artery.

Posterior arch

- unites the transverse processes and pedicles posteriorly;
- carries inferior articular facet anteriorly at its junction with pedicle;
- spine is bifid.

Thoracic spine

Body

- heart-shaped (looking down on it); bodies
- become larger from T1 to T12. Typical vertebra has
- two demifacets for synovial joint with head of rib,
  —superior lies just in front of pedicle,
  —inferior in front of inferior vertebral notch.

Pedicles

- attached to posterosuperior angle of body just behind rib facet;
- unites body with lamina;
- forms superior border of inferior vertebral notch.

Transverse process

- thick and strong. Each
- arises at junction of pedicle and lamina, and
- has facet on anterior surface of tip for synovial joint with tubercle of rib, except eleventh and twelfth vertebrae.

Articular processes

Superior
- from junction of lamina and pedicle;
- flat surface;
- facet looks backward, and slightly up and laterally.

Inferior
- from junction of pedicle and lamina, below and just posterior to plane of superior facet;
- facet looks forward, slightly medially and downward;
- forms posterior wall of inferior vertebral notch (body forms anterior wall);

- pedicle of vertebra below forms inferior margin of notch (now called intervertebral foramen, through which the nerve root escapes from vertebral canal).

Laminae

- wide and strong, and
- overlap each other like roof tiles (shingles).

Spinous process

- long, narrow, slopes down and back.
- on anteroposterior (AP) x-ray, tip of spinous process appears opposite body of vertebra below (confusing when confirming levels by x-ray during surgery).

Vertebral canal

- narrow, circular.

Peculiar thoracic vertebrae

- first thoracic vertebral body has 1½ articular facets for ribs; tenth, eleventh, and twelfth thoracic vertebral bodies have one complete facet each, and eleventh and twelfth have no facets on transverse processes;
- posterior facet joints, transverse processes and spines of eleventh and twelfth thoracic vertebrae are transitional between thoracic and lumbar vertebrae.

Lumbar spine

Body

- large, strong and heavy; bodies
- increase in size from above down.

Pedicles

- short and thick, project back from proximal half of body and
- join body to lamina;
- form superior border of inferior intervertebral notch.

Transverse processes

- from base of pedicles, increase in length from first to third, then decrease; they are
- thin and weak compared with the rest of the vertebra except the fifth which has short, thick, strong processes.

Articular processes

Superior

- from junction of pedicle and lamina superiorly;

- facet is concave and looks medially and backwards.
Inferior
- from junction of pedicle and lamina inferiorly;
- facet is convex, looks laterally and forwards, and locks with superior facet of vertebra below;
- forms posterior margin of inferior vertebral notch. Superior surface of pedicle below turns the notch into the intervertebral foramen through which the nerve root escapes.
Pars interarticularis
- the junction of superior and inferior facets, the pedicle and the lamina;
- stresses thus concentrate here.
- defect or fracture here (spondylolysis) may allow the proximal vertebra to slide forward on the distal one (spondylolisthesis). The
- pars is seen clearly on an oblique x-ray,
  —"Scotty dog" head is transverse process, eye is the pedicle,
  —ear is superior articular process, neck is pars interarticularis,
  —front leg is inferior articular process, body is lamina. A
  —"collar" around the neck denotes spondylolysis.

Laminae

- short, thick and strong, and
- do not overlap with those above and below.

Spinous process

- short, thick and strong, and
- projects straight backwards.

Spinal canal

- triangular,
- larger than thoracic canal, smaller than cervical canal;
- may be narrowed laterally by thickened base of lamina or abnormally short pedicles, spinal stenosis.

Joints

Cervical spine

Typical cervical vertebrae C3 to C7

- the intervertebral joints are three at each level and form a triangle, base posteriorly.
Intervertebral disc
- a fibrocartilaginous joint (see lumbar spine);

- allows limited AP flexion, extension, lateral flexion and rotation.
- no disc between occiput, atlas and axis.

Posterior joints
- Synovial joints between superior facets of lower vertebra and inferior facets of upper vertebra.
- allow AP flexion, extension, lateral flexion and rotation.

Ligaments
- capsule around the synovial joints;
- anterior (in front of bodies) and posterior (behind bodies) longitudinal ligaments, broad opposite the discs and attached to them, narrow opposite the bodies and not attached.
- ligamentum flavum (yellow)
  —attached near anteroinferior margin of proximal lamina, runs downward to attach to superior border of adjacent lamina below;
  —elastic tissue, allows movement between vertebrae;
  —protects spinal cord posteriorly between laminae.
- interspinous ligament—weak,
- supraspinous ligament—strong;
- ligamentum nuchae, from occiput to spine of C7, weak in humans, strong in giraffe!
- intertransverse ligaments—strong.

Atlantooccipital joint

Synovial joints
- two joints, one on either side, placed laterally;
- large and oval in AP direction;
- foramen magnum medially and vertebral artery laterally and posteriorly;
- mainly flexion and extension (nodding the head).

Ligaments
- capsule around the joints;
- anterior and posterior atlantooccipital membranes (thin and membranous) attach to superior border of respective arches of atlas and superiorly to margins around foramen magnum.

Atlantoaxial joint

Odontoid process
- articulates with anterior arch of atlas (in front) and transverse ligament of atlas (behind), by synovial joints;

- posterior to transverse ligament is vertebral canal with spinal cord.

Synovial joints

- synovial joints between articular facets allow rotation between axis and atlas (shaking the head); surrounded by capsule.

Ligaments

- apical ligament from tip of dens to anterior margin of foramen magnum;
- alar ligaments, one on each side, run from side of apex of dens laterally to occipital condyles;
- accessory ligaments from lateral side of base of dens to lateral mass of atlas close to attachment of transverse ligament;
- cruciate ligament consisting of vertical band from back of body of axis, upwards to transverse ligament (the horizontal band), thence to superior surface of basiocciput just in front of foramen magnum;
- membrana tectoria is posterior to these ligaments, is continuation of posterior longitudinal ligament of the vertebral column from axis to basiocciput;
- ligamentum flavum between posterior arches.

Stability

- short paravertebral muscles and ligaments between axis, atlas and skull stabilize this occipitoatlantoaxial articular system.

Movements

- flexion (atlantooccipital), 70°;
- extension (atlantooccipital), 70°;
- rotation (atlantoaxial), 70° to each side;
- lateral tilt (C3 to C7), 45° to each side.

Thoracic spine

Intervertebral disc

- between adjacent bodies (see lumbar spine).

Posterior joints

- synovial joints almost in coronal plane, to allow flexion, extension and rotation.

Ligaments (see cervical spine)

- capsule around posterior joints;
- ligamentum flavum (elastic);

- anterior and posterior longitudinal;
- interspinous, supraspinous and intertransverse.

Movements

- limited flexion, extension and rotation.
- the rib cage stabilizes the thoracic spine and limits its mobility.
- the most mobile segments of the spine are C5 to C6, D12 to L1 and L5 to S1 (where a stiff segment joins a mobile one).

Lumbar spine

Intervertebral disc

- similar at all vertebral levels; lies
- between adjacent vertebral bodies.

  Vertebral end plates

  - plate of hyaline cartilage covering the inferior and superior surface of each vertebral body;
  - before the end of growth, periphery of plate is surrounded by growth cartilage (ring epiphysis).

  Nucleus pulposus

  - forms center of disc;
  - soft, gelatinous, spherical;
  - composed of collagen fibers and cells in a ground substance rich in mucopolysaccharides, glycoproteins and water.
  - hydrophilic (attracts water) but loses this property with age and becomes desiccated and atrophic.

  Anulus fibrosus

  - fibrocartilage;
  - surrounds the nucleus pulposus;
  - strong anteriorly and laterally, weak posterolaterally. Posteriorly, strengthened by posterior longitudinal ligament.
  - made of concentric lamellae of collagen fibers in a ground substance containing less water than the nucleus, (76% as against 86% at 30 years of age).
  - fibers cross each other obliquely to form a lattice work and are firmly anchored in the cartilaginous end plates;
  - this lattice work allows compression (e.g., flexion, extension, lateral flexion) but not shear (e.g., rotation).
  - the collagen fibers (made by fibroblasts) are composed of three polypeptide chains rich in proline, hydroxyproline and glycine.

Posterior joints
- synovial, curved, lock into each other.

Ligaments
- similar to thoracic spine but
- oblique lumbosacral joint, where shear stress is maximum due to 45° forward tilt, is stabilized by very strong
- iliolumbar and lumbosacral ligaments.

Movements
- flexion and extension possible, but shape of posterior articular facets
- prevents rotation and thus
- protects intervertebral disc, especially the anulus fibrosus.

MUSCLES

Cervical spine

Deep, intrinsic muscles
- origins and insertions within the occiput, cervical and thoracic spine complex, posterior, lateral and anterolateral;
- anteriorly, prevertebral fascia separates the muscle groups (provides relatively bloodless plane for dissection).
- nerve supply is segmental.
- these muscles
  —flex, extend and
  —rotate the head and neck.

Superficial (extrinsic) muscles
- origin or insertion outside the spine.
  Trapezius
  - see Chapter 2.
  - flexes head and neck laterally when shoulder is fixed.
  Scalenes
  - see Chapter 1.
  Sternocleidomastoid (SCM)
  - from mastoid process
  - to medial end of clavicle (clavicular head) and by tendon into superior surface of manubrium (sternal head);
  - innervated by accessory nerve (C1 to C5);
  - action is
    —rotation of head to opposite side, and

—lateral flexion of head to same side (look up and over th opposite shoulder);

—both contracting together flex the neck.

important relations:

—carotid sheath lies behind the lower part and along anteric border of upper part of muscle;

—accessory nerve runs through its upper part;

—brachial plexus appears in posterior triangle behind poste rior border of muscle.

Thoracolumbar spine

Deep (intrinsic) muscles

- origins and insertions within the spine/sacrum complex;
- nerve supply is segmental;
- action is flexion, extension and rotation.

Superficial (extrinsic) muscles

- origin or insertion outside the spine

  Trapezius and latissimus dorsi
  - see Chapter 2.
  - flex the spine laterally if the shoulder is fixed.

  Intercostals and abdominals
  - acting
    —bilaterally, flex the spine forwards,
    —unilaterally, flex it laterally.

  Psoas
  - see Chapter 6.
  - action, with hip fixed, is
    —forward flexion of spine when acting together, or a
    —combination of forward and lateral flexion when acting unilaterally.

  Quadratus lumborum
  - from posterior part of iliac crest
  - to inferior surface of twelfth rib and tips of first four lumba transverse processes;
  - nerve supply, D12 to L1;
  - action is lateral flexion of lumbar spine.

BLOOD SUPPLY

Cervical spine

- spinal branches of vertebral arteries enter vertebral canal throug

intervertebral foramina at every level; divide into branches which
- supply all parts of the vertebrae,
- anastomose above and below with other spinal branches and with the
- anterior and posterior spinal arteries to supply the spinal cord.

Thoracic spine

- descending thoracic aorta gives off segmental, intercostal arteries; these divide into two rami in front of head of rib; the
  —anterior, follows the intercostal space, and the
  —posterior, which gives a spinal branch through intervertebral foramen to canal, supplies the vertebrae, anastomoses, and the spinal cord (anastomoses with anterior and posterior spinal arteries of the cord).

Lumbar spine

- four segmental lumbar arteries, from abdominal aorta, in series with intercostal arteries;
- run laterally and posteriorly, on vertebral bodies beneath psoas and crus of diaphragm, then
- divide into two rami
  —anterior continuing in abdominal wall,
  —posterior entering intervertebral foramen to supply vertebrae and cauda equina.

IMPORTANT RELATIONS

Cervical spine (Fig. 10.1)

- carotid sheath anterolateral to bodies;
- vertebral artery enters vertebral foramen of C6 and runs up through foramina to C1. Vertebral vein descends lateral to artery and leaves cervical spine at C6 or C7;
- esophagus in midline, lies directly on anterior surface of vertebral bodies;
- trachea in front of esophagus, with recurrent laryngeal nerve following the posterolateral border of trachea;
- thyroid gland wrapped around trachea at C6 and C7;
- phrenic nerve, C3, C4, C5, lies in front of scalenus anterior.

Thoracic spine

T1 to T4

- left common carotid and subclavian arteries anterolateral on left,

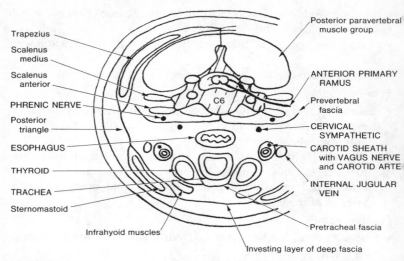

Figure 10.1. Transverse section of neck through the sixth cervical vertebra.

- brachiocephalic arterial trunk anterolateral on right, and arc of aorta anterior to T4.
- esophagus and trachea anterior, in superior mediastinum.

T5 to T12 (Figs. 10.10 and 10.14)

- descending aorta is anterolateral on left, goes through diaphragm at T12;
- azygos vein is anterior with thoracic duct on its left, both go through aortic opening of diaphragm at T12 on right side of aorta;
- esophagus anterior (in posterior mediastinum), goes through diaphragm at T10;
- vagus nerves anterolateral, pass through diaphragm with esophagus;
- sympathetic chain laterally;
- heart just anterior to these structures, and lungs anterolaterally

Lumbar spine (Fig. 10.2)

- abdominal aorta anterolaterally on left side, divides into
- common iliacs in front of body of L4;
- common iliac veins slightly below, behind and to right of common

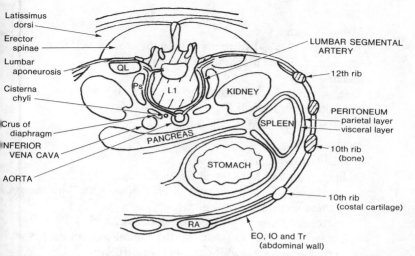

Figure 10.2. Transverse section of the abdomen through the first lumbar vertebra. *EO*, external oblique; *IO*, internal oblique; *Ps*, psoas; *QL*, quadratus lumborum; *RA*, rectus abdominis; *Tr*, transversus abdominis.

iliac arteries, unite to form inferior vena cava in front of and to right of body of L5;

- inferior vena cava anterolateral to vertebral bodies on right, passes up behind liver, through opening in diaphragm at level of T8, thence into right atrium;
- renal arteries and veins at L2;
- psoas muscles laterally with lumbar plexus and ureters.

SPINAL CORD AND NERVE ROOTS

Position of spinal cord
- length of cord is
- from foramen magnum to:
  —full length of vertebral canal in 3-month fetus,
  —L3 at birth,
  —lower border of body of L1 at end of growth.
- filum terminale is a fibrous cord (continuation of pia mater) descending in middle of cauda equina from tip of spinal cord (the conus medullaris) to end of sacral canal; tethers cord.

Enlargements

Cervical

- from third cervical vertebra to second thoracic vertebra;
- contains cells for brachial plexus nerves.

Lumbar

- from ninth thoracic vertebra to first lumbar vertebra,
- for lumbar and sacral plexuses.

Columns of spinal cord (Fig. 10.3)

Sensory fibers

Conscious sensations (afferent)

- heat, pain and light touch fibers
  —synapse in posterior horn of gray matter, and the axons of these second order neurons
  —cross at same level to opposite side of cord and
  —ascend to the thalamus by the lateral and anterior spino thalamic tracts (white matter) (Fig. 10.4);
  —other neurones go from thalamus to cortex.
- vibration, deep touch, pressure, spatial discrimination and conscious proprioception
  —ascend in posterior tracts (white matter) to medulla oblongata. Here they

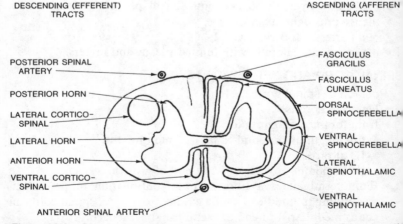

DESCENDING (EFFERENT) TRACTS

ASCENDING (AFFERENT TRACTS

POSTERIOR SPINAL ARTERY

POSTERIOR HORN

LATERAL CORTICO-SPINAL

LATERAL HORN

ANTERIOR HORN

VENTRAL CORTICO-SPINAL

ANTERIOR SPINAL ARTERY

FASCICULUS GRACILIS

FASCICULUS CUNEATUS

DORSAL SPINOCEREBELLA

VENTRAL SPINOCEREBELLA

LATERAL SPINOTHALAMIC

VENTRAL SPINOTHALAMIC

Figure 10.3. Diagrammatic transverse section of the spinal cord at T6 to show the major long tracts.

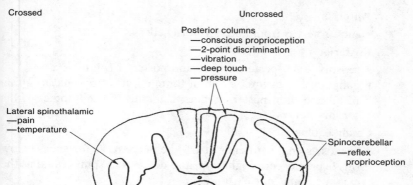

Figure 10.4. Sensory modalities of ascending columns in spinal cord.

—synapse with secondary neurons whose axons then
—cross, and ascend to thalamus;
—thalamus then projects to cortex.

Unconscious proprioception (afferent)
• from muscles, tendons and joints, ascend in anterior and posterior spinocerebellar tracts of same side to cerebellum of same side.

Motor fibers (efferent)
• from cortex, descend to
—medulla where most cross and descend in lateral corticospinal tract, then
—synapse with anterior horn cells in the gray matter;
—axons of these cells exit in the anterior root of spinal nerves.
• uncrossed motor fibers from cortex
—descend in anterior corticospinal tract and
—cross in the cord itself to reach anterior horn cells.
—most of these fibers go no further than upper thoracic cord.

Other descending tracts
• from other centers and nuclei; modify motor and sensory impulses.

Nerve roots
• these are peripheral nerves.

Anterior

- motor nerves from anterior horn cells.

Posterior

- sensory, enter posterior horn and posterior columns;
- ganglion lies in intervertebral foramen, just proximal to unio of anterior and posterior roots. Contains the cell bodies of th sensory nerves.

Cauda equina

- because spinal cord ends at L1, the nerve roots for levels belov this leave the cord higher up, and descend in spinal canal as th cauda equina (horse's tail).

Spinal nerves

- formed by union of anterior and posterior nerve roots in th intevertebral foramen;
- one pair for each vertebral level (but eight cervical);
- anterior horn cells of
  - —D5 nerve root are opposite the fourth thoracic vertebra;
  - —D11 opposite ninth thoracic vertebra;
  - —L1 opposite tenth;
  - —L3 opposite eleventh;
  - —L5 opposite twelfth thoracic vertebra;
  - —S1 to S5 opposite the first lumbar vertebra (important i examination of patient with spinal injury or spinal cor disease or tumor).

Sympathetic trunks and ganglia

Efferent sympathetic fibers

- small, myelinated fibers
- arise in lateral horn of thoracic cord,
- leave the cord by anterior nerve roots of all thoracic and firs two lumbar roots and enter corresponding spinal nerves;
- leave the spinal nerves just lateral to intervertebral foramen, b white ramus communicans, and synapse in the corresponding sympathetic ganglion;
- unmyelinated efferent fibers then travel up or down sympatheti trunk, or return to same spinal nerve through gray ramus.
- every spinal nerve (C1 to S5) receives a gray ramus communi cans by which it receives sympathetic fibers.

Sympathetic ganglia
- 3 cervical ganglia,
- 11 or 12 thoracic ganglia (lower cervical and first thoracic ganglia usually fused to form the stellate ganglion), and
- 5 lumbar and several sacral ganglia.

Sympathetic plexus
- hypogastric and pelvic plexuses (see Chapter 6).

Membranes

Pia mater
- closely invests the cord and nerve roots as far as conus medullaris;
- continues distally as filum terminale;
- forms the dentate ligament laterally, between the anterior and posterior nerve roots, fixing the cord to the dura.

Arachnoid mater
- outside the pia; encloses a space between itself and the pia, the subarachnoid space, which
- contains the cerebrospinal fluid (CSF);
- arachnoid mater (with subarachnoid space and CSF) surrounds the nerve roots as far as intervertebral foramina (blends with roots just before they join to form spinal nerves) and the cauda equina as far as S2 (lumbar puncture is safe between L3 and L4 or L4 and L5).

Dura mater
- loosely surrounds arachnoid from foramen magnum to S2 and along nerve roots;
- blends with filum terminale at S2 and with the sheaths of spinal nerves at the intevertebral foramina.
- subdural and extradural spaces contain fat and vessels besides nerve roots.

Blood supply of cord
- precarious especially in thoracic region.

Anterior spinal artery
- formed by union of branch from proximal end of each vertebral artery, then
- descends on front of cord, along the anterior median fissure.
- reinforced by segmental branches from

—vertebral and ascending cervical arteries in the neck,
—intercostals in thorax, the first two from costocervical trunk of subclavian artery, the rest from aorta, and
—lumbar, iliolumbar and lateral sacral arteries in abdomen and pelvis.
- supplies anterior two thirds of cord,
  —ventral corticospinal and
  —medial two thirds of lateral corticospinal tracts,
  —spinothalamic and
  —ventral spinocerebellar tracts, and almost all the
  —gray matter (Fig. 10.5).

Posterior spinal arteries

- one on each side, from vertebral artery;
- descends on posterior surface of cord, lateral to midline;
- reinforced by segmental branches, similar to anterior spinal artery.
- supplies posterior third of cord,
  —posterior columns,
  —lumbar root area of lateral corticospinal tract,
  —dorsal spinocerebellar tract and
  —apex of posterior horn.

Great radicular artery (Adamkiewicz)

- largest segmental artery. Occurs usually on
- left side, between
- T7 and L4, most often between T9 and T11. Artery
  —runs proximally for two or three segments, then

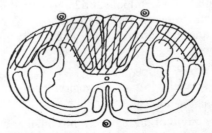

Figure 10.5. Diagram similar to Figure 10.3, to show arterial territory in spinal cord. *Crosshatched area* is supplied by posterior spinal arteries (mainly sensation), the remainder is supplied by the anterior spinal artery (mainly motor).

    —turns sharply down in a hairpin curve to enter
- anterior spinal artery.

Surgical Exploration of Cervical Spine

INDICATIONS

Posterior
- cervical fusion for instability
- open reduction of fracture or dislocation
- exploration of the spinal canal and cord.

Anterior
- cervical fusion
- biopsy of vertebral body
- tuberculosis of body
- excision of tumor
- removal of cervical disc.

SURGICAL APPROACHES

Posterior approach (Figs. 10.6 and 10.8)

Position
- prone,
- head supported on a movable ring (in traction if cervical spine is unstable),
- occiput shaved.

Incision
- midline, from occiput to T1, or any part of this incision, centered over the lesion.

Dissection
- sharp dissection in midline (bloodless plane) to spinous processes (bifid);
- gentle subperiosteal dissection of posterior paravertebral muscles from spines and laminae as far laterally as the posterior joints. Laminae are thin and break easily. Laterally,
- beware of vertebral arteries!
- for exposure of vertebral canal and spinal cord, careful resection of ligamentum flavum and partial or total laminectomy is necessary. Beware dura mater and cord, immediately under the ligamentum and lamina.

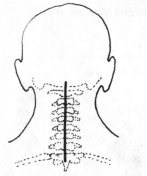

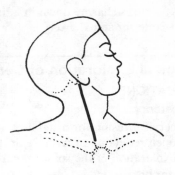

Figure 10.6. Posterior approach.   **Figure 10.7.**   Anterior approach.

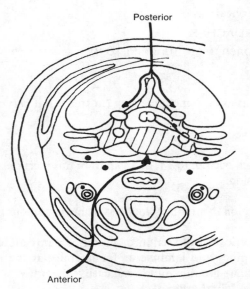

Figure 10.8.   Section similar to Figure 10.1.

Figures 10.6 to 10.8.   Surgical approaches to the cervical spine.

- levels can be confirmed by palpating spine of C7 (large), posterior arch of atlas (no spine), or by making lateral x-ray with needle in a spinous process.

Anterior (Bailey and Badgley) C3 to T1 (Figs. 10.7 and 10.8)

Position

- supine,
- sandbag between the shoulder blades,
- head turned to opposite side,
- in traction if unstable.

Incision

- along anterior border of right SCM from 2 cm distal to its origin, to insertion, or any part of this incision.

Dissection

- incise platysma in line with skin incision.
- incise pretracheal fascia in same line, where it lies over sternohyoid and sternothyroid muscles, protecting carotid sheath with a finger;
- separate anterior border of SCM from adjacent structures by blunt dissection; then, again by blunt dissection,
- gently dissect the plane between trachea, esophagus and thyroid gland in midline and the carotid sheath laterally. Retract these structures gently in opposite directions (carotid sheath one way, midline structures the other).
- ligate and divide middle thyroid vein.
- to expose C7 and T1, ligate and divide inferior thyroid vessels (do not injure recurrent laryngeal nerve in distal end of wound).
- incise prevertebral fascia and anterior longitudinal ligament in midline.
- confirm levels by metal marker and x-ray.

Surgical Exploration of Thoracic and Lumbar Spine

INDICATIONS

Posterior

- posterior fusion
- posterolateral fusion (lumbar area)

- scoliosis surgery—Harrington instrumentation and fusion
- excision of herniated disc
- open reduction and internal fixation for fracture or dislocation
- exploration of spinal canal, cord and cauda equina
- laminectomy and posterior decompression, e.g., spinal stenosis.

Anterolateral—costotransversectomy (Seddon)

- paravertebral tuberculous abscess (Pott's disease).

Anterior

- Pott's disease
- anterior interbody fusion
- anterior decompresion of cord
- scoliosis surgery—Dwyer instrumentation and interbody fusion
- tumor—biopsy or excision biopsy.

SURGICAL APPROACHES

Posterior (Figs. 10.10 and 10.16)

- similar to posterior approach to cervical spine, but note the follow ing points:
- operate with patient on bolsters or in knee-chest position to reduce blood loss by avoiding abdominal compression;
- confirm levels with x-ray;
- subperiosteal dissection (reduces blood loss);
- use wide-ended periosteal elevator (large Cobb is best) to avoid plunging into cord or cauda equina, into pleura (thoracic region) or into retroperitoneal space (lumbar region);
- do not injure capsule and ligaments around posterior joints unless they are to be fused;
- when removing ligamentum flavum, never lose sight of end of knife (to avoid cutting the dura);
- if epidural veins bleed, pack tiny gauze or cotton sponges, with black threads attached, up and down the canal;
- when handling a nerve root, do so VERY GENTLY, and
- treat the spinal cord as though it were made of nitroglycerine!

Costotransversectomy (Seddon) (Figs. 10.9 and 10.10)

- an anterolateral approach.

Position
- prone, with

- bolsters to avoid compression of thorax (Pott's kyphosis patient already has diminished vital capacity).

Incision

- curved, convex laterally
  —from third spinous process proximal to apex of kyphosis laterally and distally for 10 cm, then distally, then
  —medially to third spinous process distal to apex of kyphosis.

Dissection

- retract skin flap medially;
- divide superficial and deep muscles transversely and retract them;

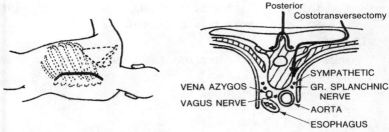

Figure 10.9. Costotransversectomy.

Figure 10.10. Section through thoracic vertebra to show costotransversectomy and posterior approach. *GR.*, greater.

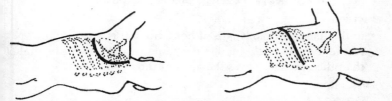

Figure 10.11. Anterior approach for C7 to T3. **Figure 10.12.** Standard thoracotomy.

Figures 10.9 to 10.12. Surgical approaches to the thoracic spine.

- expose medial 8 cm of three or more ribs, together with transverse processes and lateral third of laminae;
- remove transverse process opposite widest part of abscess, and medial 6 cm of that rib subperiosteally (do not perforate pleura! If you do, close the hole as soon as possible). Head of rib is removed with gouge.
- if greater exposure is required, remove another transverse process and proximal end of rib.

Anterior C7 to D3 (Fig. 10.11)

Position

- lateral,
- arm free above the patient's head.

Incision

- curved, down medial border of scapula, then curving anteriorly for 6 cm below inferior pole of scapula.

Dissection

- incise latissimus dorsi, trapezius, rhomboids and serratus anterior in line of incision;
- retract scapula superiorly;
- identify and resect third rib;
- incise bed of rib and underlying pleura;
- ligate and divide intercostal vessels near their origins from aorta. Closure as for standard thoracotomy.

Anterior D4 to D11 (Fig. 10.12)

- standard thoracotomy.

Position

- lateral, left side up, arm above head,
- table broken beneath chest to facilitate exposure.

Incision

- in the line of whole length of bony rib that is opposite the apex of the kyphus in the midaxillary line (usually two ribs higher than the one that leaves the apex of the kyphus).

Dissection

- superficial muscles divided in line of skin incision,
- periosteum divided along length of bony rib;

- excise the rib subperiosteally from its head to the costochondral junction,
- incise the periosteal bed of the rib and underlying pleura and
- retract the lung.
- incise the pleura parallel with and just posterior to aorta;
- mobilize aorta GENTLY and retract it anteromedially.
- ligate carefully and divide the intercostal vessels along all vertebrae to be exposed, and retract aorta further anteriorly.

Closure

- pleura must be closed with lungs under positive pressure, and underwater seal chest drain inserted;
- broken table reversed to facilitate closure of rib cage;
- rib periosteum and muscles closed in layers;
- postoperative x-ray on table to look for pneumothorax.

Anterior D9 to L2 (Figs. 10.13, 10.14 and 10.16)
- thoracoabdominal approach.

Position

- lateral, left side up (aorta is easier to repair than the vena cava!).

Incision

- along tenth rib and
- across subcostal margin;
- continue in same line across abdomen to lateral margin of rectus abdominis;
- can continue distally along lateral border of rectus if greater exposure is required, to reach L3 and L4.

Dissection

- incise superficial muscles in line of skin incision (latissimus dorsi, serratus anterior and external oblique);
- resect the tenth rib subperiosteally and
- incise the bed of the tenth rib, but stay extrapleural;
- incise the cartilage of the costal margin;
- incise the abdominal muscles as far as the rectus abdominis;
- mobilize the peritoneum and retract it anteromedially to remain retroperitoneal;
- reflect kidney forwards.
- place two marking sutures in posterior part of diaphragm, then

- divide diaphragm all the way round, 2 cm from its peripheral attachment, and retract medially;
- divide psoas transversely and retract it distally;
- ligate segmental lumbar vessels (artery and vein at each level, similar to intercostals) and divide them;
- mobilize aorta anteriorly to expose vertebral bodies.

Closure

- diaphragm must be accurately resutured (hence marking sutures);

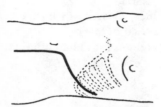

Figure 10.13. Thoracoabdominal approach for T9 to L4.

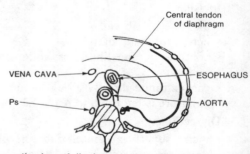

Figure 10.14. Diagrammatic view of diaphragm, seen from the abdominal cavity, to show incision in diaphragm. *Ps*, psoas.

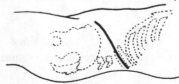

Figure 10.15. Renal approach for L2 to L4.

Figures 10.13 to 10.15. Surgical approaches to the lower thoracic and lumbar vertebrae.

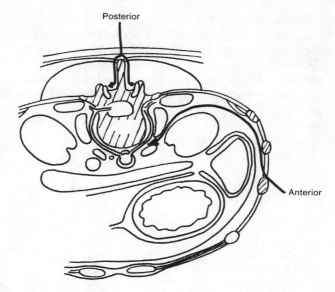

Figure 10.16. Section similar to Figure 10.2, to show the anterior surgical approach to the spine from D9 to L2. Posterior midline approach is also shown.

- wound closed in layers, approximating ribs with towel clips to facilitate closure.

Anterior L2 to L4 (Fig. 10.15)

- renal approach.

    Position

    - left side up,
    - table broken to facilitate exposure.

    Incision

    - along the twelfth rib, which is removed;
    - continue in same direction across abdomen to lateral border of rectus abdominis.

    Dissection

    - divide superficial and deep muscles in line of skin incision,
    - push peritoneum gently forward to expose vertebral bodies (kidney is posterior);

- reflect ureter forwards; then
- ligate and divide segmental vertebral arteries and veins close to their origin along all vertebrae to be exposed, and mobilize aorta anteriorly.
- to reach L5 to S1 area, continue medial part of incision distally as routine paramedian approach, down lateral border of rectus abdominis.

Closure

- reverse break of table;
- close carefully in layers, and
- drain.

GENERAL SURGICAL PATHOLOGY FOR ORTHOPAEDIC SURGEONS

chapter 11

Respiratory Physiology

Control of Breathing

RESPIRATORY CENTER

- situated in medulla oblongata
- consists of two parts (Fig. 11.1)

  Inspiratory center (IC)

  - sends impulses down
    —phrenic nerve, C3, C4, C5, to diaphragm, and
    —intercostal nerves to intercostal muscles.
  - this center is responsible for continuous, spontaneous respiration;
  - interaction between inspiration and expiration centers is responsible for rhythm of respiration.

  Expiration center

  - when lung is stretched during inspiration, proprioceptive stretch receptors in lung send impulses up vagus nerve (tenth cranial). These impulses stimulate the
  - expiratory center which then sends inhibitory impulses to inspiratory center and inspiration stops;
  - expiration then occurs passively through elastic recoil of lungs;
  - this is called the Hering-Breuer reflex.

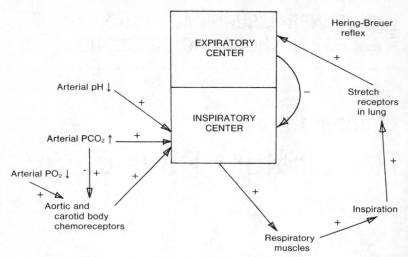

Figure 11.1. Major chemical and neural pathways that control normal breathing.

CHEMICAL CONTROL OF VENTILATION

• rate and depth of respiration mainly controlled by following three factors:

Arterial CO_2 tension ($PaCO_2$)

• increase in $PaCO_2$
  —stimulates directly the inspiratory center (IC)
  —stimulates the aortic and carotid body chemoreceptors, which then stimulate the IC.
• decrease in $PaCO_2$ below normal inhibits the IC if the arterial oxygen (PaO_2) tension is high.
• IC is very sensitive to small alterations of $PaCO_2$.

Arterial oxygen tension (PaO_2)

• fall in PaO_2 by 25% to 40% stimulates directly the IC.
• fall in PaO_2 stimulates the aortic and carotid body chemoreceptors which then stimulate the IC.
• the IC is not sensitive to small alterations of PaO_2

Arterial blood pH

• decrease in pH (i.e., increase in acidity and H^+ ions) of arterial blood stimulates directly the IC.

Ventilation

NORMAL RESPIRATORY WORK

Inspiration

- work is done during normal tidal inspiration to overcome the
  —elastic recoil of the lung (like blowing up a child's balloon), and
  —resistance to gas flow in the major airways (trachea, bronchi, bronchioles);
- this work is performed by respiratory muscles
  —diaphragm and
  —intercostal muscles (D1 to D12 nerve roots);
  —with increased demand for ventilation, accessory muscles of respiration are activated.

Expiration

- during normal tidal ventilation, expiration is a passive movement, due to elastic recoil of the lungs. No active work is necessary unless there is increased resistance to expiratory gas flow.

Oxygen requirements

- at rest, normal breathing takes 2% of total body oxygen requirement
- during heavy exercise, oxygen requirement for breathing is 20% of total body needs.

FACTORS THAT INCREASE RESPIRATORY WORK

- airway obstruction, in trachea, bronchi or bronchioles, may be due to
  —inability to clear normal secretions,
  —edema or excessive secretions,
  —spasm,
  —external pressure;
- this increases work of
  —inspiration, and also demands work for
  —expiration (abdominal muscles);
- chronic lung disease (emphysema) increases in particular the work of expiration.

NATURE OF INCREASED WORK LOAD

- when work of breathing is increased (as in problems cited above), respiration may require considerable proportion (20% or more) of total body oxygen needs;

- increase in tidal volume (depth of respiration) requires more energy than an
- increase in respiratory rate;
- thus, in early respiratory failure, patient attempts to conserve energy and compensates by
  —increase in rate, not depth, with the result that respiration is
  —rapid and shallow;
- rapid, shallow ventilation is inefficient and is a sign of incipient respiratory failure;
- excessive load is placed on the heart to deliver this oxygen to respiratory muscles;
- oxygen cost of breathing at rest may thus be very high, and leaves no reserve.
- these patients may need prophylactic mechanical ventilatory support after major surgery, but
- mechanical ventilation can eliminate need for
  —inspiratory work, but
  —not for expiratory work;
- airway obstruction in these patients must therefore be avoided by
  —repeated suction,
  —avoiding laryngeal and bronchial spasm, and using
  —bronchodilators.

NORMAL DISTRIBUTION OF VENTILATION

- distribution of inhaled air in the lung is influenced by:
  Gravity
  - influence of gravity is partly due to
    —weight of lung, and partly due to
    —deforming force of abdominal contents on diaphragm, and is
  - different at the top and bottom of the lung.
  Compliance of lung (Fig. 11.2)
  - compliance of the lung is the relationship between the
    —volume of the lung and the
    —pressure required to blow the lung up to that volume, and is
  - dependent on the elasticity of the lung.
  - compliance equals

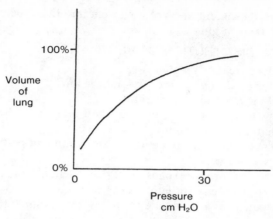

Figure 11.2. Relationship between pressure and volume of lung. Compliance decreases as volume increases.

    —volume change in liters divided by pressure change in cm of H_2O
- compliance
  —decreases with inflation; i.e., as the lung inflates (increases its volume), progressively greater pressure is required to increase its volume by a given amount. Like a
  —balloon, the more you blow it up, the harder it becomes to blow it up more.
- in the standing patient, alveoli are
  —larger at the top of the lung (compliance is low) and
  —smaller at the bottom (compliance is high).

Other factors
- these include
  —vertical height (length) of lung (this is different if patient is standing or lying),
  —position of diaphragm, and
  —interaction between air and blood pressures in lung.

Result
- result of above factors is that
  —more air flows into

—lower, dependent areas of lung than into the upper, nondependent areas of lung.

ABNORMAL DISTRIBUTION OF VENTILATION

- if dependent areas of lung are
  —collapsed (atelectasis), or compliance is low,
  —air will move preferentially into
  —nondependent areas (i.e., more air will move into the top of the lung than into the bottom.) This
  —changes the relationship between ventilation and perfusion of the lungs (see below).
- obesity prevents proper expansion of dependent alveoli, thus causing a mismatch between ventilation and perfusion;
- an obese patient is a candidate for respiratory failure after surgery.

LUNG VOLUMES

Spirometry

- subdivisions of normal lung volumes are shown in Figure 11.3
- spirometric examination includes
- resting tidal volume
  —the volume of a normal breath at rest;
- inspiratory reserve volume
  —the volume that can be inspired after normal tidal inspiration;
- expiratory reserve volume
  —volume that can be expired after normal tidal expiration;
- vital capacity (VC)
  —the three volumes above added together;
  —restrictive pulmonary or thoracic disease, e.g., scoliosis and kyphosis, reduces the VC;
- ratio of resting tidal volume to VC should be 4 to 10 or less, and gives a rough estimate of respiratory reserve of the patient.
- first-second VC is the
  —volume that can be expired in 1 second after maximum inspiration,
  —normally is 70% or more of VC;
  —obstructive disease reduces this, e.g., emphysema.

Dead space

- physiological dead space consists of
  —nose, nasopharynx and oropharynx,

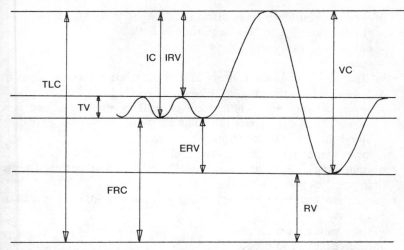

Figure 11.3. Subdivisions of normal lung volumes. *TV*, tidal volume (volume of inspired air in regular breathing) (average 500 cc); *IRV*, inspiratory reserve volume (2000 cc); *ERV*, expiratory reserve volume (1300 cc); *RV*, residual volume (lung volume left after complete, forced expiration) (1600 cc); *TLC*, total lung capacity (this average 5,400 cc); *IC*, inspiratory capacity (2,500 cc); *FRC*, functional residual capacity (lung volume at end of normal expiration) (2,900 cc); *VC*, vital capacity (maximum volume of air that can be inspired after complete, forced expiration) (3,800 cc).

- —trachea, bronchi and bronchioles and has a
- capacity of about 150 cc;
- air in these passages is
  - —functionally useless for ventilation because it
  - —never reaches alveoli;
- thus, of normal
  - —tidal volume of 500 cc, only
  - —350 cc are available for gas exchange at each inspiration.

Perfusion

NORMAL DISTRIBUTION OF PERFUSION

- perfusion refers to blood flow through pulmonary vascular bed;
- regardless of position, standing, supine or lying on the side, perfusion

of the lung is subject to the effect of
—gravity modified by the magnitude of both
—pulmonary artery and
—venous pressures;
- interaction of pulmonary artery and alveolar air pressures varies in different parts of the lung, as follows:
  —upper, nondependent lung receives little or no blood, and is a physiological dead space (alveolar air is not oxygenated here);
  —blood flow in midlung is phasic (intermittent);
  —lower, dependent lung is always perfused with blood. In
- normal lungs, dependent areas are ventilated and perfused more than nondependent (higher) regions, and
- ventilation and perfusion are normally well matched, i.e., the area of lung that
  —receives the most air also
  —receives the most blood.

ABNORMAL LUNG PERFUSION

- left ventricular failure increases atrial blood pressure which causes fluid to flow
  —from the intravascular
  —to the extravascular (interstitial) space, causing
  —pulmonary edema and
  —impairing lung perfusion;
- this occurs mainly in dependent areas of lungs,
  —the bases in the standing or sitting patient,
  —the posterior portions in the patient lying in bed on his back,
  —the lower lung in the patient on his side, e.g., for certain operations
- decreased pulmonary artery pressure, as in hypovolemia with shock
  —alters perfusion pattern in lung, and causes
  —hypoxemia and
  —hypercapnia.
- to compensate for this, an increase in tidal volume is required.

Blood Gas Exchange

- in the short time that blood passes the alveoli of the normal lung (less than 1 second),
  —carbon dioxide is removed and

—oxygen is taken up in fast and efficient manner;
- this gas exchange depends upon a nice balance between the distribution of ventilation (V) and the perfusion (Q) of the lung;
- if the V/Q ratio is altered, then oxygen and carbon dioxide removal will be altered too.

OXYGENATION

- partial pressure of oxygen in alveolar inspired air (PAO_2) is normally greater than in the pulmonary arterial blood (PaO_2) (Table 11.1)
- this pressure gradient means that
  —oxygen diffuses from the alveolar air into the blood.
- oxygen uptake by pulmonary capillary blood is diminished if
- certain perfused areas of the lung are poorly ventilated because of
  —airway obstruction,
  —alveolar collapse and
  —marked hypoventilation, or
- ventilated areas of lung are poorly perfused due to
  —pulmonary embolus,
  —hypotension or
  —fall in cardiac output.

CARBON DIOXIDE REMOVAL

- the partial pressure of CO_2 in the pulmonary arterial blood ($PaCO_2$)

Table 11.1
Partial Pressures of O_2, CO_2 and N_2 in Inspired and Alveolar Air, Pulmonary Arterial and Pulmonary Venous Blood

	Inspired Air at STP	Alveolar Air	Pulmonary Arterial Blood (Deoxygenated)	Pulmonary Venous Blood (Oxygenated)
O_2	21% 157 mm Hg	14% 100 mm Hg	40 mm Hg	93 mm Hg
CO_2	0.04% 0.3 mm Hg	5.6% 400 mm Hg	46 mm Hg	40 mm Hg
N_2	79% 593 mm Hg	80% 570 mm Hg		

STP, standard temperature and pressure.

is normally greater than that in the alveolar inspired air ($PACO_2$) (Table 11.1);

- this pressure gradient means that
  —CO_2 leaves the blood to enter the alveolar air;
- removal of CO_2 from pulmonary capillary blood is impaired if
  —some areas of lung perfused by blood are not ventilated or
  —some areas of ventilated lung are not perfused, as above.

Oxygen and Carbon Dioxide Transport

OXYGEN TRANSPORT

- oxygen that diffuses from alveolar air into the pulmonary capillary blood is carried both
  —attached to hemoglobin in the blood, and
  —in solution in the plasma.

  Oxyhemoglobin

Formation of oxyhemoglobin (Fig. 11.6)

- oxygen diffuses
  —from the plasma,
  —across the red cell membrane
  —into the red cell where it
  —combines with free hemoglobin to form oxyhemoglobin (HbO_2) as follows (Equation 1)

$$O_2 + HHB \rightleftharpoons H^+ + HbO_2 \qquad (1)$$

- hemoglobin is made of a porphyrin pigment which contains 4 iron atoms and is called heme. This is attached to a globin molecule;
- 1 molecule of oxygen combines loosely with 1 atom of iron;
- 1 gm of Hb combines with 1.34 ml of O_2;
- O_2 saturation of Hb (i.e., maximum amount of O_2 normally carried by Hb) is 20 volumes percent (i.e., 20 ml of O_2 per 100 ml of blood).

Oxygen dissociation curve (Fig. 11.4)

Characteristics

- at an oxygen tension (partial pressure) of 97 mm Hg, the Hb is 97% saturated with O_2.

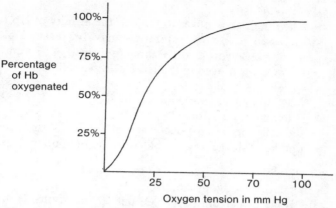

Figure 11.4.   The oxygen dissociation curve at 37° C and pH 7.4.

- the flattening of upper part of curve means that a
  —large fall in alveolar (and thus blood) oxygen tension can occur
  —without a large drop in the percent saturation. At a tension of 60 mm Hg, HbO_2 saturation is still 90%. Thus
  —large variations of alveolar oxygen tension can occur with
  —minimal variations in total oxygen load of arterial blood. This is an important built-in safety factor.
- the steepness of the lower part of the curve means that when O_2 tension is low (as in tissues), O_2 dissociates itself from the Hb. This is an advantage because free O_2 is required in the tissues for cellular metabolism.

Shift to the right

- when the curve shifts to the right, oxygen leaves the Hb more easily, e.g., at an O_2 tension of 60 mm Hg, saturation of Hb with oxygen may only be 80% instead of 90%.
- the curve is moved to the right by *increase* in
  —partial pressure of carbon dioxide (PCO_2),
  —hydrogen ion concentration and
  —temperature of blood.
- PCO_2, H^+ ion concentration and temperature are all increased in the tissues and, by moving the O_2 dissociation curve to the right, favor the release of oxygen to the tissues (Fig. 11.5)

Shift to the left
- when the curve moves to the left, the affinity of Hb for O_2 is increased, and 97% saturation may be reached at an O_2 tension as low as 85 or 90 mm Hg instead of 97 mm Hg.
- the curve is moved to the left by *decrease* in
  —PCO_2
  —H^+ ion concentration, and
  —temperature of blood.
- these factors are all decreased in the lungs, and thus favor uptake of oxygen by the blood in the pulmonary capillaries

Oxygen in solution
- O_2 in solution in the plasma is
  —0.3 volumes percent (0.3 cc O_2 per 100 cc of blood) in arterial blood, and
  —half this (0.15 volumes percent) in venous blood.
- it is this oxygen that exerts the partial pressure (tension, or PO_2)

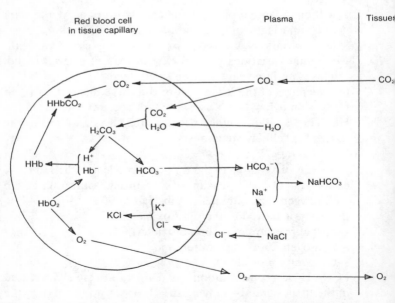

Figure 11.5. Gas and ion exchange in blood in tissue capillaries.

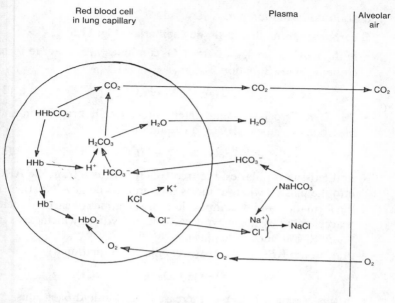

Figure 11.6.   Gas and ion exchange in blood in lung capillaries.

of oxygen in the blood, because O_2 combined with Hb cannot exert pressure.

CARBON DIOXIDE TRANSPORT (Figs. 11.5 and 11.6)

• carbon dioxide is an end product of aerobic metabolism in the tissues; this gas
   —diffuses from the tissues,
   —through the plasma and
   —into the red cell as free CO_2 in solution, because tension of CO_2 in the tissues is greater than that in capillary blood (Table 11.1). The CO_2 diffuses across a pressure gradient.
• in the blood,
   —two thirds of the CO_2 is transported as bicarbonate in the plasma and
   —one third as carbaminohemoglobin and bicarbonate in the red blood cells (RBC).

Bicarbonate formation and dissociation

Bicarbonate formation in tissue capillaries (Fig. 11.5)

- in the RBC in the tissues, free CO_2 combines with water to form carbonic acid (Equation 2):

$$CO_2 + H_2O \rightarrow H_2CO_2 \qquad (2)$$

- this then dissociates immediately into a free hydrogen ion and bicarbonate radical (HCO_3^-) (Equation 3)

$$H_2CO_3 \rightarrow H^+ + HCO_3^- \qquad (3)$$

- in the tissue capillaries, the free HCO_3^- diffuses from the RBC into the plasma where it forms sodium bicarbonate ($NaHCO_3$)
- the formation and decomposition (dissociation) of carbonic acid is accelerated by the enzyme carbonic anhydrase which exists in the RBC but not in the plasma;
- thus, in the RBC in the tissue capillaries (Equation 4)

$$CO_2 + H_2O \rightleftharpoons H_2CO_3 \rightleftharpoons H^+ + HCO_3^- \qquad (4)$$

- in this reaction, if CO_2 is increased and the hydrogen ions are removed by buffers, the reaction will be driven to the right;
- this is exactly what happens in the tissues, where
  - CO_2 in the RBC is increased by diffusion across the pressure gradient from the tissue cells as a result of aerobic respiration, and
  - oxyhemoglobin (HbO_2^-) is reduced to O_2 and Hb^-, and the Hb^- is then available to combine with the free hydrogen ion, and thus remove it from the above equation (4) as follows (Equation 5)

$$H^+ + Hb^- \rightarrow HHb \qquad (5)$$

- HHb then combines with free CO_2 to form carbaminohemoglobin ($HHbCO_2$, see below)

Bicarbonate dissociation in the lungs (Fig. 11.6)

- the reverse occurs in the lungs, where the reaction (Equation 4) is driven to the left by
  - an increase in oxygen in solution in the RBC which displaces the CO_2 and H^+ from carbaminohemoglobin ($HHbCO_2$) to form HbO_2^- (Hb has a greater affinity for O

than it does for CO_2), thus increasing the number of H^+ ions present; and

—a decrease in the free CO_2 in solution as this diffuses out of the blood and into the alveolar air across the pressure gradient.

Overall equilibrium—the isohydric shift

- the overall equilibrium is called the isohydric shift and is shown in Equation 6:

$$CO_2 + H_2O + HbO_2^- \underset{\text{lungs}}{\overset{\text{tissues}}{\rightleftharpoons}} HCO_3^- + HHb + O_2 \qquad (6)$$

- this equation is driven
    —towards the right in the tissues and
    —towards the left in the lungs. Thus
    —CO_2 increase drives O_2 out of the blood, and
    —O_2 increase drives CO_2 out of the blood.
- the pH of plasma changes very little because the negative ions
    —HbO_2^- on the left and
    —HCO_3^- on the right are balanced by presence of positive ions, mainly K^+ inside RBC and Na^+ outside it.

Carbaminohemoglobin

- in the RBC in the tissue capillaries, HbO_2^- dissociates to release oxygen which then diffuses out of the RBC, through the plasma and into the tissues (Equation 1).
- the free hemoglobin is reduced by combination with an hydrogen ion released from the dissociation of carbonic acid (Equations 3 and 5, and Fig. 11.5)
- free CO_2 then combines with amino acids of the globin part of reduced Hb (HHb) to form carbaminohemoglobin (HHbCO₂, Fig. 11.5)

Chloride bicarbonate shift (Figs. 11.5 and 11.6),

- Cl^- and HCO_3^- ions pass freely through the RBC membrane;
- cations (K^+ within the cell, Na^+ outside it) do not.
- when blood is in tissue capillaries, HCO_3^- ions pass out of the RBC into the plasma, but
- K^+ cation cannot pass out of the RBC to balance this shift, and the RBC is left with an overall positive charge. This attracts Cl^- ions which move from the plasma into the cell, (the chloride shift).
- this process is reversed in the lungs.

chapter 12

Metabolic Response to Tissue Injury

Catabolic Phase

- in these notes, the term "tissue injury" includes both trauma and surgery.

CHANGES IN BIOCHEMISTRY, METABOLISM AND VISCERAL FUNCTION (Fig. 12.1)

Protein catabolism

- after injury, protein is catabolized, but no new protein is synthesized, so there is
  —overall N_2 loss in urine, a
  —negative nitrogen balance. This is the
  —key sign of the catabolic phase.
- 70-kg adult has roughly 30 kg of muscle mass.
- 1 gm of nitrogen is equivalent to
  —7 gm of protein and
  —35 gm of muscle. So
- 1 kg of muscle is equivalent to
  —220 gm of protein and
  —30 gm of nitrogen;
- after moderate tissue injury, the total muscle mass lost may be 1 kg or more, but
- each muscle cell and its neuromuscular endplate remain intact;
- metabolic products of cellular lysis enter the extracellular fluid (ECF)
  —some of these products enter cells to be converted to glucose and burned in the citric acid cycles (Fig. 12.2), but most of the
  —nitrogen is excreted in urine as urea, and
  —creatine and creatinine are also excreted in urine;

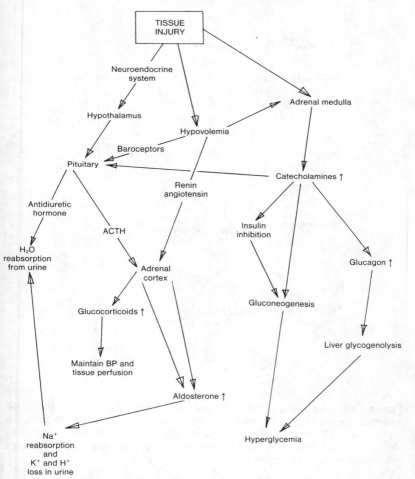

Figure 12.1 Diagram showing endocrine and metabolic responses to tissue injury in acute phase.

—potassium, phosphate and sulphate, normally intracellular, enter ECF and then the urine;
- this obligatory protein catabolism does not affect tissue healing, provided that this phase is not prolonged, e.g., by starvation;
- muscle may eventually recover its former size and strength;

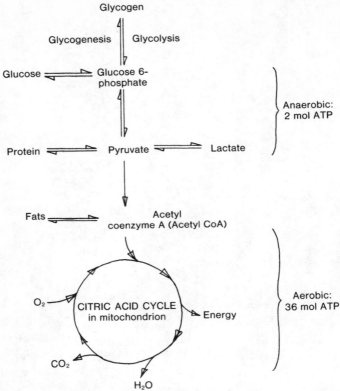

Figure 12.2. Metabolic pathway of glucose, protein and fat. This shows the anaerobic pathway (pyruvate-lactate) which produces only 2 molecules of adenosine triphosphate (ATP) and 18,000 calories of energy and creates a metabolic acidosis with lactic acid buildup. The aerobic pathway (citric acid) produces 18 times more energy and no metabolic acidosis.

- protein loss from muscle cells can be partially prevented by
  —active exercises and
  —even passive stretch exercises every day (all the more reason for daily physiotherapy for every surgical patient!);
- during this phase there is marked loss of depot fat, as this is converted to energy (see below), but
- other organs, e.g., brain, heart, lungs, kidneys, liver, are not catabolized.

Conservation of extracellular fluid (ECF) and sodium

- water is conserved in the body by
  —indirect means, through sodium conservation, and by
  —direct means;
- water conservation takes precedence over all other metabolic responses.
- interstitial component of ECF (i.e., water that is neither in the cells nor in the blood vessels) is available to replace plasma volume after hemorrhage. So ECF conservation after tissue injury is very important.

Sodium conservation

- sodium concentration in ECF determines the volume of water in the ECF;
- after tissue injury, sodium concentration is reduced in
  —urine (due to increased secretion of aldosterone)
  —saliva and
  —sweat;
- reabsorption of sodium in the distal ileum is increased;
- water loss is consequently decreased in these body fluids and in gastrointestinal juice too.

Direct water conservation

- absolute loss of water is reduced by increased reabsorption in distal renal tubule (action of antidiuretic hormone (ADH));
- urine osmolality is increased, in spite of sodium retention, due to excretion of other ions, e.g.,
  —phosphate
  —potassium
  —urea.

Sodium and water administration postoperatively

- if large quantities of sodium-containing fluids are given to the postoperative patient, the excess will be retained, and the patient will develop
  —relative hypoproteinemia and
  —edema of lungs, brain and periphery because the sodium automatically causes water retention;
- if excessive water is given, patient develops
  —hypoproteinemia, with edema as above, and
  —relative (dilutional) hyponatremia (low serum sodium);

- the normal, healthy body would excrete excess salt and water without difficulty, but the injured patient cannot;
- for the postoperative or posttrauma patient,
  —replace fluid losses, but
  —do not drown the patient!

Change in energy sources

- in the first few hours after tissue injury,
- glycogen stores are mobilized for conversion to glucose,
- protein from muscle also supplies some glucose, but
- body fat is the main source of energy (Fig. 12.2);
- ability to use these endogenous energy sources has developed because the badly injured animal is unable, in nature, to find exogenous food, and is in a state of "starvation," and also because the
- brain is an obligate glucose metabolizer; i.e., the brain's sole source of energy is glucose because it cannot metabolize anything else. The body therefore places a priority on maintaining an adequate blood glucose level.
- these changes are wrought by
  —catecholamine and
  —glucagon secretion, and
  —insulin inhibition.
- The serum glucose level rises, but in spite of this the secretion of insulin, which would normally be increased in response to this, is inhibited by catecholamines, and hyperglycemia persists.

Plasma pH

Alkalosis

- initial extracellular alkalosis develops because
  —sodium bicarbonate excretion in urine is reduced to conserve sodium,
  —transfused citrate (the anticoagulant in blood) is oxidized,
  —acidic gastric juice is removed by nasogastric tube (loss of H ions), and the
  —patient may hyperventilate (loss of CO_2) due to hypoxia or under anesthesia.
- mild, transient alkalosis is normal and does no harm.
- if alkalosis is marked, or prolonged, adverse effects may appear
  —oxyhemoglobin dissociation curve moves to left, causing mild

       tissue hypoxia,
—increased demands on cardiac output,
—hypokalemia (K^+) and
—cardiac arrhythmias.

Acidosis

- if patient becomes hypovolemic, with low perfusion of muscle,
  —tissues become hypoxic,
  —lactic acid builds up, and
  —original alkalosis becomes
  —acidosis.

Cardiac output

- this is increased, due to
  —catecholamines,
  —increased demands of hypoxic tissues,
  —increased work of breathing and
  —fever;
- if patient has chronic coronary artery insufficiency or other heart disease, this increased demand on the heart may cause
  —acute congestive heart failure or
  —cardiac arrhythmia, resulting in
  —cerebral and renal insufficiency.

Renal function

- hypoperfusion of kidney
  —activates renin-angiotensin system which causes
  —vasoconstriction of afferent arteriole with further
  —decrease of glomerular filtration rate (GFR) and
  —relative ischemia of proximal tubule which impairs resorption of Na^+; this
  —further stimulates renin release!
- angiotensin II also stimulates aldosterone production;
- aldosterone and
- ADH produce maximum resorption of salt and water in tubules and thus attempt to
  —restore circulating blood volume and renal perfusion. If
- GFR falls below 20 ml/minute, kidney becomes vulnerable to damage by
  —globin pigments and
  —drugs, with possibility of renal insufficiency;

- kidneys can be protected by
  —adequate hydration and
  —osmotic load (mannitol, glucose or salts).

Gastrointestinal tract

- automatic response to injury anywhere is
  —decreased peristalsis and
  —decreased absorption.
- if peritoneal cavity is injured, this response results in
  —paralytic ileus, and
- feeding the patient at this time may result in
  —abdominal distension,
  —decreased diaphragmatic movement,
  —vomiting and aspiration.
- stress ulcer or
- diffuse hemorrhagic gastritis may also occur.

ENDOCRINE CHANGES (Fig. 12.1)

Catecholamines

- these are epinephrine and norepinephrine
- increased secretion of these hormones is the body's emergency response to tissue injury
- initially they are advantageous, but prolonged increase in secretion causes exhaustion of the body's resources and ischemia through vasoconstriction.

Stimulus to secretion

- epinephrine secretion is stimulated by
  —all kinds of tissue injury,
  —hemorrhage,
  —hypovolemia and
  —psychological stress (fright, fight, flight).

Effects

Vasomotor

- requires presence of glucocorticoids for vasomotor responses;
- epinephrine is secreted only by adrenal medulla and stimulate beta receptors, causing vasodilation or mild vasoconstriction depending on circumstances;
- norepinephrine is secreted by adrenal medulla and all nerve

synapses. It causes vasoconstriction everywhere except in myocardium.

Metabolic

- release glucagon which stimulates glycogenolysis in liver, metabolizing liver glycogen stores. This glycogen is converted to pyruvate and glucose and burned in the citric acid cycle to produce energy (Fig. 12.2);
- stimulate directly the hydrolysis of fat with release of free fatty acids. These are converted to acetyl-COA and metabolized in the citric acid cycle.

Hormonal

- inhibit insulin secretion, with resultant liberation and metabolism of
  —amino acids from muscle, and
  —fatty acids from stored fat;
- stimulate pituitary to secrete
  —adrenocorticotropic hormone (ACTH) and therefore increase secretion of
  —glucocorticoids and
  —aldosterone.

Insulin, glucagon and growth hormone

- after tissue injury the increase in catecholamine production
  —inhibits insulin production,
  —decreases peripheral effect of insulin and
  —increases glucagon production.
- insulin
  —favors the use of glucose as the major metabolic fuel and
  —discourages the use of proteins and fat as fuels by
  —inhibiting the release of amino acids from muscle and preventing the
  —hydrolysis of fat; when
- insulin production is inhibited,
  —protein (mainly from muscle) is broken down to amino acids and
  —fat from fat deposits is hydrolyzed to fatty acids;
  —these amino acids and fatty acids are oxidized in the citric acid cycle to produce energy and
  —fat becomes the main energy source.

- glucagon increases the release and metabolism of glycogen from the liver stores.
- growth hormone normally diverts small nitrogen compounds toward protein synthesis in muscle (actin and myosin); this action is
  —suppressed after injury.
    —suppressed after injury.

Glucocorticoids

Stimulus to secretion

- trauma stimulates
- hypothalamus through the
  —peripheral nerves and
  —catecholamines; by
- humoral mediators the hypothalamus stimulates
- pituitary gland which then produces ACTH. This stimulates
- adrenal cortex to produce and secrete cortisol;
- level of cortisol in plasma, then regulates secretion of ACTH (negative feedback mechanism).

Effects

- essential for maintenance of blood pressure and adequate tissue perfusion;
- if patient is unable to produce cortisone, e.g., Addison's disease, the patient may rapidly become
  —shocked and will
  —die if not treated with
  —cortisone.

Aldosterone

Stimuli to secretion

- blood loss, with resultant isotonic hypovolemia, is the most potent stimulus;
  —low flow state through kidneys increases secretion of the enzyme renin by juxtaglomerular cells. Through cascade effect,
  —renin increases formation of angiotensin II which stimulates the adrenal cortex to produce aldosterone.
- urine sodium increase stimulates renin production and thus aldosterone secretion. The sensors lie in the macula densa, a region of specialized cells in the distal tubule wall, next to the juxtaglomerular apparatus.

- ACTH secretion by pituitary is stimulated by low right atrial pressure. This
  —stimulates adrenal cortex to produce aldosterone as well as glucocorticoids.
- hyponatremia and hyperkalemia increase aldosterone secretion.

Effects

- conserves sodium by
- increasing reabsorption of sodium bicarbonate in renal tubules;
- sodium ion is replaced by K^+ and H^+ ions which are excreted in urine;
- aldosterone thus indirectly conserves water because increased interstitial sodium automatically means increased interstitial water;
- overall effect of aldosterone secretion is to
  —maintain ECF volume and thus the
  —plasma volume.

Antidiuretic hormone (ADH)

Stimulus to secretion

- ADH is produced by the hypothalamus but is secreted by the posterior pituitary gland;
- secretion is increased by
  —trauma,
  —isotonic hypovolemia and
  —hypertonic plasma;
- blood volume and/or pressure receptors in left atrium regulate the secretion of ADH. Fall in atrial pressure increases ADH secretion.

Effects

- increased water reabsorption in renal tubules;
- postoperative patient has decreased free water excretion for hours or days. Administration of sodium free water at this stage will produce a relative hyponatremia.

RESPONSE TO DIFFERENT ASPECTS OF ACUTE INJURY

Tissue injury

- the tissue injury initiates catabolic response by pathways which include
  —neuroendocrine system and

—catecholamine secretion.

Wound closed primarily

- clean soft-tissue wound that has been closed heals sufficiently during the catabolic phase that the wound no longer needs external support, e.g., sutures, and function can be resumed;
- metabolic changes continue in the wound for many months afterwards, and
- bone healing continues well into the anabolic phase.

Open wound

- where a large area of skin is lost, e.g., through burns or the degloving injury of a lower limb, the tissue soon becomes chronically infected and acts as a
  —protein
  —electrolyte and
  —fluid sink!
- this large and chronically infected open wound inhibits the anabolic phase, and the patient remains in the catabolic phase becoming
  —emaciated
  —anemic
  —hypoproteinemic
  —hypovolemic;
- this state continues until either the patient
  —dies from complications or
  —the wound is closed.
- as soon as the wound is closed, e.g., by skin grafting, the change is quick and dramatic, with
  —positive nitrogen balance and
  —protein synthesis, restoring muscle and plasma proteins, and
  —hematopoiesis, restoring blood and its components to normal values.

Prolonged hypoperfusion

Compensated hypovolemia

- tissue injury may be associated with blood or other fluid loss, resulting in
- low blood volume;
- if blood volume is reduced by less than 15%, and not lost too quickly, then

- the body can usually compensate by
  —water and salt conservation,
  —transfer of interstitial fluid across the capillary walls and into the blood stream within 18 to 24 hours (transcapillary filling) and
  —other manifestations of the metabolic response to injury already mentioned.

Decompensated hypovolemia

- but if decrease of blood volume is marked or occurs rapidly
  —low flow state will be prolonged,
  —hypoperfusion and
  —hypoxia of tissues will occur, and
  —the body can no longer compensate physiologically. This low flow state is called
  —shock and is characterized by
  —alteration of metabolism of all cells which are anoxic or hypoxic with
  —deterioration of cellular metabolic function.
- prolonged hypoperfusion is the strongest single stimulus to the metabolic response to tissue injury.

Starvation

- this term means no food intake, whether for a day, week or longer.
- after tissue injury, a patient is often unable to eat, and fluid replacement is intravenous;
- during this period the patient is in a state of starvation;
- this probably increases certain of the metabolic responses to tissue injury, e.g., conversion of fat and amino acids to glucose.

Infection

Contamination and infection

- presence of bacteria on a wound surface is contamination. This is not infection and does not necessarily lead to infection.
- infection implies
  —invasion of tissues by microorganisms,
  —tissue destruction and
  —systemic response.

Etiopathology

- infection may be caused by
  —normal bacterial inhabitants of the human body appearing in

an abnormal site, e.g., inhabitants of the colon transferred to the peritoneal cavity; or
—normal bacterial inhabitants of increased virulence being transferred to another patient (nosocomial infection); or
—alteration of normal flora by prolonged antibiotherapy; or
—bacteria which do not normally inhabit the body, e.g., gonococcus and tubercle bacilli.
- local and systemic effects differ according to the nature of the invading organism;
  —loss of nitrogen from an infected burn wound may surpass obligatory catabolic nitrogen loss in the urine, and the local protein loss may be massive; whereas
  —a small, apparently insignificant local infection may also have marked systemic effects (tetanus!);

Stimulus to metabolic response
- systemic effects of infection exaggerate the metabolic response to tissue injury, especially responses mediated by catecholamine secretion; muscle wasting may be extreme. When
- severe injury is followed by infection, catabolic response with extreme and rapid muscle wasting is more severe than in any other surgical problem;
- catabolic phase usually ends, and the patient enters the anabolic phase, as soon as the
  —infection is controlled, by
  —antibiotics,
  —abscess drainage or
  —amputation of gangrenous limb.

Drugs
- administration of drugs may alter the metabolic response to injury in many ways.

Analgesics
- morphine
  —stimulates secretion of ADH,
  —depresses respiratory center, and may worsen hypoxic state.
- aspirin
  —interferes with blood clotting and
  —may cause gastritis with gastrointestinal hemorrhage.
- phenacetin damages kidneys (the "phenacetin kidney").

Anesthetics

- these stimulate catecholamine secretion.
- halothane
  —may cause liver damage.
- spinal anesthesia
  —stops afferent impulses from area of trauma to brain, and thus
  —impairs the metabolic response by preventing some of the information about the injury from reaching the brain. Also produces
  —peripheral vasodilation with relative hypovolemia and hypertension.
- neuromuscular blocking agents cause
  —hypotension through vasodilation.

Antibiotics

- are immunosuppressive by
  —killing sensitive bacteria and thus preventing the immune apparatus from contacting the antigen; or by
  —inhibiting protein synthesis or
  —producing leukopenia.
- alter flora by
  —killing some organisms; this
  —allows other organisms unrestrained growth, e.g., elimination of *Staphylococcus*, allowing overgrowth of *Pseudomonas*. Or
  —favoring growth of mutants, and resistant strains and L-forms.
- potassium penicillin salts may cause
  —hyperkalemia, with cardiac complications;
- specific organ damage,
  —kanamycin is toxic to the kidneys and
  —chloramphenicol may cause agranulocytosis.
- may lull the surgeon into a false sense of security by
  —masking the symptoms and signs of infection, thus prolonging the catabolic phase.

Psychological factors

- psychological stress influences the metabolic response, and includes
  —fear of pain and of malignant disease,
  —isolation from family environment, and
  —lack of sleep;

- most of these factors can be reduced if the doctors and nurses
  —talk to the patient,
  —explain the illness, treatment and prognosis, and
  —answer all questions. Do not forget that
  —relatives may be more concerned than the patient, so
  —talking with them is important, and
  —talking to the parents of a child is essential.

Convalescent Phase

- recovery from tissue injury is a dynamic process, and the patient's physiological status changes from day to day;
- be aware of the normal physiological progress of recovery because
  —failure to progress and thrive or
  —a change in the wrong direction generally signifies that something has gone wrong. The alert surgeon
  —recognized this early and can
  —institute appropriate measures before it is too late.

TURNING POINT

- the patient enters the anabolic phase, the major metabolic change of which is a
  —positive nitrogen balance, the urinary excretion of nitrogen being reduced, even without an increase in nitrogen intake, secondary to
  —reversal of the metabolic and endocrine changes that occurred immediately after the acute injury.
- other signs include
  —return of peristalsis and passage of gas,
  —return of appetite,
  —a bright, alive look in the eyes,
  —increased interest in the surroundings,
  —desire to talk and see relatives and
  —renewed interest in the opposite sex (a KEY sign).

ANABOLIC PHASE

Positive nitrogen balance

- this phase is characterized by prolonged positive nitrogen balance, more nitrogen being retained than excreted, until the total nitrogen

loss has been replaced. This phase lasts 3 to 50 days or more, depending upon
—extent of injuries,
—age and physiological status of patient and
—diet.
- during this phase the patient requires
—high protein and
—high calorie diet with
—vitamins B and C added.
- rate of anabolism is
—3 to 5 gm of nitrogen per day in the adult, and the
—patient requires 150 calories for every gram of nitrogen. Thus if the
- patient with moderate injury has
—lost a total of 1 kg of muscle mass (30 gm of nitrogen), the
—anabolic phase will last at least 6 days, and
—4,500 calories will be needed to convert this nitrogen into muscle; if the
- patient with severe injury has
—lost 2½ kg of muscle (75 gm of nitrogen), the
—anabolic phase will last 15 days or more, and
—11,250 calories will be needed for protein synthesis alone; if
- severe injury is combined with major infection, then the
—total muscle mass lost may be 10 kg (300 gm nitrogen) or more, the
—anabolic phase will last 60 days or more, and
—this protein synthesis will require 45,000 calories.
- during this phase
—muscular strength and energy return, and
—function improves, e.g., walking.
- positive nitrogen balance is essential for rehabilitation of the patient, but
- weight gain is slow, about 1 kg/week.

Endocrinology

- actions of insulin are no longer inhibited, with the result that
—protein and fat are no longer metabolized, the
—liver glycogen stores are restocked, and the
—blood sugar level returns to normal.

activity of growth hormone directs nitrogen to muscle for muscle protein synthesis.

Inhibition of protein anabolism

- normal nitrogen anabolism is inhibited by
  —infection,
  —large untreated wounds,
  —intestinal fistula and
  —rapid, continued malignant growth;
- it may be slowed down if
  —patient resumes physical activities too soon (e.g., returning to work) because this
  —uses calories for other purposes instead of protein building.

FAT GAIN PHASE

- when nitrogen balance has been restored, i.e., nitrogen intake and loss are equal, this signifies that normal muscle mass has been regained.
- body now starts to replace the fat depots that were depleted in initial acute phase to provide endogenous calories, and the
- patient is in positive caloric balance (more calories are retained than are used in energy).
- this phase may last weeks or months, depending on the
  —severity of injuries and
  —normal shape of patient!
- if the patient has insufficient exercise during this period, the patient may become obese. This must be avoided.

chapter 13
Normal Fluid, Electrolyte and Acid-Base Metabolism

Body Water

- 60% of the body weight of a young man is water (75% to 80% in a newborn infant)
- average man has 42 liters of water

DISTRIBUTION

- 40% intracellular fluid (ICF)
- 20% extracellular fluid (ECF) divided into
  —15% interstitial fluid
  —5% intravascular fluid
- 40% solid compartment, not readily available for fluid exchange.

DAILY WATER BALANCE

- figures are for a 70-kg man on an average day
  Intake
  - 1,000 ml as liquid
  - 1,200 ml in food
  - 300 ml metabolic water, result of oxidation of food
  - 2,500 ml total
  - this averges 40 ml/kg body weight, but the
  - infant requires 100 ml/kg because of higher metabolic rate and increased surface area relative to body mass.
  Output
  - 1,500 ml in urine (760 ml is obligatory)
  - 850 ml as insensible loss in expired air and transpiration from skin
  - 150 ml in feces
  - 2,500 ml total.

FACTORS INCREASING DAILY WATER NEEDS

- during hot summer, water loss is much greater than this due to heat and perspiration. Water lost as sweat may be as much as 5,000 ml.
- other factors are
  —fever (250 ml/day/° C rise of temperature),
  —diarrhea and vomiting and
  —pooling of secretions, e.g., in bowel in intestinal obstruction.

Solutes and Osmotic Pressure

SOLUTES

- a solute is a dissolved particle (Fig. 13.2)

  ECF

  - main solutes in ECF are
    —sodium, Na^+
    —chloride, Cl^- and
    —bicarbonate, HCO_3^-

  ICF

  - main solutes in ICF are
    —potassium, K^+
    —magnesium, Mg^{++}
    —phosphates, HPO_4^-
    —proteinates, Pr^-
  - sodium is kept out of the cells by active pumping at the cell wall. This uses energy.

OSMOTIC PRESSURE

What is osmotic pressure?

- concentration (number of particles per liter) of solutes is always equal in all fluid compartments, e.g., ECF and ICF. It may be
  —abnormally high, as in dehydration, or
  —low, as in water overload, but the concentrations are equal.
- those particles which cannot pass from one fluid compartment to the other across the semipermeable membrane of the cell wall exert an osmotic pressure; i.e., they attract water;
- if two fluid compartments, e.g., ECF and ICF, are separated by a semipermeable membrane, e.g., the cell wall, which allows water to cross it but not certain electrolytes (e.g., Na^+ in ECF, K^+ in

ICF) or large, uncharged particles (e.g., glucose, proteins), then
   —the compartment with the higher concentration of solutes will
      exert a greater osmotic pressure and will therefore
   —attract water across the membrane from
   —the compartment with the lower concentration until
   —the concentration of solutes in the two compartments is equal.
- the two compartments are then in osmotic equilibrium because the
  osmotic pressure is the same on both sides.
- osmotic pressure is the sum of the total number of individual
  electrolyte and nonelectrolyte particles in solution;
- it is not changed by
   —the size of the particles or by
   —their electrical charges.

Measurement of osmotic pressure

- the osmotic pressure exerted by a substance is measured in milliosmoles (mOsm);
- osmoles and milliosmoles refer to the actual number of osmotically
  active particles present in solution.
- 1 mM of protein does not dissociate, and
   —contributes 1 mOsm;
- 1 mM of KCl dissociates into
   —K^+ and Cl^- and contributes
   —2 mOsm.
- 1 mM of Na_2PO_4 dissociates into
   —$Na^+ + Na^+ + PO_4^=$ and contributes
   —3 mOsm.
- in clinical medicine, osmotic pressure is used to express total body
  water excess or deficit. It is not a true chemical measurement.

Osmotic pressure of fluid compartment

Blood

- plasma proteins are mainly responsible for osmotic pressure of
  plasma; this is called the
- "colloid osmotic pressure" of plasma.
- water, salts and small proteins filter out of the arterial end of
  the capillary bed into the interstitial fluid and are reabsorbed
  back into plasma at the venous end (Fig. 13.1); this
- constant movement of fluid and other substances is a result of
  changing balance between

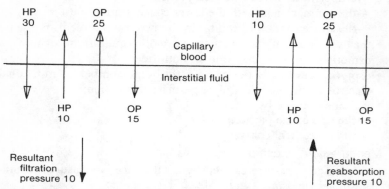

Figure 13.1. The Starling principle showing balance between hydrostatic (*HP*) and osmotic pressures (*OP*) in millimeters Hg between capillary blood and interstitial fluid. Water, salts and protein are filtered out of blood at the arterial end of the capillary and reabsorbed at the venous end. Pressures are average and vary according to circumstances.

> —hydrostatic and
> —osmotic pressures of
> —plasma and
> —interstitial fluid;

- but it is the colloid osmotic pressure of plasma which prevents overall loss of fluid from capillaries into the interstititial compartment.

Interstitial fluid

- sodium ions are major osmotically active particles in this compartment.

Intracellular fluid

- principal cation is K^+ and contributes the major portion of osmotic pressure within cells.

ADMINISTRATION OF ELECTROLYTE SOLUTIONS

Isotonic solutions

- this is a solution whose solute concentration and osmotic pressure are the same as plasma, about 285 mOsm/liter.

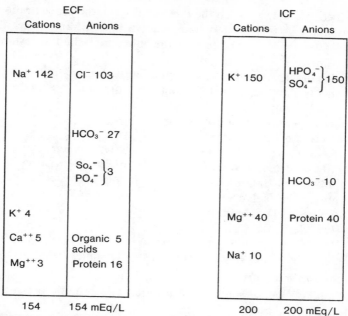

Figure 13.2. Gamblegrams showing electrolyte concentrations in ECF and ICF. All values are in milliequivalents per liter (mEq/L).

- these solutions include
  —lactated Ringer's solution,
  —0.9% physiological (normal) saline, has 308 mOsm/liter, and
  —5% dextrose in water (D5W), 278 mOsm/liter
- IV administration of these does not cause fluid shifts;
- safe rate of IV administration is less than 10 ml/kg/hour in adult. Rates faster than this require close monitoring of patient.

Hypertonic solutions

- a hypertonic solution is one whose concentration of solutes, and therefore osmotic pressure, is greater than that of plasma.
- if mannitol or dextran is administered IV, it
  —raises the concentration of particles in the plasma, and therefore
  —raises the osmotic pressure of plasma;
  —water then passes from the interstitial fluid to the plasma until osmotic equilibrium is reached. In doing so, plasma volume is increased.

—because water has left the interstitial fluid, the concentration of solutes in this fluid is high relative to ICF, and water then leaves the cells and enters the interstitial fluid to establish osmotic equilibrium;

—this movement of water continues until all three fluid compartments have equal solute concentrations and are in osmotic equilibrium.

- other hypertonic solutions are
  —3% and 5% saline,
  —5% dextrose in 0.9% saline (D5S), 586 mOsm/liter,
  —10% dextrose in water (D10W), 556 mOsm/liter.
- rapid administration of hypertonic solutions causes cellular dehydration. This is dangerous.
- safe rates of IV administration in the adult are
  —D5S, less than 8 ml/kg/hour
  —D10W, less than 5 ml/kg/hour;
- reduce these rates for children and small people.

Hypotonic solutions

- a solution whose solute concentration and osmotic pressure are lower than plasma;
- these include
  —0.5% saline, 165 mOsm/liter, and
  —half-strength lactated Ringer's;
- these fluids should be given cautiously because if rate is too rapid,
  —water will pass from ECF to ICF, creating intracellular edema, pulmonary edema and hypoxia, and
  —red blood cells will hemolyze (absorb water, expand and burst) with resultant hypoxemia, hemoglobinemia, hemoglobinuria and possible renal failure.
- hypotonic solutions are more dangerous than hypertonic ones.

Electrolytes

MEASUREMENT

Milliequivalents

- electrolytes are electrically charged particles, and their concentration in body fluids is measured in milliequivalents (mEq) because

this measurement takes into account
  —osmotic activity (osmolality),
  —concentration of particles (molality) and
  —electric charges (valence), and
- 1 mEq of any substance will combine chemically with 1 mEq of any other substance.
- the equivalent of an ion is
  —that weight in grams which will combine with or replace 1 molecular weight of hydrogen; another way to define equivalent weight is
  —the atomic weight of the substance in grams divided by its valence.
- a milliequivalent is that figure expressed in milligrams. For example, the
- equivalent weight of K^+ is the
  —atomic weight 39 divided by 1, which equals
  —39 gm, and 1
  —mEq is 39 mg;
- equivalent weight of Ca^{++} is the
  —atomic weight 40 divided by 2, which equals
  —20 gm, and 1
  —mEq is 20 mg;
- when using milliequivalents, the
  —number of cations (positively charged particles) always
  —equals the number of anions (negatively charged) in the solution (Fig. 13.2).

Millimoles and milligrams
- substances that are not ionized are measured in
  —millimoles (mM) per liter of water or
  —milligrams (mg) per 100 ml of water.
- a mole is the molecular weight of a substance expressed in grams (millimoles in milligrams); e.g., the atomic weight of
  —Na^+ is 23 and of
  —Cl^- is 35; so the molecular weight of
  —NaCl is 58; therefore 1
  —mole of NaCl is 58 gm and 1
  —mM is 58 mg.

CATIONS

Sodium (Na$^+$)

Body content

- makes 92% of all cation particles in ECF (Fig. 13.2) and is
- very important in fluid balance of patient.
- total sodium content in a 70-kg man is
  - —4,500 to 6,300 mEq or
  - —40 mEq/kg.
- distribution is
  - —50% in ECF,
  - —10% in ICF and
  - —40% in bone, nonexchangeable
- normal concentration in ECF is 138 to 152 mEq/liter

Intake and output

- average daily intake is a little more than 1 mEq/kg or
  - —100 mEq total and is
  - —much greater than normal daily requirements.
- kidneys carefully regulate output to equal intake;
- absolute minimum daily output in urine is
  - —1 mEq and
- maximum daily urinary output in the normal adult is
  - —200 mEq. This equals the
  - —maximum daily tolerance.
- in very hot climate, sweat may contain
  - —70 mEq/liter, and
  - —total daily loss in sweat may equal the average daily intake.
- some sodium is also lost in feces through gastrointestinal (GI) secretions.

Regulation of sodium metabolism

- sodium content in fluid compartments is regulated by
  - —aldosterone which increases tubular reabsorption of sodium and by
  - —antidiuretic hormone (ADH) which increases tubular reabsorption of water and thus dilutes sodium in ECF and ICF.

Potassium (K$^+$)

Body content

- makes 75% of all cation particles in ICF (Fig. 13.2).

- total exchangeable potassium content in a 70-kg man is
  —3,500 mEq
- 98% of total body K^+ is in ICF
- normal concentration in ECF is 3.5 to 5.0 mEq/liter.

Intake and output

- average daily intake is
  —1 mEq/kg, or
  —50 to 100 mEq/day total; this is
  —much greater than normal daily requirements.
- excretion normally equals intake;
- minimum daily urinary output is
  —30 mEq. So
- minimum daily need is
  —0.4 mEq/kg, or
  —30 to 40 mEq total.
- maximum daily tolerance is
  —400 mEq total.
- renal conservation of K^+ is less efficient than Na^+ conservation;
  —1 molecule of K^+ is excreted for every N^+ molecule reabsorbed, and
  —aldosterone increases this excretion. If
- IV therapy replaces the patient's Na^+ without replacing K^+, then
  —serious K^+ depletion may occur.
- after moderate tissue injury, and especially if intestinal or biliary fistulae are present, the patient may lose
  —60 to 120 mEq of K^+ per day, and after severe trauma, daily loss may be
  —200 mEq, three times the average daily intake.
- most IV solutions contain too much Na^+ and not enough K^+.

Regulation of potassium metabolism

- K^+ metabolism is regulated indirectly by
  —aldosterone, which preserves Na^+ at the expense of K^+, and by the
  —pH of plasma, an increase of 0.1 pH causing a decrease of 0.6 mEq/liter of K^+, and vice versa.

Calcium (Ca^{++})

- total body content is 1,000 to 1,200 gm.

- more than 90% of the body's Ca^{++} is in bones and is exchangeable; i.e., it can be easily withdrawn and replaced if plasma Ca^{++} level falls.
- plasma calcium level is 5 mEq/liter or 9 to 11 mg/100 ml and is very carefully regulated by
  —diet,
  —acid-base balance,
  —parathyroid hormone and
  —thyrocalcitonin.
- normal daily intake is 1 to 3 gm, much more than the
- daily normal requirement for the average adult, which is
  —0.25 mEq/kg or
  —5 mg/kg.
- abnormalities of calcium metabolism are rarely a problem in the postoperative patient.

ANIONS

Chloride (Cl^-)

- chloride and bicarbonate (HCO_3^-) are the major anions in ECF;
- normal plasma concentration of chloride is 95 to 105 mEq/liter;
- fall in plasma chloride concentration is usually accompanied by rise in HCO_3^- concentration, and vice versa.
- daily ingestion of chloride is in the form of Na^+ and K^+ salts; thus
- intake and output of Cl^- depends on intake and output of
  —Na^+ and K^+;
  —depletion of these cations as well as depletion of H^+ (e.g., in severe vomiting), automatically
  —reduces Cl^- too, and
  —HCO_3^- usually rises, causing
  —metabolic, hypochloremic alkalosis. Correct this by administration of
  —KCl as well as NaCl, and the
  —kidney will restore the H^+ ions.

Phosphate (HPO_4^-)

- the major anion in ICF.
- normal plasma concentration is 1.7 to 2.3 mEq/liter and is
- regulated by
  —diet,
  —acid-base balance and

—endocrine glands.

Bicarbonate (HCO_3^-)

• the other major anion in ECF.

Acid-Base Balance

pH OF BODY FLUIDS

• pH is the
  —negative logarithm of the H^+ ion concentration in a fluid. If the
• H^+ ion concentration is
  —$10^{-7.0}$ Eq/liter, then the
  —pH is 7.0. When the
• H^+ ion concentration is
  —$10^{-6.0}$ Eq/liter, then the
  —pH is 6.0, and the acid is
  —10 times stronger than one of pH 7.0.
• neutrality is the pH of plain water, 7.0;
• body fluids are slightly alkaline, pH 7.4, because of the bicarbonate content;
• pH of blood must be maintained within very narrow limits.

BUFFERS

Buffers in body fluids

• a buffer system consists of a weak acid or base and its salt;
• the base combines with a strong acid to form a weak acid and thereby prevents large fluctuations in pH.
• similarly, when a strong base is added, this is buffered and a weak base is formed.
• buffers usually work in pairs;
• the major buffer pair in the ECF is
  —bicarbonate (HCO_3^-) and carbonic acid (H_2CO_3), but
• in the red blood cells, the major pair is
  —ionized hemoglobin (Hb^-) and unionized hemoglobin (HHb).
• major intracellular buffers are
  —proteins and
  —phosphates

How the HCO_3^- buffer pair functions

• H^+ ions are strongly acidic, and when

- added to blood, e.g., from hydrolysis of water during normal cellular metabolism (Equation 1), they combine with bicarbonate ions (Equations 2 and 3) to form carbonic acid in the presence of enzyme carbonic anhydrase

$$H_2O \rightleftharpoons H^+ + OH^- \tag{1}$$

$$NaHCO_3 \rightleftharpoons Na^+ + HCO_3^- \tag{2}$$

$$H^+ + HCO_3^- \rightleftharpoons H_2CO_3 \tag{3}$$

- carbonic acid is a much weaker acid than hydrochloric acid, HCl (Equation 4).

$$HCl + NaHCO_3 \rightarrow NaCl + H_2CO_3 \tag{4}$$

- in the lungs, carbonic acid forms carbon dioxide and water (equation 5), and these escape in exhaled air

$$H_2CO_3 \rightarrow H_2O + CO_2 \tag{5}$$

- but because some of the HCO_3^- has been used up, the blood is a little more acidic than before, but not as acidic as it would have been if the H^+ ions had not been "buffered."

Replacement of bicarbonate ions

- the blood remains mildly acidic until the kidneys replace the HCO_3^- ions by
  —reabsorbing Na^+ and HCO_3^- and
  —excreting H^+ ions in the urine;
- the kidneys can excrete a urine of pH 4, much more acidic than the blood.

Elimination of acids

- volatile acids are eliminated by the lungs, e.g.,
  —H_2CO_3 is eliminated by lungs as CO_2 and H_2O (Equation 5);
- nonvolatile acids, e.g.,
  —phosphoric,
  —sulphuric and
  —lactic acids, are excreted in the urine, by exchanging the H^+ ions for Na^+ ions.

chapter 14

Acute Fluid, Electrolyte and Acid-Base Imbalance

Acute Fluid and Electrolyte Imbalance

EVALUATION OF PATIENT

- evaluation and correction of fluid, electrolyte and acid-base imbalance are just as essential before surgery as they are during or after it.

History and physical examination
- there are never any short cuts
- you must
  —always take a good history and do a
  —complete physical examination.

Laboratory examinations
- serum electrolytes, Na^+, K^+, Cl^-, HCO_3^-
- BUN, hematocrit and plasma proteins, and
- urinalysis with
- urine electrolytes if indicated;
- plasma pH and blood gases as well, if an acid-base problem is suspected.
- if results of some of these laboratory tests are not available, then
- base your conclusions on clinical evidence alone (not difficult to do) and treat the patient accordingly, monitoring the patient's vital signs
  —pulse rate,
  —blood pressure and
  —urine output throughout treatment
- looking for reversal of signs of electrolyte or acid-base imbalance.

CLASSIFICATION

- volume abnormalities
  —extracellular fluid (ECF) deficit (water and electrolytes)
  —ECF excess (water and electrolytes)
- concentration abnormalities
  —hyponatremia (water intoxication)
  —hypernatremia (water depletion)
- mixed, paradoxical volume and concentration abnormalities
  —ECF and Na^+ deficit
  —ECF and Na^+ excess
- composition abnormalities
  —acid-base imbalance
  —hypokalemia
  —hyperkalemia
- though each is a separate entity, the categories may overlap.

ACUTE ECF DEFICIT (WATER AND ELECTROLYTE DEPLETION)

- this is volume deficit, the most common fluid disorder in a surgical patient.

Etiopathology

- burns,
- intestinal obstruction, gastric suction,
- peritonitis, diarrhea and vomiting,
- diabetic acidosis,
- chronic renal failure and
- excessive sweating.
- water and electrolytes are lost almost entirely from ECF.

Clinical features

- in all degrees of severity, concentration of serum sodium may be near normal, even though there is an absolute decrease in body sodium content;
- hematocrit increases with severity.
  Mild
  - 8% to 16% of ECF loss produces
  - 2% to 4% of body weight loss,
  - thirst and
  - decrease of eyeball tension and of
  - tissue turgor.

Moderate
- 20% to 24% of ECF loss produces
- 5% to 6% weight loss,
- oliguria,
- tachycardia,
- collapsing veins and pulse,
- postural hypotension,
- sleepiness, apathy and anorexia.

Severe
- 28% to 40% ECF loss produces
- 7% to 10% weight loss,
- hypotension,
- hypoperfusion and
- severe oliguria;
- death may ensue.

Treatment
- replace losses with physiological isotonic solution of electrolytes in water

  0.9% saline
  - this contains
    —Na^+, 154 mEq/liter
    —Cl^-, 154 mEq/liter
  - this is called "physiological" or "normal" saline, but
  - it is not physiological because it contains
    —too much Na^+,
    —much too much Cl^-, and
    —does not contain
    —K^+ or
    —HCO_3^-;
  - it is isotonic; i.e., it has nearly the same osmotic pressure as ECF:
  - when using this, add
    —one part of sodium bicarbonate solution, 44 mEq of $NaHCO_3$ in 250 ml, to
    —two parts of saline;
  - for vomiting, add
    —potassium as well—KCl, 40 mEq/liter

Ringer's lactate

Contents

- this contains
  - Na^+, 130 mEq/liter
  - Cl^-, 109 mEq/liter
  - K^+, 4 mEq/liter
  - Ca^{++}, 3 mEq/liter, and
  - lactate, 28 mEq/liter.
- this solution is similar to ECF and is much more physiological than "normal" saline.
- lactate is converted to bicarbonate in the body and helps correct the metabolic acidosis resulting from tissue hypoxia of hypoperfusion.

Contraindications

- old patient, especially if he
  - fails to increase urine output or the
  - central venous pressure (CVP) rises during administration of Ringer's lactate;
- congestive heart failure;
- acute renal failure, unless dehydration and electrolyte losses are severe.
- Ringer's must not be used as a substitute for maintenance therapy.

Protein loss

- this may produce edema once water and electrolyte balance is restored; so
- treat this with
  - serum albumin or
  - plasma or
  - whole blood.

ACUTE ECF EXCESS (SODIUM AND WATER OVERLOAD)

Etiology

- usually iatrogenic (your fault!), a result of
- excess administration of saline solution, especially in a patient with chronic disease of the
  - kidneys, with diminished ability to excrete Na^+; of the
  - heart, with fall in glomerular filtration rate (GFR) and reflex increase in Na^+ reabsorption; or the

—liver with decreased plasma proteins, decreased circulatory volume, secondary aldosteronism and increased Na^+ reabsorption; or of
- prolonged steroid therapy.

Clinical features and treatment

- may cause
  —congestive heart failure (CHF) and
  —pulmonary edema.
- treat by
  —restriction of fluid administration!
  —digitalization and diuretics may also be necessary for CHF and pulmonary edema.

ACUTE HYPONATREMIA (WATER INTOXICATION)

Etiopathology

- nearly always iatrogenic, i.e.,
  —too much fluid and too little Na^+ postoperatively, e.g., 5% dextrose in water (D5W), especially if the patient has
- acute or chronic renal insufficiency and cannot conserve Na^+ efficiently. When
- serum sodium is less than 130 mEq/liter,
- excess fluid is excreted in urine if the patient is healthy; but
- if the patient is
  —old, or has
  —cardiac disease, overload may cause
- pulmonary edema and
- CHF.

Clinical features and treatment

- signs of increased intracranial pressure due to cerebral edema,
- generalized edema, and
- oliguria progressing to anuria and death.
- treat by
  —water restriction and,
- in severe cases, give
- 150 to 300 ml of hypertonic (5%) saline to pull water out of cells into ECF. But
- too much 5% saline will expand circulatory volume and cause CHF and pulmonary edema!

ACUTE HYPERNATREMIA (WATER DEPLETION)

Etiology

Reduced intake

- coma,
- patient too young, too old or too ill to ask for water,
- esophageal or pyloric obstruction,
- nasogastric tube feedings rich in salt and protein (thick soup) but deficient in water.

Increased loss

- fever,
- hot, dry climate or environment (e.,g., boiler stoker in an iron foundry),
- copious diarrhea (hypotonic),
- diabetes insipidus (deficiency of antidiuretic hormone (ADH) secretion) or
- diabetes mellitus (causes osmotic diuresis due to glycosemia).

Pathology

- decrease of water in all fluid compartments because water is freely diffusible
- results in
  - —increased osmolality (hypertonicity) with increased concentration of
  - —electrolytes and
  - —proteins in all fluid compartments.

Clinical features

- these are most severe if dehydration is acute, not chronic;
- major symptom is thirst!
- dry, sticky mucous membranes in the mouth;
- body temperature may rise to a lethal level;
- with 5% body water loss (3 to 4 liters in adult)
  - —eyeball tension and
  - —tissue turgor are reduced.
  - —10% loss of fluid without electrolyte loss causes
  - —dangerous rise in electrolytes with
  - —restlessness, weakness, personality changes and
  - —difficulty in swallowing;
- serum Na^+ of 170 mEq/liter produces unconsciousness;

- serum Na^+ of 200 mEq/liter causes death from circulatory failure.

Diagnosis

- loss of 1 liter of water reduces body weight by 1 kg in the adult;
- measurement of acute weight loss provides an estimation of acute fluid loss, e.g., in the postoperative patient;
- this presupposes that the patient was weighed before surgery, which should be done whenever possible, especially with children.

Treatment

- replace pure acute water deficit with
- D5W (5% dextrose in water) slowly as follows:
  —one third in 6 hours
  —one third from sixth to twenty-fourth hour
  —one third from twenty-fourth to forty-eighth hour
- at the same time, daily minimum requirements must be administered. Adults need 35 to 40 ml of fluid per kg of body weight per day as
  —1,000 ml of Ringer's solution, or normal saline, and
  —1,500 ml of D5W for daily maintenance.
- if loss is mainly due to sweating or diarrhea, replace this with
  —0.2% saline solution, or
  —5% glucose in 0.2% saline.
- chronic deficit can be replaced more slowly.

MIXED, PARADOXICAL VOLUME AND CONCENTRATION ABNORMALITIES

- these are paradoxical because the combination of abnormalities is the opposite of what one would expect.
- caused by
  —disease or
  —inappropriate IV therapy.

ECF deficit and Na^+ deficit (hyponatremia)

- produced in patient who is
  —losing gastrointestinal (GI) fluids and
  —drinking only water, and also
- postoperatively when
  —GI losses are replaced with
  —D5W or
  —hypotonic saline only.

ECF excess and Na^+ excess (hypernatremia)

- produced when
  - excess sodium salts are administered with
  - restricted water intake, and also by
- replacing pure water losses with saline solutions only.

Clinical features

- these are a composite of the features of each individual state; i.e.
  - similar features of each state will be additive
  - opposite signs will cancel each other out; e.g., a fall in temperature caused by ECF deficit will cancel the rise in temperature caused by hypernatremia, and the patient's temperature may remain normal;
- normal kidneys may compensate for these changes, but in th presence of
- renal insufficiency, mixed abnormalities are particularly likely t develop

HYPOKALEMIA

- serum K^+, less than 3 mEq/liter
- more common than K^+ excess.

Etiology

- prolonged low potassium intake;
- vomiting
  - loses K^+ and
  - causes alkalosis through loss of HCl. To compensate,
  - H^+ moves out of cells and
  - K^+ moves into cells to replace H^+, thus causing hypokalemia Also
  - excess K^+ in preference to H^+ is excreted in urine in exchang for Na^+ which is reabsorbed;
- respiratory and metabolic alkalosis, with K^+ being excreted in th urine to preserve H^+ ions. Potassium normally competes with th hydrogen ion for renal tubular excretion in exchange for th sodium ion;
- diarrhea;
- sodium depletion, because kidneys reabsorb more Na^+, to conserv it, in exchange for K^+;
- steroid therapy;

- diuretic therapy increases KCl loss in urine;
- renal disease.

Clinical features

- alkalosis may occur because
  —kidney reduces excretion of K^+ in an attempt to conserve it and excretes H^+ instead;
  —H^+ moves into cells to replace the K^+ loss.
- arrhythmias and
- ECG changes
  —flat T waves and
  —depressed S-T segment;
- muscle weakness progressing to flaccid paralysis and
- paralytic ileus.

Treatment

- K^+ is given as
  —KCl, in a concentration of
  —40 mEq/liter or less, and
  —no more than 0.5 mEq/kg/hour, to a
  —maximum of 240 mEq/24 hours.
- if the patient has not lost excessive quantities of K^+, administration is not necessary in the first 48 hours after surgery, in spite of the increased urinary excretion of K^+, because
  —K^+ is released into ECF from cells in injured tissues and
  —tissue catabolism is increased secondary to starvation (starvation in this context means no food for 2 or 3 days, fasting);
- do not give K^+ to the oliguric patient, i.e., the patient whose urine output is less than 500 ml of urine daily;
- give supplemental oral K^+ to patients on diuretics.

HYPERKALEMIA

- serum K^+, more than 5 mEq/liter

  Etiology

  - acute or chronic renal insufficiency
  - excess release of intracellular K^+ in extensive
    —burns
    —crush injury
    —major surgery or
    —infection;

- severe metabolic acidosis, K^+ leaves cells for ECF.

Clinical features
- hyperactive reflexes and increased muscular excitability;
- ECG changes progress from
  —peaked (pointed) T waves,
  —wide QRS,
  —depressed S-T segment and
  —P-R interval prolonged, to
  —arrhythmias,
  —heart block and
  —ventricular fibrillation.
- GI system
  —nausea and vomiting,
  —colic and diarrhea.

Treatment

Reduction of K^+ in ECF
- to lower K^+ in ECF, give the patient IV over 30 minutes
  —200 to 300 ml of 25% dextrose containing
  —80 mEq of sodium lactate or sodium bicarbonate, with
  —regular insulin, 1 unit/5 gm or more of glucose (too much insulin will produce hypoglycemia. Do not add to the patient's problems!).
- dextrose and insulin stimulate synthesis of glycogen, resulting in K^+ uptake and a reduction of K^+ in the ECF;
- sodium lactate raises the pH (more alkaline) and pushes K^+ out of the ECF into the cells;
- cation-exchange resin, e.g., Kayexalate, can control a serum K^+, rising by less than 1 mEq/day.
- peritoneal dialysis may be used as a last resort

Treatment of myocardial toxicity
- if ECG changes occur or
- arrhythmia is present, give
  —10 to 30 ml of 10% calcium gluconate or chloride IV over 5 minutes under ECG control immediately, followed by
  —dextrose, insulin and sodium lactate as above.

Acute Abnormalities of Acid-Base Balance

- a few hours after a change in pH, the body normally starts to compensate and tries to return the pH to normal.
- compensation is never complete unless the cause of the a-b imbalance is removed.

METABOLIC ACIDOSIS

Etiopathology

- acidosis with normal serum Cl^- is caused by
  —diabetic acidosis, uremia,
  —tissue hypoxia, e.g., hypovolemic shock,
  —aspirin excess and
  —starvation;
- base bicarbonate is lost and serum Cl^- is raised by
  —diarrhea and
  —renal tubular acidosis;
- all result in
  —excess of H^+ ions in plasma with
  —lowered pH and
  —decreased plasma HCO_3^- (bicarbonate ion) because it has been used up in buffering (Table 14.1).

Table 14.1
Metabolic Changes in Acute Acid-Base Imbalance

	Metabolic acidosis	Metabolic alkalosis	Respiratory acidosis	Respiratory alkalosis
pH	↓	↑	↓	↑
$PaCO_2$	–	–	↑	↓
Plasma HCO_3^-	↓	↑	–	–

$PaCO_2$, partial pressure of carbon dioxide in arterial blood.

Compensatory mechanisms

- lungs compensate initially;
- buffer system exchanges a weak acid for a strong one, and plasma HCO_3^- is decreased;
- H_2CO_3 (carbonic acid, a weak acid) is increased, and through hyperventilation this is excreted by the lungs as CO_2 and H_2O vapor.
- renal compensatory mechanisms develop 12 to 24 hours later; in the renal tubular cells the following reactions occur:

$$H_2CO_3 \xrightarrow{\text{carbonic}~\text{anhydrase}} H^+ + HCO_3^-$$

—H^+ ions are excreted in acid urine (with K^+) and

—HCO_3^- and Na^+ are reabsorbed into circulation.

- renal insufficiency will interfere with this important compensatory mechanism, and acidosis will progress rapidly. The
- liver metabolizes lactic acid.

Treatment

- correct underlying disorder;
- correct
  —metabolic defect and replace
  —lost H_2O and electrolytes by
  —Ringer's lactate or
  —0.9% saline with $NaHCO_3$ added if acidosis is severe, but if
- too much HCO_3^- is given, metabolic alkalosis may result, and patient will be no better!
- with correction of acidosis, K^+ will move back into cells, serum K^+ will fall and hypokalemia may develop.

METABOLIC ALKALOSIS

Etiopathology

- caused by loss of fixed acids,
  —vomiting or gastric drainage with loss of H^+ and Cl^-; or by
- gain of base,
  —excessive administration of $NaHCO_3$,
  —multiple blood transfusions with sodium citrate converted to bicarbonate in the body,
  —potassium depletion causing increased H^+ ion excretion in urine which increases HCO_3^- reabsorption.

- alkalosis is aggravated by an already-existing potassium deficit.
- metabolic abnormalities in blood include
  —elevated pH and
  —excess of HCO_3^-. The
- kidney compensates if it can by excreting excess HCO_3^- ions.

Complications

- hypokalemia because
  —K^+ enters cells in exchange for H^+ and
  —K^+ is excreted in urine in exchange for Na^+.
- tissue hypoxia because
  —O_2 dissociation curve is shifted to the left, which
  —limits ability of Hb to release O_2 in tissues.
- tetany because
  —amount of ionized Ca^{++} in alkaline serum is decreased.

Treatment

- replace water, K^+ and Cl^- with
  —simple Ringer's solution or
  —0.9% saline and KCl;
- do not give
  —Ringer's lactate or
  —K^+ as the bicarbonate.

RESPIRATORY ACIDOSIS

- result of hypoventilation due to
  —airway obstruction, pneumothorax, hemothorax,
  —atelectasis, pneumonia, emphysema, asthma,
  —thoracotomy, laparotomy or thoracic spine surgery,
  —central respiratory depression due to anesthetic or narcotics,
  —inadequate ventilation during anesthesia, or
  —muscular weakness as in polio.
- pH is low, arterial partial pressure of carbon dioxide ($PaCO_2$) is high, and plasma HCO_3^- is near normal.
- usually accompanied by hypoxia unless patient is breathing O_2.
- compensatory mechanisms are similar to metabolic acidosis (above).
- treatment includes
  —assisted ventilation and
  —correction of the underlying condition (see Chapter 23, "Postoperative Respiratory Insufficiency").

RESPIRATORY ALKALOSIS

- result of hyperventilation due to
  - —fear, anxiety, pain
  - —mechanical ventilator maladjusted
  - —hepatic coma
  - —brain injury or
  - —Gram-negative bacterial infection.
- arterial $PaCO_2$ is decreased with the increase of plasma pH.
- treat the cause.

Summary of IV Therapy

MAINTENANCE

- patient's normal daily requirements per kilogram are
  - —water, 40 ml
  - —glucose, 12 gm
  - —Na^+, 1.0 mEq
  - —K^+, 1.0 mEq
  - —Cl^-, 1.0 mEq
  - —HCO_3^-, 5 mEq
- these can be supplied by
  - —5% dextrose with
  - —electrolytes in low concentration (lower than 0.9% saline or Ringer's) or
  - —5% dextrose in
  - —2% saline, adding
  - —20 to 35 mEq/liter of KCl (but do not add KCl in first 3 postoperative days unless the patient has abnormal K^+ losses);
- do not use the following for more than one third of daily needs:
  - —0.9% saline or
  - —Ringer's, because these carry too much sodium, or
  - —D5W because this has no electrolytes.

REPLACEMENT

Isotonic fluid loss

- if fluid lost is similar to ECF in electrolyte content, and the patient's serum Na^+ is normal, then Ringer's lactate is a good replacement fluid, but

- stop administration of this and other replacement fluids if the patient remains oliguric, and
- give instead a fluid without K^+, to avoid hyperkalemia.

Hypotonic fluid loss

- if fluid lost was hypotonic; i.e., patient is hyperkalemic and hyper-natremic, give
  —D5W or
  —0.45% saline or half-strength Ringer's solution;
- if fluid is lost through vomiting, give
  —solutions high in Cl^- (KCl) and H^+ (NH_4) because gastric juice contains HCl.

Hypertonic fluid loss

- hyponatremia
  —restrict water intake if mild; give
  —0.9% NaCl if the loss is moderate, or give M/6 (one-sixth molar) sodium lactate if acidosis is present too; give
  —150 to 300 ml of 5% NaCl if losses are severe, or give molar sodium lactate when acidosis is present too.

DROWNING VERSUS DEHYDRATION

- the postoperative patient may suffer just as easily from
  —too much fluid (drowning!) as he may from
  —too little (dehydration);
- remember that
  —too much too soon is no better than
  —too little too late!

chapter 15

Surgical Aspects of Body Temperature

Physiology

NORMAL VALUES

- oral temperature is
  - —36.5° C to 37.5° C or
  - —97.7° F to 99.5° F;
- average is
  - —37° C or
  - —98.6° F;
- rectal temperature is about
  - —1° F higher than oral and
- axillary is
  - —1° F to 3° F lower;
- temperature normally has diurnal variation, at evening is 1° F higher than early morning temperature.
- to convert Fahrenheit to centigrade
  - —subtract 32 from degrees F,
  - —multiply by 5 and
  - —divide by 9;
- to convert C to F
  - —multiply degrees C by 9,
  - —divide by 5 and
  - —then add 32.

HEAT PRODUCTION AND HEAT LOSS

Production

- in the body at rest, heat is produced by the contents of the
  - —head (brain),
  - —thorax (lungs and heart) and
  - —abdomen (viscera);

- this central "core" is the heat generating plant;
- metabolic activity of an adult at rest produces 1,400 to 1,800 calories a day.
- heat is also gained from
  —hot food and drink, and
  —the environment when the external temperature is greater than the body's.

Loss

Skin

- when air temperature is below 36° C
- the skin, especially that of exposed areas, loses heat by
  Radiation
- 65% of heat is lost this way.
  Evaporation
  - when water evaporates it removes heat from the skin;
  - 15% to 20% of total heat loss is by water vapor passing through intact skin (insensible transpiration);
  - this is not sweat, and no salt is lost this way;
  - this is a passive method, dependent on atmospheric conditions, and not under body's control.
  - heat loss is increased by sweating;
  - sweat contains NaCl 5 to 100 mEq/liter, depending on climate;
  - hot dry climate, man acclimatizes by reducing amount of NaCl in sweat.

  Conduction and convection
  - 10%

  Amount of heat loss
  - this depends on
    —temperature of skin, which is controlled by vasomotor activity; vasodilation increases heat loss, vasoconstriction decreases it. Also depends on
    —environmental (ambient) temperature, and
    —movement of air over skin, heat being lost by conduction to adjacent air, and then carried away by convection currents or breeze.

Air and food

- inspired air is heated in the air passages and
- 5% to 10% of heat is lost by adding water vapor to expired air.

- feces and urine remove heat too.

Heat transfer

- heat is carried from the "core" (generator) to the shell (cooler) by

Convection

- blood is
  —heated in the core, then travels to the
  —shell where it loses heat to the cooler air surrounding the skin;
- this transport of heat by movement of body fluid is called
  —convection.

Conduction

- heat is moved through the solid body tissues, from core to shell, by transfer from one atom to an adjacent atom;
- to be efficient, this method requires a high temperature gradient, i.e., high central temperature, low peripheral temperature.

BODY TEMPERATURE CONTROL

- maintenance of body temperature within narrow range is necessary for normal function;
- the temperature of hypothalamus is maintained within very narrow limits, and this is probably where the control mechanism is situated;
- this control center responds to changes in temperature of blood perfusing the brain.

Thermal neutrality

- when air temperature is 29° C to 30° C.
  —heat loss equals
  —heat production of body at rest. This is
- thermal neutrality, and body temperature is
  —well controlled by small changes in vasomotor tone of skin vessels, thus
  —increasing or
  —reducing heat loss by radiation.

Ambient temperatures above neutrality

- air temperature above 30° C invokes
- sweating. The higher the temperature, the more the skin sweats. This lowers peripheral temperature by
  —evaporation.
- salt is lost as well.
- air temperature above 36° C, the body can lose heat only by

sweating because radiation no longer occurs.

Ambient temperatures below neutrality

- with air temperature of 28° C or below, maximum peripheral vasoconstriction occurs, and below 27° C shivering occurs in effort to increase heat production, but these mechanisms are
  —inefficient;
  —more heat is still lost than can be produced, and so hairless human
  —puts on clothes, lights a fire and builds a house.
- men and women can withstand warm climates much better than cold ones because our physiological mechanisms for
  —losing heat are more effective than those for
  —producing and conserving it.

Fever and Disease

DEFINITION

- fever (pyrexia) is elevation of body temperature secondary to disturbance of regulatory mechanism;
- above 40.5° C (105° F), it is called hyperpyrexia.
- fever is generally of no advantage and may be harmful except in
  —virus infections when larger amounts of
  —interferon are produced at high temperatures.

ETIOLOGY

- many diseases raise body temperature, e.g.,
  —bacterial and viral infections
  —ischemia and infarction
  —tumors, Ewing and Hodgkin's disease
  —hemorrhage, severe anemia
  —brain damage
  —acute gout and
  —acute rheumatic fever
- common factors among them are
  —tissue injury and
  —inflammation.
- the thermostat (central control in the brain that decides what the body's temperature shall be) is set at a higher level than normal, resulting in

—increased heat production by shivering, a chill, a rigor, and
—decreased heat loss until temperature of body reaches new level.
- alteration of the thermostat is probably partly due to
  —pyrogens, produced either by
  —invading organisms themselves or
  —mononuclear cells reacting with antigen, or from
  —damaged leukocytes and tissue cells.
- pyrogens of Gram-negative bacteria are lipopolysaccharide endo-toxins from the cell walls; they cause
  —fever and leukopenia,
  —alterations in coagulation of blood, and in large doses can cause
  —shock and death.
- other causes of fever include
  —dehydration and hypernatremia
  —acute endocrine stimulation, e.g., thyroid storm, and
  —loss of normal cooling mechanisms, e.g., paraplegic or quadriplegic patient loses vasomotor control and ability to sweat.

PATHOLOGY

- increase in body temperature
  —raises the metabolic rate which
  —increases energy consumption. This in turn
  —increases oxygen and fuel consumption.
- to provide more oxygen to the tissues,
  —respiratory rate and depth and
  —cardiac output are increased, which themselves increase demand for oxygen and energy.
- to provide more energy
  —muscle protein is broken down, the quantity increasing with the height of the fever. This protein catabolism is in addition to the
  —catabolic response to tissue injury.

Body Temperature during Surgery

HYPOTHERMIA

- hypothermia is defined as body temperature below 35° C (95° F)
  Grade 1
  - 37° C to 32.2° C (98.4° F to 90° F)
  - normally body reacts vigorously to increase heat production with

—violent shivering and cutaneous vasoconstriction,
—tachycardia, increase of blood pressure (BP) and
—tachypnea.

Grade 2

- 32.2° C to 24° C (90° F to 75° F)
- metabolic rate depressed with associated
  —bradycardia, hypotension and sometimes
  —ventricular fibrillation;
- respiration rate slows, with resultant
  —respiratory acidosis;
- certain neurosurgical procedures use hypothermia in this range because
  —circulation to brain can be stopped for
  —8 minutes at 30° C,
  —45 minutes at 15° C (59° F), without brain damage; but
  —convulsions may occur!

Grade 3

- less than 24° C (75° F)
- temperature regulating center stops functioning and
- heat is lost as from inanimate object.

HYPOTHERMIA DURING SURGERY

Etiology

- body temperature during and after surgery falls because
  —large skin area is exposed to the cool air of operating room,
  —skin prepared with alcohol cools as the alcohol rapidly evaporates, and
  —big incision and long operation leave large areas of tissues exposed and thus increase evaporation from these;
  —IV solutions and blood are not often warmed before infusion. Bottled blood is especially cold when just removed from the refrigerator;
  —anesthesia prevents shivering and vasoconstriction, so patient cannot increase heat production nor decrease heat loss during surgery;
- intraoperative hypothermia is most marked in
  —aged, because heat production is poor, and in
  —infants, because surface area is large in proportion to mass, the temperature-regulating system is not well developed, and total

body heat content is small;

- postoperatively, when consciousness returns, the patient starts shivering to increase heat production. If shivering is violent, it may impair ventilation and increase hypoxia.

Prevention

- prevention, as always, is easier and more effective than treatment. Use following measures:
- record patient's temperature frequently during surgery,
- maintain air temperature of operating room (OR) between 22° C and 24° C,
- warm IV fluids by allowing IV tubing to lie in bowl of warm water, and reheat the water as necessary;
- wrap parts of patient not having surgery in something that will reduce heat loss, e.g., cloth, wool.

Treatment

- rewarm the patient gently and slowly, but NEVER put any heat source, e.g., hot water bottle, on the skin because you will always burn the patient!
- excessive shivering can be prevented by promethazine (Phenergen) or meperidine (Demerol).

HYPERPYREXIA DURING ANESTHESIA

- called "malignant hyperpyrexia"
- rare complication of general anesthesia
- occurs during or at end of anesthetic
- fatal in 70% of cases

Etiology

- etiology is unknown, but is probably a
  —dominant, genetic, metabolic defect, and so is
  —hereditary.

Physiopathology

- at 41.5° C, cells begin to degenerate;
- when body temperature reaches 43°C (110° F), the metabolic rate has doubled, and the
- temperature-regulating center no longer functions when the hypothalamus becomes this hot, with the result that
  —sweating stops, and the

—patient's uncontrolled temperature rises rapidly; death follows.

Clinical features

- patient is usually young and healthy; there is an
- increase in muscle tone and pulse rate;
- body temperature rises by $1°$ C every 10 to 15 minutes, and the
- skin rapidly becomes hot;
- tissue hypoxia occurs secondary to increased oxygen consumption due to increased metabolic rate, with resultant
- severe metabolic acidosis followed by
- convulsions and death.

Treatment

- stop anesthetic immediately and
- reduce body temperature by external means using
  —water,
  —ice,
  —alcohol and
  —fans to evaporate the liquid quickly;
- cool IV solutions;
- prevent shivering because this would increase heat production, and
- combat severe acidosis with
  —hyperventilation,
  —oxygen and
  —$NaHCO_3$.

Temperature and the Metabolic Response to Tissue Injury

INFLUENCE OF INJURY ON TEMPERATURE CONTROL

- during first 12 to 36 hours after surgery or trauma
  —heat production is reduced and
  —core temperature may fall;
- when catabolic phase starts, after this initial period, temperature
  —returns to normal and
  —may go higher, due to
  —increased protein breakdown and
  —increased metabolic rate.

ENVIRONMENTAL TEMPERATURE AND THE METABOLIC RESPONSE

- when environmental temperature is in the thermoneutral zone, i.e., 28° C to 30° C (or 82° F to 86° F),
  —protein breakdown of the catabolic phase is reduced,
  —less nitrogen is lost in urine and
  —plasma protein metabolism is more normal; with
- environmental temperature between 20° C and 21° C (or 68° F to 70° F), the
  —catabolic phase is increased with
  —greater protein breakdown and nitrogen loss; the
- lower temperature benefits hospital personnel but not the postoperative patient!
- ideally, the
  —intensive care and
  —recovery rooms should be heated to a thermoneutral zone, 28° C to 30° C, an
  —intermediate care area to 25° C (77° F), and the
  —wards to 20° C.
- in the summer it may be necessary to
  —cool these areas to these temperatures, because an
  —environmental temperature too high is just as injurious as one too low.

BURN INJURY AND METABOLIC RESPONSE

- after severe burns the metabolic response is particularly marked and prolonged with increased
  —metabolic rate,
  —protein breakdown and
  —fever;
- this response can be diminished by
  —decreasing evaporation of water from burn wound with plastic wrapping, thus reducing heat loss, and by
  —increasing ambient temperature.

Postoperative Fever

BACTERIAL ORIGIN

Etiology

- postoperative fever of 38° C (or 100.4° F) is usually caused by bacterial infection of the
  —lung, e.g., atelectasis with pneumonia,
  —urinary tract often after urethral catheterization,
  —thrombophlebitis usually due either to an IV needle in the arm or venous stasis in the legs, or infection of the
  —surgical wound.

Clinical stages

Cold stage

- while the fever is rising, the patient
  —feels cold, shivers, the teeth chatter, and there is
  —peripheral vasoconstriction;
- this increases body temperature;
- pulse rate rises 18 beats/minute for every 1° C rise in temperature (10 beats for every 1° F rise).

Hot stage

- as body temperature reaches a new level set by the brain's thermostat, the
  —skin vessels relax, and the
  —patient feels warm and dry;
- heat gain equals heat loss.

Stage of sweating

- when thermostat lowers the heat level, the
  —patient sweats profusely and
  —feels very hot (the "crisis" in patients with pneumonia in preantibiotic era);
- body temperature falls to new level.

Clinical investigation

- postoperative fever must be
- investigated by careful
  —history
  —physical examination and appropriate
  —radiological and

—laboratory examinations, e.g., white cell count, blood cultures taken at fever peaks, culture of sputum, urine and wound drainage.

Treatment

- locate the source of infection,
- identify the agent and give appropriate
- local (surgical) and systemic (chemotherapeutic) treatment;
- prompt abscess drainage is mandatory;
- identification of the bacteria and antibiotic sensitivity tests must be done in all cases, and
- antibiotics selected on this basis;
- if temperature rises very high, the patient must be cooled to prevent cellular damage, especially of brain cells. Temperature can be lowered by
    —salicylates and
    —water, alcohol and fans on the skin;
- reduction of temperature also diminishes metabolic demands on
    —lungs and
    —circulatory system, reduces
    —oxygen and energy consumption, and diminishes the severity of the
    —catabolic phase.

NONBACTERIAL ORIGIN

- burns may produce fever within 2 to 4 days, before wounds become infected;
- neurosurgery near the base of the brain may disturb or inactivate the temperature control center.

chapter 16

Surgery and Nutrition

Nutrients

NUTRIENT COMPOSITION AND REQUIREMENTS

- nutritional status of patient is important because
  —preoperative malnutrition and undernutrition
  —increase postoperative morbidity and mortality, and
  —preoperative fasting followed by the
  —catabolic response to surgery may aggravate an already poor nutritional status.
- the causes of inadequate nutrition are
  —dietary ignorance (common in North America!),
  —poverty, and
  —the disease process itself, e.g., chronic osteomyelitis or tuberculosis.
- body composition of an average 70-kg man includes
  —water and minerals, 48 kg,
  —fat, 16 kg and
  —protein, 6 kg, and his average
- daily requirements of nutrients are
  —water, 1,500 to 2,500 cc,
  —calories, 1,800 to 2,100,
  —protein, 70 to 140 gm, mainly muscle,
  —carbohydrate and fat 150 gm each. After
- tissue injury these
  —requirements may be
  —doubled.

CALORIC VALUE OF NUTRIENTS

- body energy is derived from metabolism of nutrient fuel through the
  —glycolytic pathway, either
  —aerobically via the citric acid cycle or

—anaerobically through the pyruvate/lactic acid pathway (Fig. 12.2).
* fat provides
  —9 calories/gm;
* protein
  —4.25 calories/gm;
* glucose
  —4 calories/gm
* 70-kg man in resting state needs about
  —1,500 calories/day; in the
* fasting state, approximately
  —1,300 calories comes from fat breakdown and
  —200 from protein catabolism, but some of this protein can be
  —spared by giving 200 gm or more of glucose a day.

Nutritional Deficiency

ETIOLOGY

Social, economic and cultural factors

* poverty;
* economically depressed geographic area usually involves
  —low food production,
  —poor storage facilities and control, and
  —inefficient distribution.
* dietary ignorance;
* religious or cultural taboos and superstitions;
* clothing which prevents sunlight reaching the skin and thus interferes with vitamin D formation, e.g.,
  —saris, chadri and veils among certain religious sects;
* elderly people, especially living alone, often eat a poorly balanced diet.

Illness

General effects

* acute infections, such as osteomyelitis and peritonitis,
  —drain the body's resources by
  —tissue destruction and loss of
  —fluid, electrolytes and proteins in the pus;
* chronic infections and malignant disease are
  —constant and long-term drains on the patient's fuel reserves;

- fever from any cause increases the
  —basal metabolic rate by 7% for every 1° F rise in temperature;
- tissue injury causes obligatory protein catabolism, and a
  —very ill patient may lose more than 1 kg of muscle tissue per day;
- chronic hemorrhage is a protein drain because
  —1 liter of blood contains 40 gm of plasma proteins;
- prolonged bed rest causes
  —protein and mineral loss from bone (osteoporosis), and
  —muscle atrophy;
- anorexia with inadequate intake of carbohydrates causes the body to use
  —protein and
  —fat as alternative fuels.

Specific problems

- gastrointestinal (GI) tract may be a source of inadequate nutrition through
  —obstruction preventing ingestion of food,
  —inflammatory disease, e.g., Crohn's, losing large amounts of protein in exudate,
  —fistula, with loss of fluid, electrolytes and protein,
  —parasitic infestation and
  —prolonged diarrhea or vomiting from any cause;
- thyrotoxicosis increases the metabolic rate and the caloric requirements;
- liver disease impairs the ability of the liver to metabolize carbohydrates, fats and proteins;
- nephrotic syndrome is a constant protein drain through damaged kidneys;
- extensive burns lose huge quantities of
  —fluid and proteins, added
  —infection will
  —increase this loss and aggravate the catabolic response;
- iatrogenic nutritional problems may be caused by
  —long-term corticosteroid therapy provoking
  —K^+ depletion,
  —Na^+ retention and
  —protein catabolism with negative N_2 balance; or by

—resection of a long intestinal segment with resultant malabsorption.

PROTEIN METABOLISM

Protein physiology

- normal daily protein turnover in a 70-kg man is
  —140 gm of wet muscle tissue, or
  —28 gm of proteins, or
  —4 gm of nitrogen (1 gm of nitrogen is equivalent to 7 gm of protein or 35 gm of muscle).
- there are no body stores of spare protein (unlike fat);
- all proteins in the body are in active use, e.g., the
  —contractile elements of muscle, actin and myosin, contain the majority of the body's proteins;
  —plasma proteins, maintaining osmotic pressure of plasma and thus blood volume, immunological proteins and hemoglobin,
  —coagulation factors, e.g., fibrinogen and prothrombin,
  —enzymes and cell walls.

Protein catabolism and deficiency

- nutritional deficiency is a lack of
  —several food substances, not just one;
- proteins and calories are the most important factors in undernutrition and malnutrition;
- protein catabolism is increased when
  —other caloric sources such as carbohydrates are missing from the diet.

Skeletal muscle

- chief source of protein lost in fasting and in the catabolic phase after tissue injury.

Plasma proteins

- 70-kg man has 245 gm of plasma proteins;
- during protein catabolism
  —1 gm of plasma protein is lost for every
  —30 gm of total body protein lost;
- similarly during anabolism
  —1 gm of plasma protein is replaced for every
  —30 gm of body protein replaced. Loss of
- albumin is more important than loss of other plasma proteins because

—albumin is responsible for 85% of the total plasma osmotic pressure and therefore
—regulates the circulating blood volume;
- loss of albumin from plasma (hypoalbuminemia) to a level of less than 3 gm/100 ml causes
—increased susceptibility to hypovolemic shock, and by itself may cause
—hypovolemia.
- immune globulins may be decreased, thus reducing resistance to infection (Fig. 16.1).

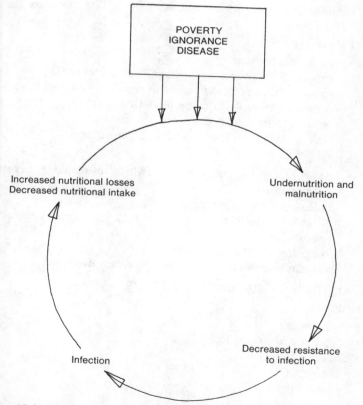

Figure 16.1. Vicious circle of nutritional deficiency and infection. Circle is driven by poverty, ignorance and disease.

Hematopoiesis

- bone marrow and lymphoid tissue activity are depressed causing
  - anemia, leukopenia and
  - increased susceptibility to infection.

Skin healing

- healing of a skin wound may be impaired if other detrimental factors are present as well, e.g.,
  - vitamin deficiency,
  - wound infection or
  - errors in technique;
- decubitus ulcers occur more often and heal more slowly; the
- catabolic phase will continue as long as large wounds remain open.

Pulmonary function

- diminished because
  - respiratory muscles are weakened as protein catabolism continues, with decreased ability to ventilate and cough, and
  - low plasma proteins cause interstitial pulmonary edema and increased bronchial secretions;
- death in starvation is usually due to pneumonia.

Liver

- liver contains 350 gm of protein, which influences many of its vital functions;
- inadequate protein intake may cause
  - decreased resistance of the liver to toxic and fatty metamorphosis, with
  - impairment of function; the
- liver can be protected by avoiding protein depletion.

EVALUATION OF NUTRITIONAL STATUS

History

- socioeconomic status,
- age, diet and weight loss;
- does the patient have
  - anorexia
  - vomiting
  - diarrhea, and
  - for how long?

Physical examination
- most inadequate diets are a mixture of
  —protein,
  —carbohydrate and
  —vitamin deficiencies, and the
- early signs are subtle and difficult to detect.
- protein deficiency almost always associated with inadequate caloric intake; signs may include
  —dry, fine, brittle hair; low weight;
  —anemia; hypoalbuminemia with peripheral edema;
  —muscle atrophy; stunted growth and development in children;
- kwashiorkor and marasmus are advanced stages of mixed protein and calorie deficiency.
- carbohydrate deficiency manifested by
  —loose skin with no subcutaneous fat, edema;
  —skin-fold thickness reduced.
- vitamin deficiencies cause
  —scurvy (vitamin C),
  —beriberi (thiamin),
  —keratomalacia (vitamin A),
  —rickets and osteomalacia (vitamin D).
- mineral deficiency includes
  —hypochromic anemia due to lack of iron, and
  —goiter due to inadequate iodine intake.

Laboratory examinations

Hematology

Hemoglobin and hematocrit
- remember that
  —people who live at 10,000 feet should have more red blood cells, more hemoglobin and higher hematocrit than
  —people who live at sea level, and
  —these measurements are changed by dehydration, overhydration and recent blood loss and may then mislead you.

Serum proteins
- measure these in patients with suspected undernutrition;
- these levels are altered by blood loss and changes in hydration;
- minimum levels are
  —total protein, 5.5 gm/100 ml

—albumin, 2.5 gm/100 ml.

Urinalysis

- look for excessive
  —protein,
  —sugar or
  —electrolyte losses.

Liver function

- liver function studies will show liver disease which may interfere
  with metabolism.

PREVENTION AND TREATMENT

- ideally, patients should be well-nourished before surgery, and any
  nutritional deficit should be corrected, but this is not always possible.
- however, it is possible, while the patient is in the hospital, to
  —prevent further nutrient loss and
  —correct some of the patient's deficiency.

Prevention

- as long as a nutrient drain remains open, e.g., a
  —fistula drains GI juice,
  —infected bone drains pus or
  —an area of skin loss remains uncovered, the patient will continue
  to
  —lose protein, fluid and electrolytes.
- plug the drain by treating the cause!
- intraoperative nutrient losses can be reduced by
  —limiting the extent of surgery whenever possible,
  —operating fast (but not too fast, surgery is not a race!), and
  keeping
  —blood and fluid loss to a minimum.
- postoperatively, patient will require a
  —high protein
  —high calorie diet with
  —vitamin and
  —mineral supplements.

Treatment

- patient for elective surgery should have his nutritional deficit
  rectified;

- replacing what is missing by oral
  —high protein and calorie diet with
  —supplements, or by
- tube feeding for patients unable to take food by mouth;
- treat anemia by
  —oral iron salts,
  —whole blood or
  —packed red cells, depending upon circumstances;
- patients should be rehydrated
  —before surgery, and adequately hydrated
  —during and
  —after surgery.

Parenteral hyperalimentation

Nutrient solution

- this recently developed technique can
  —provide the patient with two to three times his daily nutritional requirements so that
  —deficiencies can be met and the catabolic phase of the metabolic response to tissue injury can be converted to the
  —anabolic phase with a positive nitrogen balance.
- nutrient solution is hypertonic, several times more concentrated than blood, and is administered directly into the
  —superior vena cava, using strict aseptic technique. The solution usually contains
  —dextrose,
  —protein hydrolysates and amino acids,
  —sodium, potassium and
  —1,000 calories/liter.
- to this basic solution can be added intermittently, according to the substance, more
  —sodium and potassium as well as
  —magnesium, calcium, iron,
  —phosphate, bicarbonate, chloride, lactate and
  —vitamins A, C, D, and K and certain essential B vitamins. The
- contents of the solution can be tailored according to the
  —particular needs of the patient, his
  —illness and concurrent disorders.

Clinical features

- hyperalimentation therapy is indicated for patients suffering from
  - gastrointestinal disorders, such as fistulae or colitis, with excessive loss of fluid and nutrients,
  - major burns, and after
  - extensive intestinal resection.
- regular evaluation of the patient's status must include measurements of
  - fluid intake and output and urine sugar two to four times a day,
  - body weight daily,
  - serum electrolytes, blood sugar and BUN daily at first, then three times a week when stable,
  - blood count, plasma proteins and serum Ca^{++}, $P^{=}$ and Mg^{++} weekly, and
  - renal and hepatic function tests once or twice a month.
- complications include
  - misplacement of the catheter or its needle,
  - infection,
  - air embolism,
  - thrombosis in the catheter (rarely of the vein),
  - hyperglycemia and hyperosmolar coma.
- parenteral hyperalimentation may be continued for many months when necessary, with excellent results.

chapter 17

Inflammation and Healing

Inflammatory Response

ETIOLOGY

- stimulus which evokes an inflammatory response may be
  —mechanical (laceration)
  —chemical (acid)
  —ionizing radiation (x-rays)
  —thermic (heat or cold)
  —ischemic (infarct)
  —living organisms (bacteria)
  —immunological.
- the basic vascular and cellular response is always the same regardless of the causative mechanism. The object is to
- localize the reaction,
- kill invading organisms, and
- remove
  —foreign material and
  —tissue debris in preparation for the
- repair process.

PATHOPHYSIOLOGY

- inflammatory reaction is usually
- beneficial, e.g., bacterial infection, but it may be
- harmful, e.g., autoimmune reaction.

Vascular phase

Vasodilatation

- initial capillary constriction is followed by release of chemical mediators, e.g., histamine, and activation of
- axon reflexes, which cause

- vasodilatation (5 to 10 minutes later) of all local
  —small vessels, with opening of
  —precapillary sphincters. The result is
- increased blood flow with an
- increase in the hydrostatic pressure of blood at the arterial end of the capillary bed and consequent
- increased exudation of serum into interstitial space (Starling's law) (Fig. 17.1). With this loss of fluid, blood becomes
- more viscous, and flow in the small vessels then slows down.

Margination of leukocytes

- blood flow through the capillary bed slows;
- red blood cells form rouleaux and occupy the center of the blood stream;
- white blood cells (WBCs) and platelets drift to the periphery of the stream;

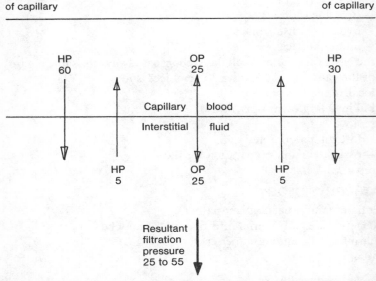

Figure 17.1. Altered balance of hydrostatic (*HP*) and osmotic (*OP*) pressures between the capillary blood and interstitial fluid in acute inflammation. Compare with Figure 13.1. Figures are approximate, with the hydrostatic pressures in particular varying with the circumstances. Pressures are in mm Hg.

- endothelial cells of the capillary and venule walls become "sticky," perhaps due to a coating of gelatinous substance, and the
- white cells adhere to these endothelial cells. This is margination.

Exudative phase

Fluid and protein exudate
- is due to
  —increased hydrostatic pressure in the capillaries and venules, forcing fluid out;
  —leak of plasma proteins through capillary and lymphatic walls and breakdown in tissue of large protein molecules into smaller ones, thus increasing the osmotic pressure of interstitial fluid and favoring the movement of more fluid into interstitial space; and
  —change in ground substance which becomes more fluid, allowing the exudate to spread more easily and thus preventing a rise in hydrostatic tension of tissue fluid.
- increased capillary and lymphatic permeability to plasma proteins may be due to an
  —increase in size of the intercellular spaces in the vessel walls due to the action of histamine; the cells become more spherical, and gaps appear at the corners.
- this protein leak brings
  —complement,
  —immunoglobulins,
  —opsonins and
  —fibrin to the injured area. The
- complement system is an enzyme cascade. It
  —increases vascular permeability,
  —induces migration of leukocytes,
  —causes lysis of bacteria and dead tissue and
  —prepares material for phagocytosis.
- fibrin
  —slows physical progress of the invading organisms,
  —augments phagocytosis by enabling white cells to trap organisms in the fibrin net,
  —plugs lymphatics and prevents lymphatic drainage, thus localizing inflammation, and provides a

—framework for eventual tissue repair by fibroblasts.

Cellular exudate

Diapedesis

- white cells, sticking to capillary walls, squeeze out of the capillaries by ameboid action, levering a space between endothelial cells with a pseudopod. This is diapedesis.
- polymorphonuclear neutrophils (PMNs) are the first to migrate, followed by
- monocytes, which become macrophages in the interstitial tissue;
- PMNs predominate at first but die within a few days, leaving mainly monocytes.

Chemotactic phenomenon

- migration of WBCs may be controlled by chemical factors,
  —bacterial substances,
  —leukotaxine (polypeptide mixture),
  —complement, which liberates two active substances, C3a and C5a; and
  —antigen-antibody complex in the presence of activated complement.

Phagocytosis

- WBCs engulf foreign matter and tissue debris in the presence of
  —nonspecific opsonins which require the presence of complement, or
  —immune opsonins;
- opsonins attach themselves to surface antigens of virulent bacteria and make the material "palatable" to the WBCs (a sort of salad dressing!);
- engulfed organisms in the PMN leukocyte are
  —enclosed in phagosomes and
  —killed, probably by chlorine or iodine which may be formed by the interaction of hydrogen peroxide and another substance in the presence of myeloperoxidase. Other bactericidal agents may also be present; then the dead orgnisms are
  —broken down and dissolved by lysosomal enzymes.
- PMNs are active early in the response, and when they die, undigested particles are released into interstitial space and are

phagocytosed by
- mononuclear cells which remain in the area much longer.

Chemical mediators
- exact mechanism is unknown, but the following substances are probably important:
- *histamine* may be liberated from mast cells under the influence of platelets and PMNs and is active in the very early phase of the inflammatory response;
- *prekallikrein* and other *similar enzymes* present in blood can liberate kinins in the plasma through a cascade system;
- *kinins*: Bradykinin is liberated from plasma globulin by kallikrein and is many times more powerful than histamine as a vasodilator.
- *plasmin*, from the plasma protein plasminogen, can
  —liberate kinin from kininogen,
  —activate prekallikrein and
  —release C3a from complement;
- *complement* and its cleavage products;
- *prostaglandins*, a group of fatty acids, may mediate a later phase of inflammation, with substances released from PMN lysosomes.

SEQUELAE
- acute inflammation may terminate in one of the following ways:

Resolution
- local infiltration with no tissue destruction;
- all debris removed by macrophages and
- tissue returns to normal.

Fibrosis
- little or no tissue loss;
- invasive agent removed, but
- removal of exudate is slow, and the fibrin network is invaded by granulation tissue which in turn is replaced by
- fibrous tissue, fibrosis.

Suppuration
- large quantity of dead cells and debris, liquefied by proteolytic enzymes released by dead PMNs. This is
- pus and contains
  —live and dead WBCs, mainly PMNs,

—live and dead organisms (when infection is present),

—edema,

—fibrin and

—tissue debris. When pus is

- trapped under pressure in an abscess cavity surrounded by
  —acutely inflamed tissue forming the
  —pyogenic membrane, the pus
- spreads along the line of least resistance and bursts into free space (unless surgically drained first). If
- pus is not under pressure, water is gradually absorbed from the pus, and the pus becomes thick and may calcify.
- when inflammatory process involves an epithelial surface, then an
- ulcer forms with a floor of dead tissue and exudate; this sloughs and the ulcer slowly heals by
- repair and regeneration.

Chronic inflammation

Etiology

- may be caused by anything that provokes an acute inflammatory response if the causative agent is not soon removed.
- agents which usually cause chronic inflammation are
  —insoluble particles, e.g., talc, asbestos,
  —mycobacteria, e.g., tuberculosis,
  —fungi, e.g., actinomycosis,
  —collagen diseases and
  —hypersensitivity reactions, e.g., contact dermatitis.

Pathophysiology

- inflammatory reaction is called chronic when
  —destruction,
  —inflammation and
  —tissue healing occur simultaneously.

  Acute inflammation
  - exudate and the presence of polymorphs are marked in chronic suppurative disease, e.g., chronic osteomyelitis and actinomycosis;
  - exudate may be rich in proteins with resultant hypoproteinemia.

Repair

- macrophages are prominent in this phase, especially marked
  —in lepromatous leprosy;
- epithelioid cells are macrophages which have either
  —digested or extruded phagocytosed material, or
  —have not been active in phagocytosis; epithelioid cells
  —cannot phagocytose but can absorb material by
  —pinocytosis. They are
  —polygonal, large and ill defined, with pale eosinophilic cytoplasm, and are typical of
  —tuberculoid granulomata.
- giant cells form when
  —macrophages meet insoluble material, e.g., sequestra, uric acid crystals, silk and catgut, and in response to organisms which cause chronic inflammation, e.g.,
  —tuberculosis, where nuclei are found in semicircle at one end of the giant cell (Langhan's giant cell).

Healing

- granulation tissue contains
  —new blood vessels and lymphatics,
  —fibroblasts making collagen (a salient feature of chronic inflammation),
  —lymphocytes and
  —plasma cells which are involved with immunoglobulin production.

Systemic effects

- localized foreign body reactions have no systemic effects whereas some
- chronic infective diseases do, e.g., tuberculosis (TB) and actinomycosis. Systemic effects may include
  —hyperplasia of the reticuloendothelial system,
  —antibody production (serological type with kala azar, cell-bound type with TB, sometimes causing amyloid disease),
  —anemia, hypoalbuminemia and raised erythrocyte sedimentation rate (ESR), and
  —"toxemia," with its symptom complex of malaise, pyrexia, headache and loss of appetite, weight and libido.

Healing in Skin

STRUCTURE

Epidermis

- germinal layer is the deepest, lying on the basement membrane, and produces new epithelial cells by mitosis;
- malpighian layer of living epithelial cells is immediately above the germinal layer;
- keratinized layer of dead cells is the most superficial, derived from maturation and keratinization of underlying epithelial cells. The epidermis
- allows passage, from the dermis to the surface, of hair follicles, and ducts of sweat and sebaceous glands.

Dermis

- fat layer beneath basement membrane allows passage of
  —blood vessels,
  —lymphatics and
  —nerves on their way to the epidermis and
- contains
  —hair follicles
  —sweat and
  —sebaceous glands
- subcutaneous tissue lies beneath the dermis.

SUPERFICIAL ABRASION

- usually involves only the epidermis;
- wound fills with inflammatory exudate, debris and blood clot (scab);
- this seals the wound and anchors the edges;
- live epithelial cells at the margins of the wound migrate laterally into the clot, beneath surface exudate and necrotic tissue;
- these cells are replaced by mitosis of adjacent cells. Direction of migration is determined by
  —orientation of the substrate (contact guidance) and
  —contact with adjacent epithelial cells (contact inhibition), sending the cell in a new direction until it touches similar cells all around its periphery.
- when a new epithelial layer covers the wound, cells proliferate to rebuild the
  —full thickness of the epithelium; the

—scab falls off and
—surface cells keratinize. A
- scar eventually is barely visible.

LACERATION

- laceration or surgical incision divides epidermis, dermis and subcutaneous tissue;
- wound healing occurs by five phases which usually overlap in time and space:

Inflammation

- this is the initial response and includes
  —fluid and
  —cellular exudate rich in protein, fibrin, polymorphonuclear leukocytes and monocytes.

Epithelialization

- may start during the preceding phase or at the beginning of the fibroplastic phase;
- epithelial cells migrate from wound edges beneath the scab, directed by contact guidance and inhibition;
- remaining hair follicles and gland ducts may provide other sources of epithelial cells;
- cells may completely cover a small open wound but may
- fail to reach the central area of a large wound, and a chronic ulcer may result unless the wound is skin-grafted.

Fibroplasia

- fibroplastic phase starts near the end of the inflammatory phase when most debris is already removed by macrophages.

Capillaries

- solid buds appear on adjacent vessels, grow into the wound, become
  —canalized, and form
  —arcades by anastomosing with other vessels. Some
- differentiate to become
  —arterioles or
  —venules.

Fibroblasts

- evolve from nearby undifferentiated mesenchymal cells, especially those associated with blood vessel adventitia, and

- migrate into the wound along strands of the fibrin network. This network is necessary because
  — fibroblasts (and epithelial cells) move by forming
  — adhesive contacts with the substratum,
  — not by ameboid cytoplasmic flow (white blood cells do this). However,
- too much fibrin is a barrier to fibroblast penetration; so
  — endothelial cells of advancing capillary buds secrete
  — plasminogen activator which releases
  — plasmin; this
  — removes the fibrin barrier.
- fibroblasts proliferate in the wound, then manufacture
- collagen. The
- replacement of inflammatory exudate, debris and blood clot is called
- organization, and the newly formed tissue is
- granulation tissue. When visible, as in an open wound, this is
- red, granular (hence the name),
- friable and
- bleeds easily.
- if an open wound is allowed to heal by itself (by secondary intention), the space
  — fills up from the bottom with granulation tissue, then
- epithelializes over the top, beneath the superficial layer of exudate and debris.

Collagen synthesis

- collagen is the body's structural protein and forms
  — one third of total protein content.
- in the fibroblast,
  — messenger RNA formed from DNA template leaves the nucleus and
  — enters the cytoplasm, attaches to
  — ribosomes along the endoplasmic reticulum and directs formation of an
  — amino acid sequence. This becomes a
  — polypeptide chain which leaves the ribosome and enters
  — cisternae (Golgi apparatus) of the endoplasmic reticulum;
  — energy for protein synthesis comes from mitochondria.

- three polypeptide chains twist around each other, attached to each other by
  —hydrogen bonds, later by stronger
  —chemical bonds formed by alteration of certain amino acids. This spiral helix then twists on itself to form a
- superhelix. This is
- tropocollagen and is
- transported outside the cell. Tropocollagen units are
  —15 Å wide and 3,000 Å long. The
- ground substance then seems to influence the combination of tropocollagen units into mature collagen fibers.
- collagen contains two unique acids,
  —hydroxyproline and
  —hydroxylysine;
- periodic banding of collagen fibers is related to overlap of tropocollagen units as they form mature fibers. The
- amount of ground substance, consisting of
  —water,
  —ions, and
  —protein polysaccharide polymers,
  —decreases as collagen increases, and tissue becomes much less vascular; the
- tensile strength of the wound increases with collagen synthesis; when
- collagen formation is sufficient, the number of fibroblasts in the wound diminishes; this marks the
- end of the fibroplastic phase.

Wound contraction
- fourth phase.
- in an open wound, about 5 days after injury, wound edges start to approach each other, and the wound gradually contracts;
- this phenomenon is probably due to the presence in the wound of myofibroblasts which carry contractile protein in their cytoplasm. A
- small wound may close completely if the adjacent skin is mobile or very little if the skin is fixed, e.g., over the anterior surface of the tibia.
- resultant contracture may be

—advantageous, e.g., over the thigh, or it may cause

—flexion contracture across a joint, e.g., neck, elbow, and may later require

—excision and a full-thickness skin graft.

Scar maturation

- the final phase.
- initially, collagen fibers have weak hydrogen bond links and are arranged in the wound at random; with time,
- new intramolecular and intermolecular covalent bonds and cross-links are made, and collagen fibers are
- reorientated, partly under the influence of stress lines in the wound, with the result that the
- tensile strength of the scar tissue increases. The
- quantity of collagen also changes by an altered relationship between
  —production by remaining fibroblasts and
  —resorption by enzyme collagenase.

FACTORS DELAYING WOUND HEALING

Local

- poor blood supply
- low tissue oxygen tension
- infection
- movement of wound edges
- ionizing irradiation which decreases vascularity and impairs granulation tissue formation and wound contraction
- irritant substances
- too frequent dressing changes by enthusiastic doctors; the fragile regenerating epithelium adheres to the dressings!
- adhesion of wound edges to bone prevents wound contraction.

General

- protein deficiency diminishes formation of granulation tissue and collagen;
- vitamin C (ascorbic acid) deficiency prevents collagen formation in wounds;
- excess steroid therapy inhibits inflammatory response and slows granulation tissue and collagen formation;
- vitamin A deficiency impairs collagen remodelling.

Fracture Healing

INFLAMMATORY REACTION

- fractured bone surfaces and damaged soft tissues bleed, and resultant
- hematoma fills the space around the fracture;
- inflammatory exudate, composed of
  —plasma and
  —white cells, invades the hematoma, and removal of debris begins;
- osteocytes in bone adjacent to the fracture die for lack of nourishment caused by rupture of haversian vessels.

CALLUS FORMATION

- callus around the outside of a fracture is called external callus, and that between bone ends and the medullary canals is called the internal (medullary) callus, though both are in continuity;
- phases of bone repair and remodelling are not clear-cut, and different phases may occur simultaneously at different sites.

  External callus

  - formed in two phases:

    Primary callus response

    - proliferation of fibroblastic and osteogenic cells starts within a few hours of fracture;
    - osteoblasts come from
      —osteoprogenitor cells of inner (cambium) layer of periosteum and
      —perhaps from osteogenic marrow cells too.
    - osteoblasts produce a
      —ground substance and construct
      —trabeculae of bone collagen along new capillaries. This is
      —osteoid tissue, the
      —organic matrix of bone, and is
      —firmly anchored to distal live ends of fracture fragments and is
      —nourished by the ingrowth of new vessels from adjacent soft tissues. If the
    - periosteal sleeve is intact, or only partially torn, primary callus bridges the gap. But if the
    - periosteum is completely torn, then

- primary callus forms around the
  —distal ends of living bone fragments, thus creating
  —two bone collars separated by a gap. This gap is closed by bridging callus.

Bridging callus response

- multipotent fibroblasts are recruited from surrounding soft tissues, and
- induced to form osteoblasts. These
- join the two collars of primary callus by diffuse osteogenic activity across the gap.
- cartilage may be formed first if
- oxygen tension is low; then when blood supply improves, bone is formed by enchondral ossification.
- initial primary and briding callus is called
  —provisional callus, consists of
  —immature, woven bone with
  —trabeculae arranged at
  —random. Callus is relatively
  —weak.
  —osteoblasts trapped in the callus become osteocytes.
  —necrotic bone ends play little or no part in callus formation.

Control of callus formation

Movement

- primary callus response is probably not controlled by mechanical factors, but a certain amount of
- movement of bone ends at the fracture site stimulates rapid formation of bridging external callus. Once formed, the
- bone bridge immobilizes the fracture. When rigid internal fixation prevents movement, little or no external callus forms. The
- purpose of external callus formation is probably to immobilize the fracture (this callus is mechanically well placed to do this).
- bridging callus response is
  —finite; if
  —movement continues indefinitely,
  —bridging fails, and the response stops.
- external bridging callus formation is probably controlled by

- a bioelectrical feedback mechanism related to movement of bone fragments.

Fragment relationship

- when fragments are
  —widely separated, or
  —soft tissue is interposed,
- bridging callus response is
  —hindered and may
  —fail.

Humoral factors

- primary callus may release chemical substances which
- trigger the bridging callus response by
- osteogenic induction.

Mineralization of callus

- this occurs within hours of formation of osteoid tissue;
- crystals of hydroxyapatite
  —$Ca_{10}(PO_4)_6(OH)_2$ are deposited on
- seeding sites in the osteoid collagen and are
- oriented in the long axis of collagen fibers.
- crystals are 400 Å to 2,000 Å long and wide, and 25 Å to 50 Å thick.

Medullary callus

- forms in a manner similar to the formation of external callus except that
  —cells originate mainly from osteogenic cells in the marrow, the
  —process is slower,
  —continues longer, and is
  —less deterred by immobilization and soft-tissue interposition.
    Formation probably is
- controlled by
  —electrical and
  —biochemical factors.

Primary bone union

- occurs when fragments are in
  —direct contact and
  —rigidly immobilized, as after compression plating.
- new haversian systems are drilled from the live bone of one

fragment to the other, through the dead ends of the fractured bone, thus
—nailing the fracture surfaces together.

- small gaps between the fracture surfaces on the side opposite the compression plate are filled with callus which then conducts haversian systems across the fracture.

- this process is similar to the physiological process of normal bone turnover and haversian system renewal which occurs continuously in the healthy skeleton.

- primary bone union is
  —very slow, particularly in the presence of extensive bone necrosis;
  —stability depends on the implant for a long time, and
  —normal strength is probably not restored as long as the implant remains.

Remodelling

- continues over ensuing months;
- provisional callus gradually is resorbed by osteoclasts and rebuilt simultaneously into
  —mature bone with haversian systems, the
  —collagen fibers being reoriented under the influence of stress.
- new haversian canals are drilled through dead cortical bone and callus by
  —osteoblastic cone or "cutter-head," and an
  —artery grows down the new canal.
- lamellae of compact bone are formed in concentric circles around the haversian canal to form an
- osteon.
- new osteons cannot penetrate fibrous tissue.
- cancellous bone has no osteons or haversian systems; because blood supply is plentiful, bone replacement occurs on the surface of trabeculae.
- useful dead bone is incorporated into the new callus, ultimately converted to living bone by haversian penetration;
- excess dead bone and callus not serving a useful purpose are resorbed, following Wolff's law (stress dictates structure).
- most of external callus is removed as remaining callus is rebuilt and strengthened; the
- medullary canal appears across the fracture site by central resorption of callus. A

- pattern of periosteal and intramedullary blood vessels is gradually reestablished.

Factors affecting fracture union

Local

- epiphyseal separation heals faster than
  —metaphyseal fracture which heals faster than
  —shaft fracture.
- healing is slower when the fracture is
  —open, by injury or by surgeon, because soft-tissue and vascular damage is greater;
  —comminuted, as this implies greater bone and soft-tissue damage;
  —displaced with gap between fragments and especially with interposition of soft tissue;
  —transverse rather than oblique or spiral, because the surface area available for healing is small;
  —segmental, because intramedullary blood supply is interrupted;
  —mobile, because mobility disrupts young vessels and callus;
  —through bone where fracture interrupts blood supply, e.g., neck of femur, scaphoid;
  —in bone where blood supply is relatively poor, e.g., distal third of tibia which has no muscle attachments; or in
  —pathological bone with tumor, especially if malignant.

General

- time for a given fracture to heal
  —increases from birth to the end of growth, then
  —remains constant to old age;
- vitamin C is necessary for protein matrix construction,
- vitamin D, for mineralization, and
- vitamin A, for remodelling;
- hypoproteinemia delays fracture healing.

BONE GRAFTING

Types of graft

Cortical

- hard and strong,
- relatively avascular and acellular,
- poorly osteogenic but

- good for fixation when combined with a plate;
- tibia and fibula are usual sources.

Cancellous

- spongy and weak,
- very vascular and cellular,
- good for osteogenesis but
- poor for internal fixation;
- iliac crest, anterior or posterior third, is usual source.

Autograft (autogenous)

- bone from same individual;
- the best graft possible.

Isograft (isologous)

- bone from genetically identical individual, e.g., identical twin, with identical histocompatibility antigens.

Allograft (homogenous or homograft)

- from same species, but genetically dissimilar;
- useful in small children, old osteoporotic patients and to fill large cavities, where sufficient autogenous bone is not available.

Xenograft (heterologous or heterograft)

- from different species.

How bone graft works

Bone formation by graft cells

- only cells in cancellous graft can form bone directly; cells in cortical graft do not.
- only the superficial cells of the cancellous graft survive;
- cells must be compatible (autograft or isograft);
- cells must be alive (transfer from donor to host site with minimum delay);
- cells must have immediate access to nutrients in host site, so graft should not be thicker than 5 mm and should be placed in a well-vascularized area in intimate contact with host bone.

Bone induction

- cancellous and cortical bone grafts can induce host bone cells to form bone;
- this may be due to proteins (humoral factors) released by the graft.

Replacement of trabeculae

- trabeculae and osteocytes of all grafted cancellous and cortical bone die;
- osteoclasts resorb one surface of trabecula while osteoblasts deposit new bone on the other surface;
- all trabeculae are thus entirely replaced, faster in cancellous (narrow trabeculae) then cortical bone (wide trabeculae).

Immunological response

Autografts and isografts

- no immunological response by host because proteins in the graft are recognized as "self" and are therefore compatible.

Allograft

- fresh allograft evokes strong immunological response;
- after two weeks, inflammatory reaction kills the graft cells and destroys any tissue that they have made,
  —the "rejection phenomenon";
- to be accepted, this graft must be modified, for example by
  —freezing or
  —freeze drying (freezing and then drying the bone graft in a vacuum).

Peripheral Nerve Healing

WALLERIAN DEGENERATION

- when a peripheral nerve is cut, the
- axons and myelin sheaths fragment and degenerate proximally for only a few millimeters but
- distally, the whole length of axon and myelin sheath degenerates (wallerian degeneration);
- macrophages enter the neural tube (endoneurium consisting of collagen and fibroblasts), and together with Schwann cells, they remove debris;
- cell body, situated
  —in anterior horn for motor nerve,
  —on posterior root for sensory nerve,
- swells, and its
- nissl granules, which are

　—endoplasmic reticulum and
　—ribosomes,
- disappear! This is
- chromatolysis and is evidence of
- dysfunction in protein synthesis.

AXONAL REGENERATION

- cell body swells over several weeks, and intracellular metabolic activity increases to prepare for regeneration of axon;
- Schwann cells in the distal end of the neural tube
　—proliferate, and if the two cut ends of the neural tube are apposed, the Schwann cells
　—move across the gap to unite the two ends of the tube and
　—form columns in the distal part of the tube to guide regenerating axon sprouts;
- endoneurium proliferates and reconstitutes the neural tube.
- after a few days, axon in the proximal stump puts out several thin sprouts; one may find its way into the distal tube and grows to the end organ at a speed of about 1 mm a day;
- proteins for new axoplasm are
　—produced in the cell body and
　—transported in vacuoles down the regenerating axon;
- Schwann cells roll themselves around new axon and coat it with myelin sheath.
- if axon reaches the
　—correct end organ, e.g., sensory axon and sensory receptor,
　—function is restored in that axon; but if axon reaches an
　—inappropriate end organ, then
　—function is lost; thus
- prognosis is better for a
　—pure motor or sensory nerve than for a mixed nerve, and for damaged axons with the
　—nerve trunk intact (axonotmesis) than for those with the nerve trunk cut (neurotmesis).
- axon may fail to reach the distal tube if the
　—gap between cut ends is too large,
　—local inflammatory and fibroplastic reaction fills the gap with scar tissue,
　—proliferation of Schwann cells is so enthusiastic that they block the distal tube, or

—regenerating epineurium hypertrophies and constricts the fascicles, thus restricting axonal growth. So
- successful neural regeneration requires
- optimum local conditions and thus depends upon
- surgical excellence.

Tendon, Ligament and Muscle Healing

TENDONS

- gap between ruptured tendon ends fills with hematoma; this is
- invaded by fibroblasts and capillaries from surrounding soft tissue as part of the normal inflammatory response;
- fibroblasts deposit collagen fibers in the long axis of the tendon, the fibers at each end uniting with those in the cut ends of the tendon;
- tensile strength of the tendon is thus reestablished.
- some adhesions form between the repair site and surrounding soft tissues. These adhesions interfere with the gliding mechanism and may impair function;
- repaired tendon gradually becomes
  —more fibrous and
  —less vascular and cellular and
- remodels to a limited extent to remove adhesions and create a gliding surface;
- collagen fibers become indistinguishable from normal tendon fibers.
- restoration of
  —continuity and
  —functions depends on
  —good surgical technique with close and accurate apposition of tendon ends because
- regeneration across a large gap is unusual, especially in flexor tendons.

LIGAMENTS

- ligaments heal in a similar manner with the addition that fibroblasts in the ligament also contribute to collagen formation and repair whereas tendon fibrocytes (tenocytes) do not.

MUSCLES

- striated, voluntary muscle heals mainly by fibrosis following normal inflammatory response;

- limited regeneration of myofibrils and production of new myocytes may occur if parts of muscle fibers remain. If
- injured muscle surfaces are
  —apposed, continuity of muscle is restored, and
  —function is generally good. But if a
- large gap fills with fibrous tissue, there is
  —no regeneration of muscle fibers across the scar tissue barrier and
  —function is impaired.

chapter 18
Cardiopulmonary Arrest

Etiopathology

- cardiopulmonary arrest is the
  —unexpected cessation of effective ventilation and circulation; the arrest may be
  —primarily cardiac, with secondary respiratory cessation after about 60 seconds,
  —or vice versa.

PRIMARY CARDIAC ARREST

- may be due to
- sudden coronary occlusion;
- reduced cardiac output secondary to
  —shock or
  —cardiac tamponade;
- hyperkalemia or acidosis from any cause;
- direct cardiac stimulation by
  —operative manipulation or
  —electrocution;
- hypothermia or hyperthermia, or
- vasovagal stimulation, e.g., tracheal suctioning in a quadriplegic.
- hypoxia from any cause makes the heart more susceptible to arrest.

PRIMARY RESPIRATORY ARREST

- may be due to
- airway obstruction from any cause;
- ventilatory failure due to
  —poliomyelitis, muscular dystrophy or
  —overdosage of paralytic drugs;

- central respiratory depression due to
  —head injury,
  —anesthesia or overdosage of narcotic drugs.

PATHOLOGY

Primary cardiac arrest

- cardiac function is inadequate when the heart is in
  —ventricular fibrillation (common after myocardial infarction) or
  —mechanical asystole.
- when circulation ceases
  —pupils start to dilate at 30 to 45 seconds and
  —respiratory drive is lost at 60 seconds due to central respiratory depression;
- cerebral cellular damage is irreversible after 4 to 6 minutes of anoxia.

Primary respiratory arrest

- circulation may continue for several minutes after the respiratory arrest, and
  —oxygen extraction by the tissues (particularly the brain) may be sufficient to sustain life during those few minutes;
- thus, irreversible brain damage may not occur for 8 to 10 minutes after cessation of ventilation.

Death

- this is always by asphyxiation, i.e., anoxia at the cellular level, no matter whether the arrest was primarily cardiac or respiratory and regardless of the cause.

Diagnosis

PRIMARY CARDIAC ARREST

During surgery

Anesthetist

- requires good light at the head of the table;
- monitors patient's condition throughout anesthetic by
- clinical evaluation including
  —carotid or femoral pulse,
  —heart sounds through thoracic or esophageal stethoscope,

—serial blood pressure readings,

—pupillary reaction,

—skin color, and by

- electrocardiographic oscilloscope, the ideal monitoring device.

Surgeon and assistants

- although the anesthetist delivers the anesthetic, the surgeon is ultimately responsible for the welfare of the patient;
- during surgery, the surgeon and assistants (including the scrub nurse) should be alert for signs of cardiac arrest which include weakening or cessation of

—aortic and iliac pulsation if the surgeon is operating in the abdomen,

—cardiac or aortic pulsations in the chest and

—carotid pulsation in the neck;

- dark, cyanotic blood, or little or no bleeding are late signs. To make the diagnosis at this stage suggests that monitoring was inadequate.
- with good monitoring and an alert surgical team,

—cardiac arrest, or its

—premonitory sign (arrhythmias) can be

—diagnosed immediately as it occurs, and treatment can be instituted

—before the brain is irreversibly damaged;

- key word for diagnosis and successful treatment of cardiac arrest in the operating room is

—vigilance.

Outside the operating room

- diagnosis is more difficult and is made on the

—absence of the carotid or femoral pulses;

- even though a systolic blood pressure (BP) of 50 mm Hg may be present when the pulses are absent, assume the heart has stopped and start treatment immediately because

—delay in starting treatment is catastrophic.

- confirmatory evidence of cardiac arrest includes

—unconsciousness,

—dilating or dilated pupils and

—pale peripheral skin and cyanosed lips.

PRIMARY RESPIRATORY ARREST

- diagnosis is usually more obvious than cardiac arrest because the patient
- stops breathing! But
- upper airway obstruction is accompanied by
  —useless, gasping movements, and
  —purple features.
- start treatment immediately if you suspect respiratory arrest, and if the heart has stopped beating, treat this simultaneously.

Basic Life Support—Initial Treatment

- the ABC of basic life support is
  —*A*irway
  —*B*reathing
  —*C*irculation.

AIRWAY

- place the patient flat on her back on hard, stable surface (floor or ground is best),
- remove foreign bodies from the mouth or throat, including false teeth,
- tilt head back and pull the jaw forward to prevent the tongue from falling back into the oropharynx and blocking the airway.

BREATHING

  Technique with an adult
  - tilt the head back and hold it back with one hand;
  - if breathing does not start spontaneously,
  - close the patient's nostrils with the other hand,
  - take a deep breath, then
  - seal the patient's mouth with your lips and
  - exhale into her mouth.
  - watch the patient's chest to see that it rises. If it does not rise, either your
    —technique is wrong or there is
    —airway obstruction which you must remove by turning the patient on the side, thumping her back, then clearing the throat again with a finger.
  - give 12 breaths/minute, allowing the patient to exhale passively

between each breath (listen to make sure that the patient does exhale).

Technique with a child

- similar to that with an adult but do not tilt the head as far back;
- if the child is small, cover the nose and mouth with your mouth and
- use smaller breaths at a rate of
- 20 a minute.

CIRCULATION

Cardiac compression

- after 5 breaths, palpate the carotid pulse. If this is absent,
- start simultaneous closed cardiac compression.
- when resuscitating an adult,
  —place the heel of one hand on the lower half of the sternum (not on the xiphisternum) and the other hand on the dorsum of the first;
  —with the elbows extended and shoulders directly above the patient (arms vertical) depress the sternum 5 cm (2 inches). This movement should be quick, not slow;
  —repeat 60 times a minute. The effectiveness of cardiac compression can be assessed by palpation of the carotid or femoral pulsation at each compression. For a
- child use
  —one hand because less force is required, and place it on
  —midsternum because the heart is higher in chest. With an
- infant
  —use only two fingers for chest compression at a
  —rate of 80 to 100 compressions/minute.
- effective resuscitation results in a cardiac output of only 30% of normal at best, and should therefore
  —not be interrupted for more than 5 to 10 seconds at a time, but
  —for tracheal intubation you may allow interruption of 20 to 30 seconds.
- if two rescuers are present,
  —one should ventilate while
  —the other does cardiac compression;
  —they should change positions every 3 to 4 minutes to reduce fatigue;

—working on opposite sides of the patient will facilitate the changeover without interruption of resuscitation.

- if only one rescuer is present, do
  —15 chest compressions, at a rate of 80 compression/minute, to compensate for time taken in ventilating, then
  —two quick lung inflations.

Complications of Resuscitation

- fractured ribs or costochondral separations due to compression of the chest wall instead of the sternum may cause pneumothorax;
- fractured sternum, from too vigorous compression, may damage the pericardium and heart muscle;
- pressure over the xiphoid process instead of the sternum may rupture the liver, rarely the stomach or spleen. These
- complications can be avoided by
  —smooth, steady action, keeping the
- hands on the distal sternum and
- off the chest wall and xiphoid.

Adjuncts to Basic Life Support

- once the patient is in the hospital, the adjuncts to initial treatment may be employed.

OPEN CARDIAC COMPRESSION

Indications

- failed closed cardiac compression,
- penetrating wound of heart,
- suspected cardiac tamponade,
- tension pneumothorax or
- thoracic deformity, e.g., scoliosis and kyphosis where closed compression would be ineffective.

Technique

- thoracotomy incision through left fifth intercostal space with the first knife that comes to hand;
- open the pericardial sac widely to allow entry of your hand; sterility at this stage is not important!
- squeeze the heart between the fingers and thumb 60 times/minute; if the

- heart is fibrillating, use defibrillator (must be DC, not AC: Plugging the patient into the light does not help!);
- in a successful but unsterile procedure, give IV antibiotics and take the patient to operating room as soon as possible for
  —irrigation of the wound and
  —suture of the thoracic wall with underwater-seal drain.

DRUGS

- IV route is best because
- intracardiac injection may cause
  —pneumothorax or cardiac tamponade, or damage the
  —myocardium or coronary vessels; but
  —cardiac compression must be effective for drugs to reach tissues.
- sodium bicarbonate is essential to combat metabolic acidosis. Dosage is
  —1 mEq/kg IV in one injection (into IV tubing),
  —then 30 mEq every 5 minutes or
  —by continuous infusion.
- epinephrine can convert asystole to sinus rhythm and improve the heart rate in bradycardia. The dosage for asystole is
  —0.5 mg of 1:1000 IV and double the dose every 5 minutes until sinus rhythm is restored, or as an
  —IV infusion of 1 to 4 μg/minute until the heart is beating spontaneously at more than 60 beats/minute.
- calcium chloride improves electrical conduction of the ventricle. Do not mix it with sodium bicarbonate (forms a precipitate) and do not use in a fully digitalized patient (may suppress sinus discharge). Dosage is
  —5 ml of 10% solution, i.e., 0.5 gm, every 5 minutes IV. If
  —calcium gluconate is used, give 10 ml of 10% solution every 5 minutes.
- atropine sulphate is used for sinus bradycardia of less than 60 beats/minute. Dosage is
  —0.5 mg IV and may be repeated every 5 minutes until either the sinus rate is above 60 beats/minute, or a total of 2 mg (four doses) have been given.
- lidocaine for arrhythmia, multifocal premature ventricular contractions, ventricular tachycardia or ventricular fibrillation occurring again after defibrillation. Dosage is

—50 to 100 mg bolus IV. This may be supplemented by
—continuous infusion of 1 to 3 mg/minute. If
—arrhythmia persists, use
- procainamide, 100 mg IV.
- continuous monitoring of the patient after successful resuscitation is vital to avoid recurrent arrest.

TERMINATION OF RESUSCITATION

- the decision to stop life support measures is the responsibility of the doctor. Base this decision on
- cerebral status:
  —fixed dilated pupils,
  —deep coma, and an
  —absence of spontaneous respiration for 15 to 30 minutes, or a
  —flat EEG, indicate that the brain is dead; and on
- cardiovascular status:
  —absence of cardiac electrical activity after 10 minutes of resuscitation signifies cardiac death.

Prognosis

- younger patients and patients who have a second arrest have a poor prognosis;
- patients with ventricular fibrillation when first seen have a better prognosis than those in asystole;
- the underlying disease, e.g., coronary artery disease, has an important influence on the prognosis.

Summary

- diagnosis, 5 seconds;
- decision to resuscitate or not, 2 seconds;
- instructions to assistants, 5 seconds; then
- continuous
  —mouth-to-mouth ventilation and
  —closed cardiac compression;
- transfer to hospital for
  —IV drugs
  —ECG and
  —defibrillation;
- decision to continue or not.

chapter 19

Hypovolemic Shock

Etiopathology

- shock may be due to
  - absolute hypovolemia with loss of extracellular fluid (ECF) as in hemorrhage and burns,
  - relative hypovolemia as in peripheral pooling after cord transection,
  - cardiogenic disorders with pump failure, such as myocardial infarction or pulmonary embolus, or
  - bacteremia causing septic shock.
- hypovolemic shock is a dynamic state associated with inadequate tissue perfusion.

HOMEOSTATIC RESPONSE

- when fluid is lost rapidly, there is
- reduction in venous return to the right side of the heart, leading to
- decrease in cardiac output and
- inadequate perfusion of tissues, with
- consequent impairment of organ function.
- the body's homeostatic mechanisms are activated by the fall in arterial blood pressure (Fig. 19.1).

Sympathetic response

- sympathetic stimulation increases
  - peripheral resistance by constricting arterioles and increases
  - cardiac output by augmenting rate and force of contraction;
- enhances effective blood volume by increasing venomotor tone. This squeezes blood from large venous reservoirs into the central circulation;
- redistributes blood volume to brain and heart by diverting it from the extremities, bowel and kidney.

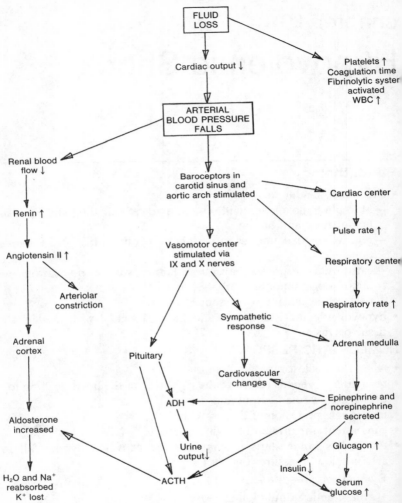

Figure 19.1. Sequence of hemodynamic and metabolic events in hypovolemic shock.

Catecholamines
- norepinephrine production is increased by
  —reduction in blood volume,
  —acidosis and
  —increase in partial pressure of carbon dioxide (PCO_2);

- epinephrine production is increased by a
  —prolonged low-flow state.
- epinephrine is an alpha and a beta stimulator,
- norepinephrine is almost purely an alpha stimulator. These substances have hemodynamic effects similar to a sympathetic response; they
  —increase cardiac output,
  —dilate arteries in striated and myocardial muscle,
  —constrict arterioles in skin, kidneys and viscera, and
  —constrict most veins. They also have
- hormonal effects; they
  —inhibit the production and action of insulin (the "banker" hormone which promotes storage of metabolic fuels),
  —increase amino acid mobilization from muscle, increasing hepatic gluconeogenesis from amino acids,
  —stimulate production of glucagon (the "spender" hormone which enhances glucose formation from liver glycogen and also through gluconeogenesis) and
  —increase ACTH production which causes the adrenal cortex to produce aldosterone.

Aldosterone

- production is increased by
  —ACTH and
  —low renal blood flow, through the renin and angiotension mechanism; the
- action of aldosterone causes
  —Na^+ retention which leads to
  —H_2O retention, and
  —K^+ secretion by kidneys

Antidiuretic hormone (ADH)

- ADH is released from the posterior pituitary by
  —increased baroceptor activity due to a fall in arterial pressure,
  —changes in plasma osmolality and
  —reduced left atrial filling pressure.
- action is to increase water resorption from urine in collecting ducts which are rendered permeable to water by ADH (countercurrent system).

CELLULAR METABOLISM

Normal Cellular metabolism

Organelles

- nucleus controls cell function;
- chromosomes contain genes which direct protein synthesis;
- mitochondria produce energy in the form of adenosine triphosphate from the breakdown of sugars, fats and amino acids;
- ribosomes create protein from amino acids, using energy from the citric acid cycle (Fig. 12.1);
- rough endoplasmic reticulum contains ribosomes, and transports protein and cell products along a canal system to the
- Golgi apparatus which packages the products of protein synthesis into vacuoles;
- lysosomes are sacs of digestive and lytic enzymes.
- the plasma or cell membrane covers the cell and is
- built of lipid and protein layers

Energy production

- glucose enters the cell and is transformed into glucose-6-phosphate (Fig. 12.2);
- this is then either
  —stored as glycogen or
  —oxidized through the citric acid cycle in the mitochondria to form energy in the form of
- adenosine triphosphate, written as
- $A - P \sim P \sim P$. The
- last two phosphate bonds are energy-rich and release 8,000 calories/mole when liberated by oxygen;
- this energy is used in
  —protein synthesis,
  —maintaining K^+ in the cell and Na^+ outside it ("sodium pump") and
  —other metabolic activities of the cell.

Cellular metabolism in hypovolemic shock

- as a result of inadequate perfusion of cells and tissues, their nutritional and metabolic needs are not met, and their normal function is impaired; the
- sequence of events is shown in Figure 19.2

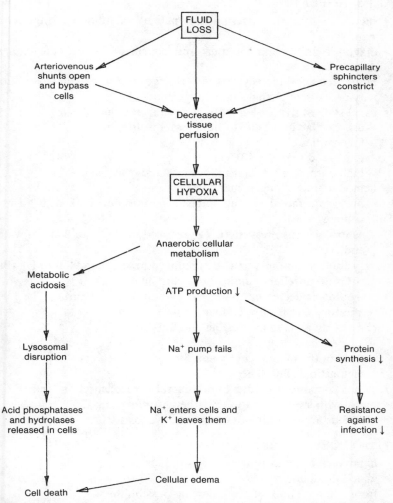

Figure 19.2. Sequence of changes in cellular metabolism during hypovolemic shock.

Clinical Features and Diagnosis

CLINICAL FEATURES

- shock is a dynamic state, and the patient's condition changes constantly;
- diagnosis and treatment must run concurrently, and the clinical features must be
- monitored continuously, because changes in the patient's condition may necessitate changes in management. The
- usual state of hypovolemic shock is clinically one of
  —low cardiac input due to fluid loss, resulting in
  —low cardiac output,
  —low blood pressure (BP) and
  —high peripheral resistance (homeostatic response).
- hemodynamic changes include a
  —pulse rate raised above 100 beats/minute but weak with a small volume, a
  —central venous pressure (CVP) reduced to less than 2 cm of water and
  —systolic blood pressure (SBP) reduced to less than 90 mm Hg (but BP is an unreliable indicator of cardiac output).
- urine flow is decreased to less than 20 ml/hour (oliguria). The
- respiratory rate is raised. Do a
- chest x-ray as soon as possible and look for
  —air or
  —fluid in the pleural cavity and for
  —mediastinal shift. The
- skin is cool and pale, due to peripheral vasoconstriction, and
- damp with sweat, due to sympathetic stimulation;
- nail beds are blue, due to peripheral cyanosis.

FLUID LOSS

- hypovolemic shock is a result of fluid loss;
- which fluid, and
- from where? Think of the following possibilities:
  —closed, multiple fractures (especially pelvis) or open fracture;
  —vascular injury;
  —intra-abdominal, intrathoracic or intrapelvic trauma;
  —gastrointestinal hemorrhage with melena or hematemesis, or peritonitis;

—massive diarrhea and/or vomiting;
—massive hemoptysis or
—extensive burns.
* blood loss in closed fractures in the adult may be
—0.5 liter with a forearm fracture,
—1.0 liter with a femoral fracture, and
—more with pelvic fractures.
* losses may be
—double or higher with open fractures.
* loss of
—20% of circulating blood volume causes mild shock with SBP below 90 mm Hg;
—30%, moderate shock with SBP lower than 70 mm Hg; and
—more than 40%, severe shock with SBP less than 50 mm Hg.
* shock is less severe when blood loss is slower.

DIFFERENTIAL DIAGNOSIS OF SHOCK

* in major types of shock
—BP and urine flow are lowered, and
—pulse rate (PR) is usually high. The
* following are distinguishing features:
* myocardial infarction may have a
—history of precordial pain and previous episodes, with
—ECG changes and
—CVP raised;
—PR may be raised or lowered.
* mediastinal shift
—the trachea is eccentric;
—physical examination and x-ray of chest will show the pathology, e.g., pneumothorax.
* peripheral pooling
—paraplegia or other etiological problems will be clinically evident.
* septic shock
—CVP is raised.
* severe brain injury
—never causes the classical shock state;
—pulse rate is slow.

COMPLICATIONS

* major complications are
* acute tubular necrosis and

- acute respiratory failure, "shock lung," with
  —pulmonary hemorrhagic edema and
  —progressive hypoxia refractory to treatment.

Treatment of Hypovolemic Shock

- it is relatively simple to treat a patient with hypovolemic shock because
- the patient has lost a certain amount of fluid which
- you must replace.

GENERAL PRINCIPLES

- you must restore
  —metabolic and
  —hemodynamic stability as soon as possible. A
- chronic low-flow state promotes failure of the
  —kidney, liver, and heart, and
  —increases susceptibility to infection and cellular breakdown.
- treatment should start at the site of the accident. Time spent
  —arresting hemorrhage by compression (not tourniquet) and
  —immobilizing fractures before the journey to the hospital may save the patient's life;
  —establish an airway and ventilate the patient with 30% oxygen by mask if possible, and
  —intravenous infusion during the journey would be very valuable.
- do not give too little treatment too late.

FLUID REPLACEMENT

Intravenous lines

- IV line by venepuncture or cutdown is urgent and mandatory. So
- do not waste time fiddling with a needle; if it will not go easily into a vein, do a cutdown. Take blood at the same time for
  —group and cross-match,
  —hemoglobin, white blood cells (WBCs) and hematocrit (Hct),
  —BUN, blood sugar and electrolytes (SMA 12 or 15),
  —pH and blood gases, and a
  —blood culture and smear for bacteria.
- establish a CVP line as soon as possible too.

Intake and output chart

- an accurate intake and output chart is the
- key

- to successful fluid replacement;
- intake includes all liquids by
  —mouth (food too; this has water content), by
  —nasogastric tube and by
  —IV infusion (all crystalloids and colloids, including blood).
- output includes
  —urine (indwelling Foley catheter mandatory), feces (these have water content), vomitus,
  —gastric aspirate, fluid loss from a fistula,
  —blood loss from a wound, and plasma and serum loss from burns;
- estimates should also be made of fluid loss by
  —sensible and insensible perspiration and
  —water vapor in expired air.

Intravenous fluids

Immediately

- 1.5 liters of crystalloid fluid
  —1,500 cc of Ringer's lactate (best) or
  —physiological saline;
- 5% glucose in water should not be used unless there is nothing else.

Followed by

- additional fluids which should consist roughly of
  —half crystalloid (as above) and
  —half colloid;
- colloidal fluids include:
  —fresh frozen plasma or albumin for peritonitis, burns and acute pancreatitis;
  —whole blood for blood loss. Give grouped or O-negative blood if the need is urgent; otherwise use crystalloids until cross-matched blood is ready. For
  —dextran, the least effective of the colloids, give no more than 1 liter a day.
- if large quantities of fluid are given, the fluid should be warmed to 35° or 38° C (90° to 99° F) by resting the IV tube in a bowl of warm water.

Speed of infusion

- in hypovolemic shock, fluids should be given IV as fast as possible until the shock begins to reverse;

- judge the speed of infusion by the clinical response of the patient, particularly the changes in
  —urine output,
  —pulse rate, blood pressure,
  —CVP and
  —pulmonary artery wedge pressure (PAWP) using a Swan-Ganz catheter. PAWP is a more sensitive index of blood volume changes than CVP.
- alter your treatment according to the patient's response.

Acid-base balance

- usually the patient is in metabolic acidosis which is
- best corrected by restoring adequate tissue perfusion;
- sodium bicarbonate is of limited value in hypovolemic shock.

DRUGS

- vasoconstrictor drugs are
  —dangerous in hypovolemic shock,
  —may mask the underlying pathology, and
  —should not be used.
- vasodilator drugs
  —have very limited indications (see below).
- steroids
  —are not helpful.
- digitalis
  —is useful, especially in the older age group when there is a history or evidence of
  —congestive heart failure, or an
  —abnormally elevated CVP, or
  —severe, persistent atrial tachycardia over 130 beats/minute.
- broad spectrum antibiotics
  —should be given.

CONTINUOUS MONITORING

- important because it guides treatment. The
- pulse rate decreases, and the volume of the pulse increases as shock is reversed;
- CVP returns towards normal;
- peripheral circulation improves as shock is reversed, shown by
  —veins filling up,
  —IV infusion running faster and

—fingertip capillaries refilling increasingly quickly.
* peripheral temperature rises toward normal with improved circulation.
* hourly urine output approaches normal which is 40 cc or more (0.5 cc/kg/hour) with improvement of renal circulation;
* serial Hb and Hct estimations are valuable for evaluating fluid replacement in case of hemoconcentration due to fluid loss, e.g., in
    —burns,
    —diarrhea and vomiting and
    —peritonitis; but
* serial Hb and Hct estimations are
    —not helpful in the early stages of shock when this is due to
    —whole blood loss.
* weigh the patient daily, to assess fluid deficit or overload.
* respiratory rate decreases and
* depth increases as hypoxia and acidosis are corrected.
* level of consciousness and mental state improve.

FRACTURES

* do not send patient to x-ray department, nor
* manipulate fractures while he is
* still in shock, because you may provoke
* profound hypotension and decompensation.
* until shock is reversed, splint the limb as it lies unless injury compromises circulation.

Recurrence of Shock

* patient may be resuscitated from original shock, withstand surgery and manipulation of fractures, then
* relapse into shock 24 to 36 hours later.
* when this happens you must reexamine the patient and make a fresh diagnosis.
* the most likely cause is hypovolemia, with diagnosis and treatment as outlined above, but consider other problems as well:
* if neostigmine and atropine are given after surgery to counteract curare-like drugs, residual effects of neostigmine may simulate shock, but
    —PR is slow;

- to treat, give 0.3 mg atropine IV slowly.
- myocardial infarction usually is associated with
  —chest pain and
  —ECG changes; but do not confuse the minor ECG changes that occur with hypotension with those of infarction.
- pulmonary embolism usually is heralded by
  —sudden chest pain with dyspnea and hemoptysis,
  —jugular vein distention, cyanosis and low BP, and sometimes a
  —history of previous thrombophlebitis;
  —bacteremic shock in its pulmonary vasoconstrictive phase can mimic this.
- bacteremic (septic) shock may have
  —pyrexia and mental confusion,
  —BP first raised, then lowered, oliguria,
  —cold and clammy skin with petechiae, and
  —cyanosis and/or jaundice.
- fat embolism syndrome may be severe with
  —marked respiratory distress and
  —hypoxemia
  —progressive anemia and
  —mental confusion or coma.

Resistant Shock

ETIOLOGY

- if patient fails to respond despite treatment, this is resistant shock and may be due to
  —inadequate fluid replacement,
  —myocardial infarction or
  —infection.

TREATMENT

- continue IV fluid until CVP reaches the upper limit of normal. If
- blood volume has been replaced, and the
- CVP is high, yet the
- shock state still persists, then
- vasoconstriction has not relaxed sufficiently, and
- vasodilator drugs may be used cautiously with continuing fluid administration. In this case, give slow IV infusion of one of the following:

- isoprenaline (Isuprel)
  - —beta-adrenergic stimulant
  - —causes increase in rate and force of contraction of heart muscle, and therefore increases the cardiac output, and also promotes
  - —vasodilation of coronary, peripheral and organ vessels; the
  - —dosage is 2 mg in 500 ml of 5% dextrose in water, run in at a rate sufficient to improve BP and urine output and reduce the CVP, but not to raise PR more than 120 beats/minute.
- dopamine (Intropin)
  - —advantages over Isuprel are that it produces renal and mesenteric vasodilation and is less likely to cause tachycardia and arrhythmia;
  - —dosage is 1 to 10 μg/kg/minute.
- phenoxybenzamine (Dibenzyline)
  - —alpha-adrenergic receptor blocker
  - —dosage is 1 mg/kg body weight until venoconstriction relaxes and CVP falls. Then
- give more fluid IV until urinary production and skin perfusion (the skin is warm and pink, the veins are filled) are restored and BP rises.
- never give vasodilator drugs if CVP is low.

Summary

- major clinical features of hypovolemic shock are:
  - —rapid, weak pulse,
  - —cold, sweaty skin,
  - —pallor or cyanosis,
  - —oliguria and
  - —mental confusion.
- major factor in treatment is
  - —rapid, adequate and appropriate fluid replacement.

chapter 20
Septic Shock

Etiopathology

- septic shock is a dynamic state associated with the inability of cells to metabolize nutrients normally (Fig. 20.1).
- diagnosis, treatment and continuous clinical, bacteriological and biochemical evaluation must run concurrently.

BACTERIA

- predisposing factors to infection include
  —diabetes mellitus, burns
  —malnutrition, hypovolemia,
  —steroids, immunosuppressive therapy, chemotherapy and radiotherapy,
  —indwelling IV or urinary catheters, tracheotomy,
  —indiscriminate use of prophylactic antibiotics and
  —intra-abdominal surgery.
- bacteria invade and multiply in the blood stream (septicemia). They may be
  —Gram-negative (commonest) or
  —Gram-positive organisms. Bacteria produce
- toxins
  —endotoxins from dead and disintegrating Gram-negative bacteria,
  —exotoxins from Gram-positive bacteria.
- normovolemic patient develops hyperdynamic shock associated with Gram-negative or Gram-positive organisms; the
- hypovolemic patient develops hypodynamic shock, usually only associated with Gram-negative organisms.

HEMODYNAMIC CHANGES

- bacteria and toxins damage cells of capillary walls and with an
- increase of the number of pores in the capillary walls, there is a

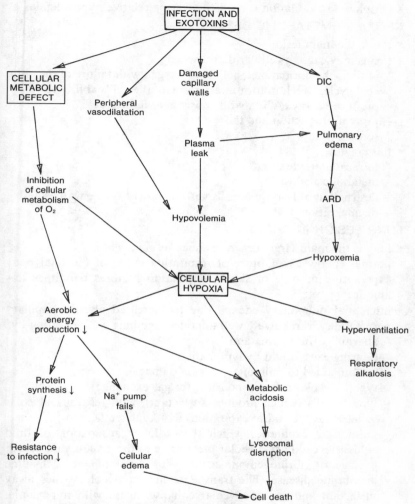

Figure 20.1. Diagram showing etiopathology of septic shock.

resultant escape of
—fluid,
—plasma proteins and
—red cells into the extracellular (third) space, creating real hypovolemia;

- peripheral vasodilation is marked, causing relative hypovolemia.

CELLULAR METABOLIC DEFECT

- this is the main lesion.
- toxins may cause a cellular defect which
  —inhibits the normal metabolism of oxygen with failure of the citric acid cycle, which in turn interferes with the cell's ability to
  —produce energy (ATP), with consequent failure of
  —protein production and the
  —sodium pump;
- this creates
  —intracellular edema,
  —metabolic acidosis,
  —destruction of lysosome walls with release of lytic enzymes and
  —disintegration of the cell.

LUNG LESION IN SHOCK

- lung is the main target organ in shock in man. The
- normal energy expenditure of respiration is 2% of the total body expenditure at rest. In shock, respiration requires ten times this amount.
- interstitial pulmonary edema, due to increased alveolar-capillary permeability, is relatively well tolerated, the lung compensating by
  —altering perfused area and
  —clearing excess fluid by lymphatics.
- infection added to pulmonary edema damages
  —type I alveolar cells (responsible for gas exchange),
  —type II cells (which produce surfactant), with resulting alveolar collapse (at the end of expiration) and hypoxemia, and
  —pulmonary capillaries which then allow transudation of fluid across the capillary-alveolar membrane to the alveoli, and permit passage of fibrinogen molecules with development of hyaline membrane disease. The transudate in the alveoli washes away surfactant and causes alveolar collapse, again with hypoxemia. The
- areas of the lung that have no ventilation are perfused, resulting in ventilation/perfusion abnormalities with
  —hypoxia resistant to treatment with 100% oxygen; this
- acute respiratory distress syndrome (ARD or shock lung) is the major cause of death among patients with septic shock.

- in survivors, healing comes from
  —type II alveolar cells, or by
  —fibrosis if damage is very severe, with
  —limitation of the lung's capacity for gas exchange.

DISSEMINATED INTRAVASCULAR COAGULATION (DIC)

- may be associated with endotoxic shock;
- formation of thrombin with deposition of microthrombi, resulting in occlusion of small vessels, may cause
  —pulmonary edema with hypoxia,
  —renal cortical necrosis, jaundice,
  —GI hemorrhage, pancreatitis with increased serum amylase and decreased serum calcium, and
  —epileptic (grand mal) seizures.
- consumptive coagulopathy may result from consumption of all clotting factors.

SUMMARY OF MAJOR PATHOLOGICAL FINDINGS

- sepsis
- plasma leak
- peripheral vasodilation
- severe hypovolemia
- cellular defect of oxygen metabolism.

Clinical Features

GENERAL

- patient is usually over 45 years old;
- two thirds of patients with septic shock develop it after admission to hospital!
- one third of patients with Gram-negative bacteremia develop septic shock;
- GU and GI tracts are commonest sites of invasion;
- shock usually lasts 2 to 3 days in survivors;
- major symptoms and signs are
  —rapid and excessive protein wasting, much more marked than in starvation,
  —pyrexia, starting with a rigor,
  —mental confusion,

   —jaundice and
   —petechiae.
- septic shock is divided into two syndromes:
  —hyperdynamic (warm) shock characterized by high central venous pressure (CVP), and
  —hypodynamic (cold) shock associated with low CVP;
  —these are further subdivided into
  —alkalotic (early) and
  —acidotic (late).

HYPERDYNAMIC SHOCK

- respiratory features are
- hyperventilation, an especially valuable sign in septic shock. Distinguish this from hyperventilation due to
  —atelectasis,
  —pneumonia,
  —pulmonary embolism and
  —myocardial infarction.
- respiratory alkalosis because CO_2 is washed out by hyperventilation (alkalotic phase).
- pulmonary edema and acute respiratory failure may develop later with resulting severe
  —cellular hypoxia and
  —metabolic acidosis (acidotic phase).
- hemodynamic effects are
- high cardiac output (hence the name hyperdynamic shock) with
- raised CVP, 12 to 13 cm H_2O;
- raised pulse rate (PR) but
- low blood pressure (BP) with consequent
- oliguria;
- peripheral skin is
  —warm, dry and
  —cyanotic;
- peripheral resistance is low due to vasodilation leading to
  —relative hypovolemia;
- damaged capillary walls leak plasma which produces
  —absolute hypovolemia; thus
- inadequate tissue perfusion causes cellular hypoxia and, together with

- deficient utilization of oxygen by cells due to cellular defect, results in later development of
- metabolic acidosis and lactic acidemia (acidotic phase);
- septic shock in the early, alkalotic phase is treatable with
    —surgery to eliminate the septic focus,
    —antibiotics,
    —fluid replacement and
    —Isuprel or dopamine (see below) to increase the cardiac output still further.
- do not allow the patient to progress to the acidotic phase because that is usually fatal! Treatment at this late stage involves
    —massive fluid replacement; and a
    —beta-adrenergic blocker may help.

HYPODYNAMIC SHOCK

- occurs in patients who have
    —hypovolemia first, followed later by
    —sepsis
- most often associated with
    —bowel obstruction or infarction, peritonitis,
    —septic abortion or
    —pyelonephritis.
- clinically it resembles hypovolemic shock;
- hyperventilation is characteristic with resultant respiratory alkalosis (alkalotic phase) which compensates for metabolic acidosis;
- hemodynamic features are
- low cardiac output (hence the name "hypodynamic"),
- low CVP, due to absolute hypovolemia and
- low BP, resulting in
- oliguria and
- inadequate tissue perfusion and low oxygen uptake, with consequent
- metabolic acidosis and compensatory
- increase in peripheral resistance with
- cold, cyanotic extremities.
- the acidotic phase is a later and terminal stage of hypodynamic shock; at this stage the patient is
    —moribund with
    —cold cynotic extremities,
    —cardiac output is low and does not respond to treatment with

drugs; there is
—severe and increasing acidosis with
—irreversible tissue hypoxia and necrosis.
- treatment must include
- antibiotics,
- surgery if necessary to eliminate the septic source and
- fluid replacement to restore effective blood volume; use
  —saline if hematocrit is more than 40,
  —blood if hematocrit is less than 40, until CVP is normal;
  —do not raise hematocrit above 40 because this will increase viscosity
   and decrease cardiac output and urine flow;
- if cardiac output is then still inadequate as shown by
  —hypotension, oliguria and measurements made through a
  —Swan-Ganz catheter, then use
- Isuprel to restore adequate tissue perfusion once cardiac filling
  pressure has returned to normal (use CVP and pulmonary artery
  wedge pressure as indices).

Prevention and Treatment

- treatment is much more difficult than that of hypovolemic shock,
  and prognosis is poorer;
- prevention is easier and has better results.

PREDISPOSITION TO INFECTION

- whether or not a patient becomes infected depends on
  —host defence mechanisms (see Chapter 17) and
  —extraneous factors.
- the major factors which predispose a surgical wound to infection are:
- age of the patient
  —the old and the very young are most vulnerable;
- potentially contaminated procedure
  —division of GI and GU tracts;
- surgical techniques
  —preservation of blood supply to healing edges,
  —elimination of dead spaces,
  —good hemostasis and
  —excision of devitalized tissue;
- duration of operation

—the infection rate increases with the length of surgery;
- presence of bacteria in the wound at the end of surgery; and
- ward environment
  —an open ward and
  —infected patients nearby increase the risk.

PREVENTION OF INFECTION IN SURGERY

Prophylactic antibiotics
- clean case, no antibiotics;
- clean but high risk, e.g., scoliosis surgery in the adult, total joint replacement with cement, GI and GU tracts divided, give antibiotics before, during and for a short time after surgery;
- contaminated or dirty wound
  —longer term antibiotics, and if wound is on a limb, then
  —leave wound open, and
  —plan delayed primary closure or secondary closure, or
  —allow nature to close the wound.

Catheters and tracheotomy
- IV, intra-arterial and urinary catheters are frequent sources of infection and septicemia;
- to avoid this
  —change IV lines every 48 hours, and for the
  —urinary catheter, irrigate regularly with antibiotics.
- tracheotomy is an excellent source of bacteria!
- regular tracheotomy toilet, changing and sterilizing the tube are essential to control local infection and prevent septicemia.

Nutrition
- some patients are
  —undernourished or
  —malnourished before surgery, and
- sepsis itself causes an extreme negative nitrogen balance with loss of proteins, which aggravates the patient's nutritional status;
- the natural resistance of these patients is lowered, and the infection rate is higher among them;
- septic complications may be avoided, or more easily treated, by vigorously correcting the nutritional status.

TREATMENT OF SEPTIC SHOCK
- two main principles of treatment are

    —antibiotics, and

    —plasma volume expansion.

- diagnose and treat infection before shock occurs;
- learn the signs of septic shock and think of it (you will not make the diagnosis if you do not think of it). Hyperventilation is a valuable early warning sign.

Antibiotics

- drain an abscess adequately to eliminate the source of infection:
- culture the wound or pus, and take
- three blood samples for culture during fever peaks.
- give antibiotics immediately the diagnosis is made if not sooner, i.e., on suspicion. It is better to overdiagnose this syndrome than to miss it;
- oral and intramuscular routes are inadequate because of poor tissue perfusion, so the
- IV route is obligatory;
- use only one antibiotic initially because combined antibiotics increase the risk of

    —side-effects, and

    —bizarre superinfections. The

- initial choice of antibiotic must be an educated guess because culture takes 2 days but death may occur within hours;
- infection of lungs, skin, heart valves, bone, joints and deep tissues is likely to be caused by
- Gram-positive organisms;
- infection of the GI or GU tract is commonly caused by
- Gram-negative organisms.

Plasma volume expansion

- restore CVP to normal
- this may require large quantities of

    —colloid and plasma volume expanders, and

    —crystalloid to fill the dilated capillary bed (capacitance vessels): monitoring is therefore essential.

- administer IV fluids rapidly and continuously until

    —urine output is adequate (key sign), the

    —skin of limbs is warm,

    —cutaneous veins are filled and

—arterial BP is stable.
- increase cardiac output with one of following beta-adrenergic stimulators:

Isoproterenol (Isuprel)
- this increases heart rate and cardiac output, and
- decreases peripheral resistance by vasodilation; the
- dosage is 1 to 5 μg/minute IV (0.25 to 1.25 ml/minute of a solution containing 2 mg of isoproterenol in 500 ml of IV fluid); the
- drawback is very rapid tachycardia and arrhythmias when dosage must be decreased or stopped.

dopamine (Intropin)
- is the immediate precursor of norepinephrine;
- improves urine flow by renal vasodilation;
- is less likely to cause arrhythmia and tachycardia than Isuprel; the
- dosage is 1 to 10 μg/kg/minute, but this must be titrated against changing signs,
  —urine output,
  —pulse rate and
  —blood pressure

Corticosteroids
- may be helpful, but
- replace fluid volume first;
- dosage is 100 to 400 mg of hydrocortisone per kg body weight IV every 4 hours for 24 to 36 hours.

Acute respiratory failure
- prevent accumulation of lung water in patients with high sepsis risk by
  —avoiding fluid and electrolyte overload,
  —frequently changing the patient's position, and
  —pulmonary physiotherapy.
- avoid microemboli from blood transfusions (a cause of ARD in itself) by using a 40-μ filter in the system when more than 5 units of blood are required;
- trachael intubation and positive pressure ventilation with 30% oxygen are helpful in treatment.

Summary

- suspect septic shock in a
  —hospitalized patient
  —over 40 who suddenly develops
  —hyperventilation,
  —fever
  —rigors,
  —mental confusion and
  —oliguria.
- treat immediately by
  —blood culture,
  —IV antibiotics,
  —massive fluid replacement and
  —abscess drainage.
- monitor continuously
  —urine output,
  —pulse rate,
  —CVP and
  —peripheral blood pressure.

chapter 21

Blood Replacement, Thrombosis and Thromboembolism

ABO and Rhesus Antigens

- the surface of the human red cell is a mosaic of antigens;
- all of these are weak except the
  - ABO and
  - Rhesus antigens;
- alloantibodies to the ABO and Rhesus groups frequently are troublesome if the blood donor and recipient are not matched;
- alloantibodies to the weak antigens occasionally cause trouble.

ABO SYSTEM

- antigens are genetically determined;
- subgroups of this system exist but will not be considered here.

Blood groups

- group A
  - red cell surface has A antigen,
  - serum has anti-B alloantibody;
  - 40% of Caucasians have this blood group.
- group B
  - B antigen,
  - anti-A alloantibody,
  - 10%.
- group AB
  - A and B antigens,
  - no alloantibodies,
  - 5%.
- group O
  - no antigen,
  - anti-A and anti-B alloantibodies,
  - 45%.

Alloantibodies

- old name was isoantibodies.
- alloantibodies can agglutinate the red blood cells (RBCs) of a person of a different blood group but cannot agglutinate the individual's own cells;
- autoantibodies can agglutinate the individual's own cells. Do not confuse the terms.
- alloantibodies are always present and are called "naturally occurring." They are mainly IgM;
- they can agglutinate RBCs in saline suspension and are called "complete."
- acquired antibodies, e.g., through pregnancy or transfusion, are immune antibodies. They cannot agglutinate RBCs in saline suspension, and are called "incomplete." They are mainly IgG, of the Rhesus type, and must be demonstrated by indirect means.

Blood grouping

- the following tests are performed to identify, and to confirm beyond a doubt, the patient's blood group:
- one drop of a 2% suspension of the patient's RBCs is mixed with one drop of potent anti-A serum, then another drop of a 2% suspension of the patient's RBCs is mixed with a drop of anti-B serum; if the
- RBCs agglutinate with anti-A serum but not with anti-B, then the
  —group is A; and if the
- RBCs agglutinate with anti-B serum but not with anti-A, then the
  —group is B; if the
- RBCs agglutinate with both sera, then the
  —group is AB; and if the
- RBCs do not agglutinate with either serum, then the
  —group is O.
- as additional safeguards, test the patient's RBCs with
  —group O serum. This contains anti-A and anti-B alloantibodies and will agglutinate all groups and subgroups except group O. Then test the
  —patient's serum with known A, B, and O RBCs to confirm the presence of expected alloantibodies in the patient's serum; this is
  —reverse grouping and should be done routinely.

RHESUS SYSTEM

Antigen

- this is a complex system of many antigens, but in practice, only the D antigen is important. The others will not be considered here.
- 85% of white-skinned people carry the D antigen on their RBCs and are termed Rh-positive;
- the remaining 15% are Rh-negative and do not carry the D antigen.

Immune antibodies

- these do not occur naturally;
- all Rhesus antibodies in Rh-negative people are acquired either by
  —transfusion with Rh-positive RBCs or by
  —pregnancy, by transplacental passage of fetal Rh-positive RBCs; the
    the fetus; these
  —antibodies may then cross the placenta, enter the fetal circulation and hemolyse the fetal RBCs, causing hemolytic disease of the newborn. An
- Rh-positive person will not make Rhesus antibodies.
- Rh antibodies are IgG, incomplete, and can be
- detected by the agglutination of Rh-positive RBCs under certain specific conditions.

Blood Transfusion

- blood transfusion is expensive and has many dangers;
- the surgeon must clearly understand the indications for transfusion.

STORAGE OF BLOOD

- stored blood may be anticoagulated using
- acid, citrate and dextrose (ACD). This consists of
  —trisodium citrate, the anticoagulant,
  —citric acid which increases the preserving power of the anticoagulant, and
  —dextrose which delays hydrolysis of phosphates. Another anticoagulant mixture is
- citrate, phosphate and dextrose. This has advantages over ACD.
- blood can be safely stored for 3 weeks at 4° C with both methods; but

—RBCs deteriorate rapidly if the temperature is above 10° C, and
—slow freezing is worse, because the RBCs hemolyze on being thawed;
- at −50° C, frozen with glycerol, RBCs survive more than a year.
- 1 unit of stored blood consists of
  —70 ml of anticoagulant
  —180 ml of RBCs and
  —220 ml plasma.
- three quarters of the RBCs stored at 4° C for 21 days survive in the recipient after transfusion. The remainder are destroyed in 24 hours;
- granulocytes die in stored blood;
- platelets are viable only in fresh blood;
- albumin, gamma globulin, fibrinogen, prothrombin and factors VII, IX and X are stable in stored blood, but
- factors V and VIII are not stable at 4° C, although they are stable in fresh frozen plasma.

BLOOD COMPONENT THERAPY

- blood is scarce!
- it consists of many components, not all of which are needed by the same patient;
- if the components are separated, they can be used to treat several patients;
- component therapy is a logical and increasingly popular trend.

Whole blood

- best replacement for sudden loss of 15% or more of blood volume and for anticipated loss of blood in major surgery, e.g., hip and spine;
- 1 unit containing 400 ml of whole blood raises the hemoglobin (Hb) of a 70 kg adult by 1 gm/100 cc of blood.

Packed red cells

- prepared by removing 85% of the plasma by sedimentation or centrifugation;
- best for correction of anemia, especially when the danger of circulatory overload exists, e.g., in an old patient or in a patient with congestive heart failure (CHF). Also in
- preparation of an anemic patient for surgery, if hemoglobin is less than 9 gm/100 ml. Note that
  —the patient with chronic (long-standing) anemia is physiologi-

cally adjusted to the new level of Hb and may not require transfusing.

Fresh frozen plasma

- prepared by removing it from fresh blood and storing at 20° C below freezing;
- once thawed, it must be used immediately and cannot be refrozen;
- used in bleeding diatheses caused by proven coagulation defects, e.g., hemophilia (factor VIII) and Christmas disease (factor IX). Note that
- coagulation factor concentrates are available; e.g., cryoprecipitate is rich in factor VIII.

Plasma fractions

- albumen is used as a plasma expander to treat hemoconcentration, e.g.,
  —burns,
  —acute pancreatitis and
  —intestinal obstruction;
- gamma globulin is useful in prophylaxis of certain viral diseases, e.g., hepatitis.
- human Rhesus immune globulin may be used in prevention of Rhesus sensitization in Rh-negative women immediately after delivery of a Rh-positive baby;
- fibrinogen carries the high risk (10%) of transferring hepatitis virus and should be used only when diagnosis of hypofibrinogenemia is certain, as in disseminated intravascular coagulation syndrome.

PREPARATIONS FOR TRANSFUSION

- blood grouping of patient and donor;
- screening of donor's blood, looking for
  —irregular blood group antibodies,
  —Australian antigen (indicates presence of hepatitis virus),
  —Wasserman reaction for syphilis, and the
  —hemoglobin level (occasionally the donor needs a transfusion more than the patient!); and
- screening the recipient's blood for
  —irregular blood group antibodies. This is particularly important for patients who will require a large volume of blood, e.g., for open heart surgery with extracorporeal circulation.
- cross-matching involves

- testing the donor's RBCs with recipient's serum to see if the latter contains antibodies against the donor's cells; if the
  —donor's serum contains antibodies against the recipient's cells, this is not important because the donor's serum is quickly diluted in the recipient's vessels.
- cross-matching before transfusing the blood is important because it will show whether the
  —recipient's serum contains antibodies other than the ABO group, and also it
  —avoids a mistake in identification.

COMPLICATIONS OF TRANSFUSION
Immediate reactions

Hemolytic reactions

- usually due to rapid destruction of the donor's RBCs by antibodies in the recipient's serum when incompatible blood is transfused;
- ABO reactions are the most common;
- usually caused by careless mistakes that result in
  —incorrect blood grouping,
  —incorrect cross-matching or
  —error in identification of the patient, a specimen of blood or the unit of blood; these mistakes are
  —preventable.
- may also be caused by
  —faulty storage,
  —old blood or
  —bacterial contamination.

Intravascular hemolysis

- due to ABO incompatibility;
- symptoms start soon after transfusion has begun and may include
  —heat and pain in transfusion vein,
  —flushing, rigor, fever,
  —loin and back pain and
  —tightness across the chest;
- signs may include
  —hemoglobinemia and hemoglobinuria,
  —oliguria and acute renal failure due to intense renal vasoconstriction,

—jaundice, which becomes apparent several hours later,

—leukopenia, thrombocytopenia and

—disseminated intravascular coagulation. This causes oozing hemorrhage and may cause death within 2 or 3 days, or

—death may follow hypotension and shock.

- in the unconscious or anesthetized patient, the only sign may be
  —inexplicable hypotension and/or
  —bleeding tendency.

- treatment
  —discontinue transfusion immediately on suspicion, check patient and bottle identification, and notify the blood bank;
  —record urine output and use an osmotic diuretic such as mannitol if the patient is oliguric;
  —treat anuria (see Chapter 24);
  —look for hemoglobinemia and hemoglobinuria, and later hyperbilirubinemia;
  —repeat cross-match and search for irregular antibodies.

Extravascular hemolysis

- usually Rhesus incompatibility;
- donor's RBCs are destroyed by the reticuloendothelial system in the liver and spleen producing hyperbilirubinemia;
- symptoms and signs are usually mild, hemoglobinemia is uncommon, and
- renal failure does not occur.

Febrile, pyrogenic

- occurs during or after transfusion and is generally not dangerous;
- usually due to white blood cell (WBC) antibodies formed by the recipient as a result of previous transfusions but may also be due to Gram-negative endotoxin if transfusion apparatus is dirty or transfusion fluid is improperly prepared;
- clinical features may include
  —fever, rigors
  —nausea and vomiting, but last
  —only a few hours;
- must differentiate this from hemolytic reaction which is dangerous.
- treat with aspirin.

Allergic reactions

- 2% to 3% of patients;
- common in recipients with hay fever or asthma and are
- usually harmless; the
- most common symptom is urticaria (itchy skin rash);
- treat with antihistamines.

Circulatory overload

- rapid increase in intravascular fluid volume due to administration of IV fluid too quickly may cause
  - —congestive heart failure,
  - —pulmonary edema and
  - —death;
- treat by
  - —slowing or stopping infusion, and
  - —treating the CHF and pulmonary edema;
- avoid by
  - —limiting transfusions and
  - —using only packed cells in susceptible patients, not more than 2 units every 24 hours, and
  - —monitoring lungs and neck veins throughout the transfusion.

Bacterial contamination

- accidental, usually during collection or storage,
- commonly cold-growing Gram-negative organisms, e.g., certain Pseudomonas and coliform organisms; may cause
- profound shock, fever, abdominal pain and usually death;
- to avoid growth of bacteria in the bottle of blood, it should be completely administered within 4 hours of leaving the refrigerator.

Citrate intoxication

- with massive or rapid transfusions, the patient's liver may not be able to metabolize the large quantity of ACD transfused;
- this results in hypocalemia; to
- avoid this, after the first 3 or 4 units, give 100 cc of 10% calcium gluconate through a different vein for every 2 units of blood transfused.

Potassium overload

- potassium levels in fresh blood are normal but increase sixfold

in banked blood 3 weeks old as K^+ leaks from the cells;
- massive transfusion of old blood, e.g., exchange transfusion or extracorporeal circulation, may cause
  —hyperkalemia with
  —ECG changes and perhaps
  —death;
- avoid this danger by using
  —fresh blood or
  —packed cells.

Hemorrhagic states

- caused by depletion of platelets, fibrinogen and coagulation factors V and VIII by progressive replacement of the patient's own blood with large volumes of bank blood, e.g., in multiple trauma, or massive bleeding during surgery;
- treat with fresh whole blood.

Air embolism

- may be introduced through poorly fitting tubing or blood administered under pressure;
- 40 cc of air may be fatal;
- plastic bags rather than bottles have all but eliminated this complication.

Delayed reactions

Sensitization

- alloantibodies formed by the recipient against antigens on the donor's RBCs, WBCs or platelets may complicate future transfusions or pregnancies.

Delayed hemolytic reaction

- if a titer of alloantibody, formed against cells of a previous transfusion, falls to undetectable levels, later transfusion of apparently compatible blood will stimulate production of these antibodies, and
- hemolytic reaction will occur 3 to 7 days after transfusion, with destruction of donor cells and jaundice.

Infections

Hepatitis
- the most important of transferred infections;
- up to 1% of the normal population is positive for HAA, the

hepatitis-associated antigen, formerly called the Australia antigen. This indicates the presence of hepatitis virus; the

- incidence of hepatitis among recipients of HAA-negative blood is 0.15%, or 1 in 700, whereas
- 50% of recipients of HAA-positive blood develop hepatitis;
- screening tests detect only 1 in 4 carriers.

Syphilis

- test donor blood for syphilis;
- *Treponema pallidum* probably does not survive 48 hours storage at blood bank temperature.

Malaria

- plasmodium survives refrigeration;
- cannot detect carriers;
- transmitted only by RBCs.

Multiple microemboli

- stored, bottled blood contains microparticles of
  —plastic from the tubing,
  —rubber from the bottle stopper,
  —glass particles from the bottle,
  —cellulose fibers and
  —clumps of platelets and WBCs.
- these can cause multiple microemboli in the lungs of a seriously ill patient, resulting in respiratory distress syndrome;
- Micropore filters should be used if patient requires more than 4 units of blood.

Thrombophlebitis

- the cannulated vein may be damaged by the needle or catheter;
- incidence increases if the catheter is left in after 12 hours and the
- incidence of septic thrombophlebitis increases after 48 hours, with the danger of fatal septicemia.
- can be avoided by
  —using careful, sterile technique for putting the needle in the vein,
  —using a plastic rather than a rubber catheter in the vein,
  —changing an indwelling catheter every 24 hours and
  —not giving autoclaved glucose solution, as this is strongly acidic and irritates the vein.

AUTOTRANSFUSION

- used for patients who will have major surgery requiring several units of blood.
- 1 unit of blood is collected from the patient 3 weeks before surgery and stored;
- 2 weeks before surgery, the unit of blood is returned to patient and 2 units are removed and stored;
- 1 week before surgery, 2 units are returned and 3 are removed.
- this has the following advantages
  —the patient's hematopoietic system is stimulated and makes up for the overall loss of 3 units of blood,
  —it avoids most complications of donor recipient transfusion, and
  —3 fresh units are available for surgery.

PLASMA EXPANDERS

- plasma is the best plasma expander!
- albumin, 1¼% in balanced salt solution, is especially useful in patients with excessive loss of plasma proteins.
- commercial high-molecular-weight (70,000) dextran, up to 1 liter/24 hours, is useful because it
  —improves tissue blood flow by reducing hematocrit and therefore
  —improves oxygen delivery. This product osmotically
  —expands plasma volume because of the large size of the molecules;
- Rheomacrodex (low-molecular-weight dextran; molecular weight, 40,000) is less efficient as a plasma expander because it leaves the vessels more easily.
- Ringer's lactate or normal saline should be started IV in all patients with impending or actual shock;
  —rapid infusion of 1 to 2 liters in 15 minutes may be given to correct reduction of extracellular fluid, but it
  —dilutes plasma proteins and may cause pulmonary edema, so do not give too much.

Phlebothrombosis and Thrombophlebitis
ETIOLOGY

Phlebothrombosis

- three factors which constitute Virchow's triad determine the occurrence of phlebothrombosis: firstly,

- intimal damage or abnormality provides focus for adhesion of platelets; secondly,
- alterations in blood flow creating eddy currents and particularly causing stasis in calves. This allows platelets to fall out of the central blood stream and reach the vessel wall. Predisposing factors are
  —low cardiac output due to hypovolemia; decreased metabolic rate (patient on bed rest!); heart failure;
  —decreased muscle activity (bed rest); and
  —external pressure from bandage, plaster cast, mattress or pillows (bed rest). Thirdly,
- constituents of blood may be altered, e.g.,
  —thrombocytosis following trauma, hemorrhage and splenectomy;
  —increased platelet adhesiveness after surgery;
  —accelerated clotting time may be caused by steroids and estrogen therapy, trauma and hemorrhage.
- other factors which increase the incidence of deep vein thrombosis are the
  —age of the patient (the older the patient, the greater the risk)
  —obesity,
  —hip and spine surgery and
  —previous episodes of thrombosis.

Thrombophlebitis

- thrombophlebitis occurs secondarily to inflammation of the vein wall. This may be due to
  —trauma,
  —chemical irritation, e.g., hypertonic dextrose solution, or
  —bacterial infection.

PATHOGENESIS

- thrombosis is the formation of an intravascular mass from constituents of the moving blood stream.

Phlebothrombosis

- platelets adhere to the damaged or abnormal part of vessel endothelium, forming the pale
- platelet thrombus. This then releases
  —ADP which causes platelets in the vicinity to aggregate, thus increasing the size of the primary platelet thrombus, and also

—platelet factor 3 (a phospholipid) which activates the clotting mechanism. This is also activated by plasma factor XII in contact with an abnormal vessel wall. The resulting

- fibrin mesh
  —covers and thus stabilizes the platelet thrombus, and
  —traps red and white cells. This is now a
- coralline thrombus, built of a series of vertical, interlacing
  —platelet laminae with interstices filled by
  —blood clot; this thrombus grows by accretion until it becomes an
- occluding thrombus, blocking the vein and thus causing complete stasis of the blood column. This then coagulates as far as the next tributary and is called the
- consecutive clot. The end may be endothelialized, or it may spread further by
- propagation which may occur by
  —continued coagulation with no further anchorage sites, thus increasing the probability of detachment and embolism, or by
  —new platelet, coralline and occluding thrombus, followed by consecutive and propagated clot. This clot is anchored at each new tributary and is less likely to become detached.
- the clot is a phenomenon secondary to venous occlusion and complete venous stasis and contains no platelet lattice. In time, the
- clot retracts and becomes dry and friable, and
- circulation may be reestablished in the vein. Blood flow may
- detach the thrombus which may then become an
- embolus travelling easily and quickly to the heart and lungs.

Thrombophlebitis

- thrombus secondary to inflammation forms in the same way, but the
  —anchorage site is very firm, and the clot is
  —not likely to propagate because blood flow is usually normal or is accelerated by inflammation. So
- detachment and embolism are rare.

CLINICAL FEATURES

- phlebothrombosis may cause
  —swelling of the limb distal to the thrombus and

—muscle pain and tenderness in the affected area and
—calf pain on dorsiflexion of the foot (Homan's sign). But
- phlebothrombosis is often
  —asymptomatic, in which case the first sign may be
  —pulmonary embolism!
- thrombophlebitis is particularly
  —painful and has local signs of
  —inflammation when the vein is superficial.
- diagnostic procedures include
  —contrast venography, the gold standard! This is difficult to do and to interpret and may itself cause thrombosis!
  —^{125}I-labelled fibrinogen scan with a hot spot over the thrombus; most sensitive in the leg;
  —ultrasound with a silent spot over the thrombus. Results vary with the experience of the technician;
  —impedance plethysmography detects venous obstruction, using electrodes which measure impedance (resistance to blood flow) in the calf. This is the most sensitive and specific test for venous obstruction in the thigh. Useful in combination with the ^{125}I scan.
- complications include
  —pulmonary embolism (see below);
  —chronic limb edema if the thrombus is organized but not lyzed and continues to obstruct the major vein;
  —varicose veins secondary to venous valve destruction after organization and recanalization of the thrombus in deep or perforating leg veins;
  —metastatic abscesses due to septic emboli.

PREVENTION AND TREATMENT

- incidence of thrombosis may be reduced by
  —daily active exercises of limbs in bed,
  —elevating legs and
  —elastic stockings or compression bandages;
- intermittent electrical stimulation or pneumatic compression of the calf during surgery may also help;
- prophylactic anticoagulation in selected patients has limited value in orthopaedic surgery but may diminish the likelihood of massive pulmonary embolism.
- clinical effects of dextran-70 and aspirin, the latter of which prevents release of ADP by platelets, are uncertain.

- surgical interruption of the inferior vena cava is rarely indicated.
- treatment of established deep vein thrombosis is by anticoagulant therapy (see below).
- treat superficial thrombophlebitis by
  —analgesics,
  —local heat (warm packs),
  —gentle compression bandage and
  —continued activity.

Pulmonary Thrombotic Embolism

PATHOGENESIS
- the most dangerous complication of thrombosis.
- massive embolus, particularly from femoral or iliac vein, may
  —fill the right ventricle and block pulmonary trunk, or it may
  —lodge at the bifurcation of the trunk or enter one of the major branches; in any case there are frequently no further embolic episodes!
- smaller emboli, e.g., from calf veins, block smaller arteries and arterioles, and patient survival rate is higher.
- pathological effects are mainly due to mechanical block but also are due to
  —reflex changes initiated by vasoactive amines, 5-HT and bradykinin released from emboli;
- preexisting heart or pulmonary disease also influences the outcome.

CLINICAL FEATURES
- phlebothrombosis with pulmonary embolism is increasing in the Western World.
- most patients have
  —chest pain with
  —dyspnea and tachycardia;
- fewer have
  —hemoptysis,
  —cyanosis and
  —hypotension.
- chest radiographs may show reduced pulmonary vascular markings at the site of the embolus and will help to exclude other pathology.
- serum LDH and bilirubin may be raised, but SGOT is not;

- pulmonary arteriography (difficult) and
- technetium-99m scan give the most reliable information about the region and extent of diminished pulmonary perfusion; if these are positive, then a
- ventilation scan with ^{133}Xe may show a ventilation/perfusion mismatch.

PREVENTION

- prevent deep vein thrombosis! Or, if this has already occurred,
- prevent its spread and embolization (see above).

TREATMENT

- anticoagulation is the best available treatment;
- heparin
  —prevents activation of the Christmas factor (IX) and
  —stops thrombin converting fibrinogen to fibrin;
  —dosage must increase coagulation time by two to three times the normal; IV initially, then subcutaneously. After a few days, start
- oral coumarin therapy and tail off heparin;
- continue coumarins for several weeks or months, depending upon clinical features and response!
- coumarins prevent formation in the liver of
  —factors VII, IX and X and
  —prothrombin. This action is
- reversed by vitamin K.
- anticoagulants
  —stop progress of propagated clot and
  —prevent further emboli from being released.
- pulmonary embolectomy is dangerous and is seldom indicated.

chapter 22

Local and Regional Anesthesia in Orthopaedic Surgery

Anesthetic Techniques

- local and regional anesthesia with local anesthetic agents is excellent for the orthopaedic and fracture surgeon because it is
  —relatively easy, safe and cheap,
  —can be administered by the operating surgeon himself, and
  —provides adequate anesthesia for almost any procedure on the limbs. However,
  —toxic reactions do occur, so monitor the patient's cardiorespiratory status and level of consciousness thoughout the procedure.

TOPICAL

- anesthetic agent is absorbed through mucous membranes and diseased skin and blocks the sensory receptors. It is
- not absorbed through intact, healthy skin unless an anesthetic ointment is rubbed in;
- provides good surface anesthesia of
  —conjunctiva and cornea,
  —oral, nasal and pharyngeal cavities,
  —esophagus, larynx and trachea, and
  —urethra and anus.

LOCAL INFILTRATION

- injected directly into the operative field, skin and subcutaneous tissue;
- blocks sensory receptors as well as terminal nerve fibers; used for
- skin surgery, such as the suture of clean lacerations.

FIELD BLOCK

- a ring of local anesthetic is injected into the tissues around the operative field;

- all sensory nerves leaving the area are blocked; a
- large volume of anesthetic is required, so use dilute solutions to avoid toxic effects. Useful for
- skin surgery and small orthopaedic procedures, such as
- release of a trigger finger (stenosing tenovaginitis).

PERIPHERAL NERVE BLOCK

- anesthetic is injected close to major nerve trunks,
- paralyzes the entire nerve, including sensory and sympathetic fibers;
- dosages quoted for specific nerve blocks in following sections are for
  —lidocaine (Xylocaine), and the
  —average 70-kg adult;
- for children, or if agents other than lidocaine are used, modify dosages accordingly.

Axillary block

- is as effective as brachial plexus block but less dangerous than it.

  Position of patient

  - supine,
  - arm in 90° abduction and 90° external rotation,
  - elbow bent 90°, back of hand resting on table.
  - useful for surgery on upper limb, particularly the lower arm and elbow; forearm and hand can be anesthetized by other methods.

  Technique

  - 20 to 50 cc of 1% solution of lidocaine with epinephrine 1:100,000 (smaller amount for children, according to weight).
  - needle is introduced through center of floor of axilla and into axillary
  - neurovascular sheath; anesthetic is injected
    —anterior and
    —posterior to axillary artery.
  - before each injection, confirm by aspiration that the needle is not in the axillary artery! This would cause seizures as well as arterial spasm, resulting in
    —ischemia of the hand and your savings account!
  - inject subcutaneously before withdrawal to block
    —intercostobrachial and medial brachial cutaneous nerves.
  - anesthesia is complete in 15 to 20 minutes and lasts about 3 hours, but analgesia lasts 4 to 6 hours;

- entire upper limb is anesthetized, both sensory and motor, except for high divisions of C5 and C6
  - —sensation over deltoid muscle and
  - —shoulder girdle muscles, and sometimes the
  - —musculocutaneous nerve; block this nerve by injecting 3 to 5 cc into the coracobrachialis muscle.

Elbow block

- provides sensory and motor anesthesia of hand, including long flexors and extensors of fingers and thumb; use
- 20 cc of 1% lidocaine with or without adrenaline.

  Ulnar nerve
  - palpate nerve in sulcus behind medial humeral epicondyle,
  - introduce needle through skin and elicit a paraesthesia; then
  - withdraw needle slightly and inject 5 cc of anesthetic.

  Median nerve
  - lies medial to brachial artery at elbow;
  - on lateral side of brachial artery is the biceps tendon which is easily palpable;
  - insert needle through skin of antecubital fossa, medial to artery,
  - elicit paraesthesias and withdraw needle slightly,
  - if paraesthesias do not occur, redirect needle until they do, then withdraw needle a little way,
  - aspirate, and if blood does not return, inject 5 cc of anesthetic.

  Radial nerve
  - insert needle through lateral aspect of skin 7 cm proximal to lateral humeral epicondyle;
  - advance needle until either
    - —paraesthesias are elicited, or
    - —needle hits bone;
  - in either case, withdraw needle slightly and inject 10 cc of anesthetic.

Wrist block

- sensory and motor anesthesia of part or all of the hand, but long flexors and extensors can still move the fingers and thumb. Not necessary to elicit paraesthesias.
- 2% solution of lidocaine with or without epinephrine, 1:100,000 concentration. Use 2 cc for each nerve.

Radial nerve

- palpate radial pulse at wrist, and introduce needle into subcutaneous tissue here;
- aspirate before injecting to avoid intra-arterial injection and disaster!
- inject 0.5 cc on medial side of artery,
- then withdraw needle to subcutaneous tissue, advance it three quarters of an inch lateral and posterior to the artery and inject 1 cc.
- inject remaining 0.5 cc as needle is withdrawn.

Median nerve

- find the palmaris longus tendon just proximal to the wrist;
- inject 0.5 cc on radial side of tendon to anesthetize the superficial sensory branch which leaves the nerve proximal to the wrist;
- then advance needle just through the fascia (you will feel it go through), but not deeper or the needle will be in the nerve (intraneural injection will destroy the nerve and your reputation!)
- inject remaining 1.5 cc.

Ulnar nerve

- small sensory branches leave the nerve proximal to the wrist.
- identify ulnar artery and tendon of flexor carpi ulnaris on its ulnar side;
- insert needle between these two structures and aspirate.
- inject 0.5 cc on medial side of artery,
- advance needle laterally beneath artery and through fascia, and inject 1 cc after aspirating again;
- withdraw needle to subcutaneous tissue, advance more dorsally through the fascia, and inject remaining 0.5 cc to anesthetize dorsal sensory branches.

Palmar digital block

General

- do not use epinephrine.
- useful for treatment of one or two injured fingers
  —lacerations,
  —fractures and dislocations,
  —removal of foreign bodies;
- if more fingers are involved, do a wrist block instead.

- each finger has four proper digital nerves
  —two palmar, one on each side, which lie beneath the palmar fascia at level of the distal palmar crease, and
  —two dorsal, one on each side, which run in dorsal subcutaneous tissue.

Technique

- use 2% solution of lidocaine without adrenaline.
- insert needle through palmar skin at level of distal palmar crease, directly over long flexor tendon,
- then angle needle laterally and advance it until you feel it penetrate the palmar fascia at the side of the tendon;
- after aspiration, inject 0.5 cc.
- withdraw needle to subcutaneous tissue, redirect it medially, push it through palmar fascia at the side of the tendon (do not go through the tendon), aspirate and inject 0.5 cc. Then on dorsum of hand
- insert needle through skin 1 cm proximal to metacarpal (MC) head;
- advance needle laterally for half an inch to radial side of MC and inject 0.5 cc after aspiration;
- withdraw needle to subcutaneous tissue, redirect it to ulnar side of MC for half an inch, and inject another 0.5 cc after aspiration.
- similarly with the thumb.
- anesthesia occurs within 10 minutes.

Sciatic nerve block

Position of patient

- on the side, with the leg to be operated on uppermost,
- lower leg straight, uppermost limb bent at hip and knee.
- can be used for surgery on leg or foot when combined with femoral nerve block.

Technique

- 30 cc of 1% lidocaine with adrenaline.
- draw a straight line between
  —upper border of greater trochanter and
  —posterior superior iliac spine, and draw a
- perpendicular line distally from the midpoint of this line;
- draw another line from greater trochanter to tip of sacrum;
- where this third line crosses perpendicular, the sciatic nerve

leaves the pelvis through the greater sciatic notch. The needle is introduced here;

- push needle in, perpendicular to skin, until either
  —paraesthesias occur or
  —needle hits bone;
- if no paraesthesias occur, withdraw and redirect needle until they do;
- as soon as the patient feels pins and needles, withdraw the needle a few millimeters, aspirate, then cautiously inject 30 cc of anesthetic.

Femoral nerve block

- 10 cc of 1% lidocaine with epinephrine.
- with patient supine, palpate femoral artery just distal to inguinal ligament, in the femoral triangle; the
- nerve lies lateral to the artery (the vein lies medial to the artery, VAN).
- push artery medially with fingers,
- insert needle perpendicular to skin and directly over nerve (lateral to artery),
- push needle through fascia lata overlying nerve and elicit paraesthesias of nerve;
- when paraesthesias occur, withdraw needle a few millimeters and inject 10 cc of anesthetic.

Ankle block

- use 15 cc of 1% lidocaine without epinephrine for nerve blocks and
- 10 cc of 0.5% lidocaine without epinephrine for circumferential skin block.
- useful for most procedures about the foot.
- not necessary to elicit paraesthesias around the ankle.

Tibial nerve

- passes 1.5 cm posterolateral to medial malleolus, deep and lateral to posterior tibial artery;
- palpate artery just above ankle joint,
- insert needle just lateral to artery, aspirate, then inject 5 cc of 1% lidocaine.

Deep peroneal nerve

- just above the ankle joint, the nerve lies lateral to the anterior tibial artery, between

—tibialis anterior and extensor hallucis longus tendons medially, and

—extensor digitorum longus tendons laterally.
- palpate tendons and artery,
- insert needle just proximal to tibiotalar joint, lateral to artery,
- aspirate, then inject 5 cc of 1% anesthetic.

Sural nerve

- purely sensory nerve, lies behind lateral malleolus;
- inject 5 cc of 1% anesthetic just posterior to lateral malleolus.

Circumferential sensory blockade

- this anesthetizes the superficial peroneal and saphenous nerves and other small branches;
- infiltrate 5 to 10 cc of 0.5% solution subcutaneously right around the ankle joint just proximal to the malleoli.

INTRAVENOUS REGIONAL ANESTHESIA

- very useful for limb surgery of less than 90 minutes duration.
- insert IV needle into vein of limb,
- empty the veins by esmarch rubber bandage,
- inflate tourniquet cuff around proximal part of limb to 250 mm Hg for the arm and 400 mm Hg for the leg. Then
- inject 25 to 40 cc of 0.5% lidocaine without adrenaline into the vein of the arm, or 40 to 60 cc for the leg, and remove the needle.
- inflate second tourniquet just distal to first and deflate first one (this step provides more comfort for the patient but is not essential).
- complete anesthesia is obtained after 5 to 10 minutes;
- sensation to pain returns 1 or 2 minutes after release of the tourniquet.
- if tourniquet is released less than 30 minutes after start, the blood level of the anesthetic rises rapidly, and systemic toxic effects are likely; so
- avoid this either by
  —leaving the tourniquet on a minimum of 30 minutes or by
  —intermittent release of the tourniquet.

Regional Anesthetic Agents

PROPERTIES

Cocaine

- naturally occurring, from the coca plant in South America. The Indians of Peru (Incas) and Bolivia chewed the leaves for pleasure (stimulates the CNS) and for sustained periods of work without eating or drinking (anesthetizes the gastric mucosa!).

Uses
- topical anesthesia only;
- used in nasal cavity surgery and is
- applied by droplet, spray or sponge.

Dosage
- used in concentrations from 4% to 10%,
- maximum safe dose is 200 mg for adults, less for children.

Advantages
- is absorbed easily through mucous membrane and
- has a strong vasoconstrictor effect, a useful hemostatic property.

Disadvantages
- must never be used with epinephrine because cocaine potentiates epinephrine;
- excites the CNS and is addicting. In the United States it is controlled by federal narcotics laws.

Procaine (Novocain)
- the prototype of synthetic local anesthetic agents.

Uses
- all methods of regional anesthesia except topical.

Dosage
- for local anesthesia, 0.5%
- for conduction anesthesia, 2.0%.
- maximum safe does for an adult is 1 gm.

Advantages
- rapid action and
- four times less toxic than cocaine.

Disadvantages
- action of short duration; so it is
- sometimes combined with epinephrine to prolong its action.

Lidocaine (Xylocaine)
Uses
- all forms of regional anesthesia including topical.

Dosage
- topical, 2% to 4%
- local, 0.5%
- conduction, 1% to 2%
- maximum dosage is 500 mg for an adult.

Advantages
- faster and longer lasting action than procaine;
- spreads well in the tissues;
- is a mild sedative;
- may be used IV as an antiarrhythmic cardiac agent.

Disadvantages
- two to three times more toxic than procaine;
- depresses myocardial and cardiac electrical conduction system;
- may stimulate or depress cerebral cortex and medulla.

Tetracaine (Pontocaine)

Uses
- all forms of regional anesthesia.

Dosage
- topical, 1% to 2%, especially for respiratory tract;
- local and conduction, 0.1% to 0.25%
- maximum dosage is 75 mg for an adult.

Advantages
- duration of action is twice that of procaine and is
- ten times more potent than procaine.

Disadvantages
- five times more toxic than procaine and has
- slow onset of action.

Benzocaine
- poorly soluble in water.

Uses
- topical, for mucous membranes and open wounds;
- is used in many analgesic ointments.

Advantages
- low toxicity and
- action lasts a long time.

Bupivacaine (Marcaine)

Uses

- local and conduction anesthesia;
- useful when prolonged sensory or sympathetic blockade is required.

Dosage

- local, 0.1%
- peripheral nerve block, 0.25% to 0.5%.

Advantages

- long duration of action, two to three times longer than lidocaine, 50% longer than tetracaine;
- speed of action similar to lidocaine, quicker than tetracaine.

Disadvantages

- six times more toxic than procaine;
- motor-blocking ability is poor.

SIDE EFFECTS OF LOCAL ANESTHETICS

Overdosage

- due to
  —too much anesthetic,
  —accidental IV injection, or
  —normal dose in old or very ill patient.

CNS stimulation

Signs of cortical irritability include

- apprehension and nervousness,
- muscle twitching and convulsions.

Signs of medullary stimulation

- increase of
  —blood pressure (BP),
  —pulse rate and
  —respiratory rate;
- nausea and vomiting.

Treatment

- every patient having large doses of local anesthetics should have an IV line in place before administration of the anesthetic. At first signs of CNS stimulation,
- stop the injection of local anesthetic,

- resuscitate with oxygen and respirator bag and
- keep airway open with oropharyngeal airway.
- for convulsions, give small doses of short-acting barbiturate IV, e.g., thiopental, 30 to 50 mgm/minute, or
- valium.
- if generalized convulsion is not relieved, give
  —succinylcholine (Scoline, Anectine).

CNS depression

Signs of cortical depression
- drowsiness progressing to
- unconsciousness,
- loss of reflexes and
- paralysis.

Signs of medullary depression
- cardiac depression and vasodilation with a
  —fall in BP and a
  —weak, slow pulse rate;
- respiratory depression with
  —slow shallow respirations;
- eventual cardiorespiratory arrest, which may occur rapidly.

Prevention
- know the relative toxicities of the anesthetic agents;
- know the safe, maximum dose, and
- use the smallest dose and lowest concentration that will be effective;
- reduce doses for children, old people and very ill patients;
- use epinephrine when possible to reduce the speed of absorption of the agent (but not in the fingers, toes or penis!).

Cardiorespiratory depression

- may be due to
  —direct action of anesthetic on heart muscle and vessels, or
  —secondary to medullary depression.
- manifested by
  —weak and ineffective myocardial activity or even asystole,
  —arterial hypotension due to vasodilation and cardiac failure, and
  —inadequate ventilation.
- treatment includes

—assisted ventilation and oxygen,

—IV fluids and

—vasopressor drugs if indicated.

Allergic reaction

- anaphylactic reaction, due to previous sensitization, or
- atopic reaction with no previous sensitization;
- signs are dyspnea and bronchospasm;
- treat with
  —oxygen,
  —antihistamines and
  —bronchodilators.

Reaction to epinephrine

- signs are
  —tachycardia which differentiates this from the usual reaction to the toxicity of an anesthetic agent,
  —increased BP, and
  —ventricular fibrillation with an extreme overdose.

chapter 23

Postoperative Respiratory Insufficiency

Etiopathology

- postoperative respiratory insufficiency is particularly likely if the surgical problem is an
  —emergency,
  —after extensive surgery,
  —if the anesthetist is inexperienced, or if the patient has
  —preexisting lung disease. The
- prevention of postoperative respiratory complications
  —starts in the preoperative period with the object of improving function as much as possible.

DEPRESSION OF RESPIRATORY CENTER

Central depression

- postoperative respiratory insufficiency is commonly due to the prolonged effect of
  —premedication or
  —anesthetic drugs, or excessive use of
  —analgesics,
- especially in the
  —very young, elderly or very ill patient, or in a patient in
  —hypotension or shock;
- major features are
  —hypoventilation with
  —hypoxia and
  —hypercapnia (CO_2 retention).

Respiratory acidosis

- respiratory acidosis due to increase in partial pressure of carbon dioxide (PCO_2) may be the result of

—inefficient absorption of CO_2 by the soda lime,
—hypoventilation during surgery, especially in the patient with distended abdomen and raised diaphragm due to intra-abdominal pathology;
- when CO_2 reaches a critical level, spontaneous respiration ceases;
- when an oxygen-rich mixture is used during anesthesia, the effects of CO_2 build-up are masked, and diagnosis may not be made until after surgery.

Respiratory alkalosis
- hyperventilation (less likely than hypoventilation) reduces PCO_2 and removes normal ventilatory stimulus;
- this may hinder establishment of spontaneous respiration postoperatively.

Reflex apnea
- may be due to
  —exhaustion of Hering-Breuer reflex after a long period of controlled respiration, or due to the
  —presence of an endotracheal tube under light anesthesia. Deflation of cuff or movement of tube usually stimulates breathing again.

PERIPHERAL NEUROMUSCULAR BLOCK
- peripheral neuromuscular blocking agents used during anesthesia to obtain muscular relaxation may cause respiratory insufficiency after surgery.

Nondepolarizers
- these are
  —tubocurarine,
  —gallamine (Flaxedil) and
  —pancuronium and may cause postoperative respiratory insufficiency in the following ways:

Overdosage
- accidental overdosage, once recognized, can be reversed by anticholinesterase, e.g., neostigmine. If the patient has
- poor peripheral circulation and poor muscular blood flow from any cause, then the dosage of relaxant should be reduced.
- some general anesthetic agents, especially ether, have a muscle relaxant effect themselves and/or potentiate the action of a

muscle relaxant like tubocurarine. The combination may cause apnea unless dosages are reduced.

- large dose of a nondepolarizing agent should not be given just before wound closure, because it will require a
- large dose of neostigmine to counteract it, and this may be dangerous.

True sensitivity

- encountered in
    —myasthenia gravis and
    —infants less than 1 month old;
- safe doses of neostigmine may have little effect, and
- controlled ventilation may be necessary for several hours before most of tubocurarine is naturally eliminated and safe doses of neostigmine become effective.

Potassium imbalance

- hypokalemia in the presence of nondepolarizing blocking agents may cause prolonged apnea; you may
- suspect this problem in an apneic patient who does not respond to
    —neostigmine and
    —adjustment of ventilation.

Antibiotics

- streptomycin, neomycin and polymyxins potentiate the
- neuromuscular blocking properties of ether and
- nondepolarizers, especially when an
- antibiotic has been used preoperatively to sterilize the gut and is then
- placed into a highly inflamed peritoneal cavity.

Depolarizers

- quaternary ammonium compounds, e.g.,
    —suxamethonium and
    —decamethonium.
- postoperative respiratory insufficiency due to

Pseudocholinesterase deficiency

- this enzyme is responsible for the breakdown of suxamethonium; the
- deficiency may be acquired by

—liver damage, malnutrition or severe anemia or may be
- familial,
  —the commonest cause of prolonged apnea following the use of suxamethonium.
- even with low levels of enzyme, suxamethonium will eventually be hydrolyzed in blood;
- meanwhile, treatment is controlled ventilation.

Dual block

- in certain instances, after
- initial depolarization, the neuromuscular endplate changes its response, and blocking agents behave like a
- nondepolarizer and can be deactivated by neostigmine.
- dual block, with slow onset of paralysis and prolonged paralytic effect, is a likely cause of prolonged apnea when the
  —patient's pseudocholinesterase is abnormal,
  —successive doses or continuous IV infusion of suxamethonium has been administered, or the
  —patient is a newborn infant with 5° F fall in temperature occurring at surgery.

RESPIRATORY OBSTRUCTION

- usually occurs within a few hours of surgery. The causes are as follows:

  Upper respiratory tract obstruction
  - tongue or false teeth blocking the airway,
  - laryngeal spasm or
  - laryngeal edema secondary to cervical cellulitis or abscess.

  Lower respiratory tract obstruction
  - excessive bronchial secretions especially with ether anesthesia;
  - preexisting lung disease,
    —unrecognized and untreated pulmonary infection with purulent secretions,
    —chronic bronchitis and
    —emphysema, especially in the
    —aged patient who has less strength to clear thick, tenacious secretions,
  - aspiration of vomit or blood;
  - bronchospasm,
  - pulmonary edema precipitated by

    —irritant anesthetic gas,

    —congestive heart failure or

    —overtransfusion;

- pneumothorax after

    —trauma, e.g., fractured ribs,

    —ruptured emphysematous bulla during ventilation,

    —surgery, e.g., Harrington instrumentation, or

    —supraclavicular brachial plexus block, and

- undiagnosed traumatic rupture of diaphragm with abdominal contents in the chest.

METABOLIC ACIDOSIS

Etiopathology

- occurs in prolonged

    —hypotension or

    —hypoxia from any cause (see Chapter 14).

- aggravated by

    —impairment of renal function, because kidney normally compensates for acidosis and maintains normal pH in plasma; and by

    —impairment of respiratory function by general anesthesia, depressant drugs or disease, because these prevent compensation by hyperventilation and elimination of CO_2.

- anerobic metabolism causes accumulation of nonvolatile acids, such as

    —lactic, pyruvic, acetoacetic and phosphoric acids; secondarily there is

- reduction in plasma bicarbonate as the carbonic acid/bicarbonate buffer system is used up, and a consequent fall in pH.

Clinical features

- following major surgery, the patient fails to respond to neostigmine given for reversal of curarization and has
- severe depression of the

    —respiratory system,

    —cardiovascular system and

    —central nervous system;

- without appropriate treatment, the patient develops

    —progressive hypotension and

—peripheral circulatory failure and
—dies.

PULMONARY COMPLICATIONS

Atelectasis

- the commonest postoperative pulmonary complication.

  Etiology

  - airway obstruction;
  - postoperative hypoventilation, as a result of the
    —residual effect of drugs,
    —immobility,
    —painful abdominal or thoracic wounds or
    —abdominal distension with elevated diaphragm;
  - ineffective cough, particularly with
    —painful wound,
    —thoracic cage trauma,
    —low vital capacity, as in spinal deformity, or
    —physical weakness or exhaustion;
  - increased viscosity of bronchial secretions due to administration of
    —atropine or
    —Demerol, especially if the patient is dehydrated.

  Pathology

  - collapse of a
    —basal segment of a lobe, or of a
    —whole lobe, or even a
    —whole lung;
  - collapsed part is airless and nonventilated but is still perfused by blood, so the
  - ventilation/perfusion ratio is altered.

  Clinical features

  - in early stages there may be
    —no physical signs, or you may hear
    —sonorous ronchi at lung bases during the first 2 postoperative days;
  - after much encouragement, the patient may cough up a plug of white or clear sputum. This is a good diagnostic sign of impending atelectasis;

- if a large area is collapsed, this may cause
  —pyrexia,
  —increased pulse and respiratory rate with dyspnea, a
  —dull percussion note and decreased or absent breath sounds over the collapsed segment and
  —mediastinal shift (look at the position of the trachea);
- x-ray will confirm the diagnosis.
- pyrexia and productive cough with yellow or green sputum are signs of infection;
- make diagnosis and start treatment before infection occurs.

Pneumonia and bronchopneumonia

- nearly always secondary to infection of atelectatic area of lung.
- clinical features are
- pyrexia with raised pulse and respiration rates,
- yellow or green sputum;
- dyspnea and cyanosis if a large area is involved,
- dull percussion note,
- scattered areas of bronchial breathing or absent breath sounds, and
- rales and ronchi;
- listen particularly to the dependent areas of the lungs,
  —posteriorly if the patient is lying on his back,
  —inferiorly if the patient is sitting,
  —both if the patient is in Fowler's position.

Aspiration pneumonitis

- especially likely during anesthesia for emergencies because the
  —preoperative preparation of the patient may be inadequate and the
  —gastric emptying time is prolonged during labor, and by fear, pain, shock and morphine;
- intestinal obstruction, hematemesis and swallowed blood from faciomaxillary injuries and ether anesthesia all increase the danger. Aspiration is usually due to
- vomiting during induction, or during the recovery period, especially after
  —ether anesthetic or
  —abdominal surgery;
- a large quantity aspirated into lungs drowns the patient!

- a small quantity causes
  - —laryngospasm or
  - —bronchospasm, with resulting
  - —acute hypoxia;
- acid gastric contents cause
  - —chemical pneumonitis, and
- particles cause
  - —atelectasis,
  - —pneumonia and/or
  - —lung abscesses.

ADULT RESPIRATORY DISTRESS SYNDROME (ARDS)

- although ARDS is not a respiratory complication of anesthesia, but rather is a complication of severe trauma and resuscitation, this syndrome is included here because it may first be clinically apparent in the postoperative period.

Etiology

- this syndrome is variously titled ARDS, congestive atelectasis, shock lung, perfusion lung, stiff lung and traumatic wet lung, and
- may occur after any severe trauma and after resuscitation;
- etiology may also include
  - —shock with sepsis, fat embolism, oxygen toxicity,
  - —vasoactive agents in circulation, intravascular disseminated coagulation, microemboli from multiple blood transfusions,
  - —neurogenic factors,
  - —effects of resuscitative fluids on lungs, particularly crystalloids, and
  - —excess fluid administration with pulmonary edema.

Pathogenesis

- injury causes mild metabolic acidosis;
- compensatory hyperventilation creates respiratory alkalosis;
- this alkalosis is aggravated by
  - —bicarbonate given during resuscitation and
  - —metabolism of citrate in banked blood which forms more bicarbonate;
- arteriovenous (A-V) shunting in the lungs and an altered ventilation/perfusion ratio cause
- arterial hypoxia;
- injury also activates coagulation, fibrinolytic, kallikrein-kinin and

complement cascade systems;
- with increasing
  - —hyperventilation and oxygen demand for increased work of breathing,
  - —alkalosis and
  - —hypoxia increase, and the patient develops
- respiratory insufficiency and increased pulmonary vascular resistance due to vasoconstriction;
- edema fluid and cellular infiltrates appear in lungs as well as thromboembolism of small vessels, causing disruption of the surfactant system, atelectasis, decrease in compliance and
- increase in A-V shunting;
- hypoxia increases;
- edema persists, producing interstitial fibrosis, and
- partial pressure of oxygen in arterial blood (PaO_2) falls further,
- cellular metabolism fails,
- cardiac arrhythmias appear with bradycardia, and death ensues.

FAT EMBOLISM SYNDROME

Pathogenesis

- this is a respiratory distress syndrome, usually associated with skeletal trauma, in which fat globules are found in the blood stream and in certain vital organs, particularly the lungs, and is more closely related to ARDS than to vascular embolic occlusion.

Physical theory

- free fat liberated from bone marrow at the site of the injury is forced into blood vessels by increased interstitial pressure;
- the fat globules form emboli which may block capillaries in the lung, while others may pass through the lung to reach the systemic circulation, brain, kidney and skin.

Physiochemical theory

- this is the more likely theory.
- fat emboli leave the marrow to reach the lungs, and at the same time the
- stability of lipids normally in the blood is altered by response to trauma, and
  - —free fatty acids, e.g., oleic acid, are formed (Fig. 23.1). These may be associated with
- alterations of the coagulation mechanism, including

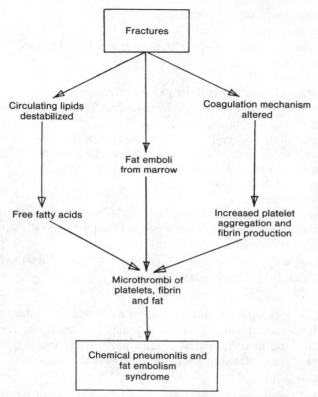

Figure 23.1.   Physiochemical theory of pathogenesis of fat embolism syndrome.

  —RBC aggregation,
  —increased platelet adhesiveness and an
  —increase in fibrin-split products with some degree of
  —disseminated intravascular coagulation. This may release
 • vasoactive substances, e.g., serotonin.
 • all these factors may act in lung by
  —disruption of capillary alveolar membranes and
  —alteration of surfactant activity which produces chemical
    pneumonitis consisting of
  —pulmonary capillary leak and edema,
  —hemorrhagic infarcts and
  —alveolar collapse.

Clinical features

Associated factor

- fractures, the most common associated factor,
  —multiple (more than 11% mortality rate),
  —femur and tibia in young adults,
  —hip in the aged.
- soft-tissue trauma
  —intrathoracic, abdominal and cranial, and
  —major arterial injuries.
- surgery
  —especially bone surgery.

Fat embolism with clinical manifestations

- incidence of fat emboli in the lungs is high after trauma, especially multiple trauma, but not all these patients develop the fat embolism syndrome.
- there are two main clinical syndromes:

  Systemic syndrome
  - spectrum ranges from
    —mild hypoxia to
    —progressive respiratory or cerebral failure and death.
  - may be fulminant with
    —marked respiratory distress,
    —shock,
    —rapid coma and
    —death,
  - or may be classical type (the most common), with following features:
  - latent period after trauma, 6 to 48 hours, then
    —rapid development of symptoms and signs which may regress, then recur;
  - cerebral damage may be secondary to
    —hypoxia or to
    —cerebral fat emboli and may cause
    —death;
  - neurological symptoms may continually change, with
    —headache, restlessness, obstreperousness, confusion, delirium and
    —coma; may have

—localizing signs, or long-tract signs or decerebrate rigidity;

—retinal hemorrhages, exudates and infarcts;

—cerebral damage may be permanent if patient survives;

- pulmonary symptoms include

  —dyspnea, cough, hemoptysis and

  —rapid respiration, 30 respirations/minute or more;

- fever is usually high, 103° to 104° F (39° to 40° C);

- pulse is very rapid, 140 beats/minute or more, and

  —blood pressure is low; the patient may go into shock;

- low hemoglobin, continually falling in spite of transfusions;

- petechiae in skin across chest, axilla, root of neck, retina and conjunctiva may appear 2 to 3 days later and

  —sometimes fade rapidly, then recur.

Cardiopulmonary syndrome

- rare

- pulmonary edema and hyperemia with

  —hemorrhagic infarcts, chemical pneumonitis, bloody sputum and

  —"snow storm" on x-ray;

- right heart dilation and myocardial ischemia.

Laboratory studies

Blood

- fall in PaO_2 is an early sign and may be less than 60 mm Hg; serial tests are useful as index of effectiveness of treatment;

- partial pressure of carbon dioxide in arterial blood ($PaCO_2$) is elevated more than 50 mm Hg;

- decrease in red blood cells and platelets (latter an important diagnostic sign); so

- hematocrit drops, sometimes precipitously;

- serum lipase is elevated in half the patients but is a late sign;

- plasma albumin levels may be low.

Urine

- free fat (triglycerides) in the urine indicates systemic fat embolism to the kidney;

- occurs from the first to the third day and is

- present in 50% of severe cases.

Radiography

- serial chest x-rays show progressive "snow storm" infiltrations;

- these changes are not specific for fat embolism syndrome,
- often occur late and
- disappear within a day or 2.

Summary of major clinical problems

- shock,
- pulmonary insufficiency,
- anemia,
- hypoxemia (this is of major clinical importance),
- mental confusion and coma.

Differential diagnosis

Posttraumatic pulmonary insufficiency

- shock lung from any cause, especially aspiration (chemical) pneumonitis,
- pulmonary contusion, and
- diffuse intravascular coagulation.

Coma after cerebral trauma

- may be difficult to differentiate this from coma due to cerebral fat embolism. The patient with
- cerebral traumatic coma usually has a
  —shorter lucid interval, the patient's
  —confusion is less marked, the
  —heart rate is slower and the
  —blood pressure is higher, the
  —respiratory rate (RR) is slower and
  —localizing signs are often present.

Management of Postoperative Respiratory Insufficiency

GENERAL

- prevention is easier, cheaper and quicker than cure and has better results!
- examine all patients carefully before surgery (not just before, but well before);
- recognize those patients most likely to develop a problem after surgery,
- discuss the problem preoperatively with the anesthetist and

—institute therapeutic measures before surgery,

—observe the patient carefully during surgery, and

—continue appropriate therapeutic measures afterwards. These are the tasks both of the anesthetist and the surgeon.

- management of respiratory insufficiency due to anesthetic or relaxant drugs is the domain of the anesthetist.

RESPIRATORY OBSTRUCTION

- usually occurs in the recovery room or ward some hours after anesthesia; the
- diagnosis is made, and the patient's life can be saved only if the medical staff is vigilant. The
- immediate treatment is
  —to establish a clear airway and
  —administer oxygen by bag and mask.
- diagnose the cause of obstruction and treat it promptly and appropriately as follows:

  Upper respiratory tract obstruction
  - elevate jaw to prevent tongue from blocking airway, insert
  - oropharyngeal airway or
  - endotracheal tube for laryngeal edema,
  - aspirate secretions and
  - remove the cause.

  Lower respiratory tract obstruction
  - aspirate secretions through endotracheal tube or nasolaryngeal catheter.
  - for aspiration of vomitus, see below.
  - aminophylline for bronchospasm;
  - thoracocentesis and chest tube for pneumothorax or hemothorax;
  - digitalis and diuretics for congestive heart failure and for fluid overload, if necessary;
  - continue assisted ventilation until the problem is solved.

METABOLIC ACIDOSIS

- this is a likely cause of impaired respiration after
  —emergency surgery for bowel obstruction;
  —cardiac arrest or
  —major tissue hypoxia.

- test the patient's pH;
- give 200 ml of a 2.74% solution of sodium bicarbonate IV in 20 minutes and
- another 400 ml over the next hour;
- adjust further infusion to clinical response; this
- alkali therapy may lower ionized serum calcium, so give 10 ml of 10% solution of calcium gluconate IV as necessary.

PULMONARY COMPLICATIONS

Atelectasis

Prevention

- preoperative assessment of pulmonary status;
- no smoking for several weeks before surgery!
- teach effective coughing before surgery (the physiotherapist should see the patient);
- treat existing upper respiratory tract or pulmonary disease.
- after surgery the physiotherapist should continue working with the patient for
  - —assisted, vigorous coughing as soon as the patient awakes from the anesthetic,
  - —postural drainage and
  - —percussion to loosen sputum;
- continue assisted ventilation if prolonged hypoventilation is likely.

Treatment

- start as soon as diagnosis is suspected;
- do not wait for signs of infection!
- use appropriate bronchodilators;
- physiotherapist should treat the patient regularly several times a day until the patient is cured,
  - —encourage deep breathing and coughing (give a mild analgesic half an hour before physiotherapist's visit);
  - —teach the patient with an abdominal or chest wound to draw the knees up, support the wound with his hands and then cough;
  - —use postural drainage in prone and lateral positions and thoracic percussion particularly to collapsed areas; if possible, the

—patient should sit out of bed for a short while the day after surgery. This change of posture and deep respirations caused by the effort are excellent measures for prevention and treatment of atelectasis;

- between the physiotherapist's visits, the medical and nursing staff should encourage
  —movement,
  —deep breathing and
  —assisted coughing;
- reduce viscosity of secretions by inhalation of water mist;
- aspirate secretions by nasotracheal catheter if necessary;
- bronchoscopy helps in
  —massive collapse or when the
  —atelectatic lobe does not respond to other measures.

Pneumonia and bronchopneumonia

- culture and sensitivity tests of sputum and
- broad spectrum antibiotics until antibiogram results are available. Then change to appropriate drug;
- deep breathing, coughing and postural drainage are very important;
- aspiration of secretions;
- tracheostomy may be necessary to
  —reduce dead space,
  —facilitate aspiration of secretions and
  —prevent death from hypoxia, CO_2 retention and respiratory failure;
- if this fails, then use
  —assisted mechanical ventilation.

Aspiration pneumonitis

Prevention

- ensure that the stomach is "empty" before anesthesia by
  —waiting 6 hours after the last meal before anesthetizing, or in the case of an
  —emergency, by emptying the stomach through a large orogastric tube or a 7-mm nasogastric tube or by employing regional anesthesia;
- use a cuffed endotracheal tube during surgery;

- hold the patient in a lateral position with pillows after surgery and
- clear the mouth and pharynx by suction.

Treatment
- head-down position immediately;
- tracheal suction and bronchial suction through endotracheal tube or bronchoscope to remove solid material;
- oxygen;
- wash trachea with 10 ml of saline,
- suction again immediately and
- repeat until aspirate is clear;
- dilute solution of sodium bicarbonate can be used if the gastric contents were aspirated;
- hydrocortisone, 100 mg IV every 6 hours for 1 to 3 days;
- aminophylline, 0.5 gm IV for bronchospasm;
- broad-spectrum antibiotics;
- give diuretics if pulmonary edema develops;
- intubation and mechanical ventilation if pulmonary edema does not respond to diuretics, and
- digitalize if cardiac failure develops.

ADULT RESPIRATORY DISTRESS SYNDROME
- assisted ventilation and
- steroids in
  - —large doses
  - —early to reduce pulmonary inflammation and pulmonary vascular resistance;
- colloid administration to restore colloid osmotic pressure of blood,
- restriction of IV fluids, especially those containing large amounts of crystalloids, e.g., Ringer's;
- heparin if disseminated intravascular coagulation is suspected;
- prophylactic antibiotics and
- prompt and proper treatment of infection.

FAT EMBOLISM SYNDROME
Prevention
- early immobilization of long-bone fractures is most important in preventing this syndrome;

- plasma albumin normally
  —binds and transports almost all the circulating free fatty acids;
  —low albumin levels allow
  —increased quantity of these acids to circulate in blood stream, thus creating
  —propitious conditions for development of fat embolism syndrome;
- maintenance of plasma albumin above 3.5 gm/100 ml during the initial 3 to 4 days after injury may reduce this risk.

Treatment

General measures

Cardiorespiratory support

- is the most important aspect of treatment;
- maintain the airway;
- give oxygen immediately, maintain PaO_2 higher than 70 mm Hg (give less than 40% oxygen; a higher percentage causes toxicity);
- endotracheal tube or tracheostomy, if necessary, e.g., if PaO_2 of 70 mm Hg cannot be maintained on safe inspired oxygen content (less than 40%); tube or tracheostomy
  —allows suctioning,
  —prevents aspiration into the lungs and
  —increases oxygenation of alveolar air by decreasing the dead space;
- PEEP mechanical ventilator may be indicated;
- digitalization if acute right heart failure is present.

Shock

- restore blood volume,
- restore fluid and electrolyte balance and
- monitor fluid replacement with central venous pressure (CVP) line to avoid overload;
- fluid replacement should be more colloid than crystalloid solution because the latter leaks into pulmonary interstitial tissue and increases the pulmonary edema;
- general care of the unconscious patient.

Fractures

- immobilize fractures to avoid further emboli;
- transport the patient gently, and only when absolutely necessary;

- reduce manipulations of injured parts to a minimum.

Specific measures

Steroids

- these improve gas exchange and reduce hypoxia by
  —stabilizing lysosomal and capillary membranes, thus
  —reducing inflammatory response and
  —decreasing capillary leaks in alveolar membranes;

Low-molecular-weight dextran

- improves microcirculatory blood flow,
- temporarily expands plasma volume and
- prevents clotting by forming a dextran-fibrinogen complex. But
- benefit in fat embolism is uncertain.
- contraindications include
  —pulmonary edema and congestive heart failure,
  —renal failure,
  —severe dehydration,
  —hypofibrinogenemia and
  —localized septic process.
- dosage is 500 ml every 12 to 24 hours by slow IV infusion.

Heparin

- lypolytic agent, and
- prevents platelet aggregation, but it
- is not recommended because the disadvantages outweigh the advantages.

Summary of treatment

- airway
- oxygen and PEEP
- blood
- steroids

Prognosis

- severe syndrome with marked pulmonary insufficiency and coma has
  —poor prognosis (50% mortality); but pulmonary lesions are
  —reversible if the syndrome is
  —diagnosed early and
  —treated promptly.
- mild syndrome has good prognosis.
- where diagnosis is made, the overall mortality rate is 10% to 15%.

chapter 24

Acute Postoperative Renal Failure

Renal Function

- kidney has three principal functions
  - —filtration, and
  - —sodium and
  - —water resorption.

HOURLY URINE VOLUME

- measurement of hourly urine volume is not, by itself, a reliable test of renal function; e.g.,
  - —oliguria in a dehydrated patient and
  - —polyuria in an overhydrated patient both show that the kidneys are functioning well. The oliguria and polyuria are both appropriate responses for the circumstances.
- normal urine volume is 30 to 60 ml/hour with proper postoperative fluid management and normal kidneys.
- inappropriate urine volume is frequently the first clinical evidence that renal failure may be developing, e.g.,
  - —oliguria in an overhydrated patient or normally hydrated patient, or
  - —polyuria in a dehydrated patient;
- wide deviation from normal range of hourly output may signify impending renal dysfunction.

FILTRATION

Physiology

- plasma is filtered through the glomerular capsule. This is an ultrafiltrate of plasma;
- volume of filtrate (glomerular filtration rate, GFR) depends on balance between the

    —hydrostatic forces of plasma in the capillary tuft and fluid in Bowman's capsule and the

    —opposing forces of osmotic pressure of plasma proteins in the capillary holding fluid back.

- normally, the hydrostatic pressure of fluid in Bowman's capsule is vented through the renal tubule, and the plasma osmotic pressure is fixed. So the
- major variable for regulation of GFR is the hydrostatic pressure within the glomerular capillary tuft;
- this hydrostatic pressure is regulated by alterations in the vascular tone of afferent and efferent arterioles;

    —vasodilation of afferent vessels and

    —vasoconstriction of efferent vessels

    —increase the intracapillary hydrostatic pressure of the glomerular tuft, and GFR will increase.

- the vascular tone of these vessels is regulated by the juxtaglomerular apparatus which secretes renin. This releases angiotensin, the active vasomotor substance.

Measurement of GFR

- creatinine is removed from the body mainly by filtration, so
- most creatinine in urine has passed through the glomerular filtrate at the concentration that exists in plasma;
- collect urine for 1 hour and

    —measure its volume and the

    —total creatinine in it;

- then calculate creatinine concentration in urine, in milligrams per 100 ml (U);
- and calculate the volume of urine excreted every minute, in milliliters (V);
- measure the concentration of creatinine in plasma, in milligrams per 100 ml (P);
- then

$$\text{GFR} = UV/P$$

- this measurement is important in the investigation of the postoperative patient who may have incipient renal failure.
- normal GFR is

    —100 ml/minute for a young adult and

—70 to 80 for the elderly;

—less than 30 ml is associated with acute renal failure.

- inulin or urea can be used instead of creatinine.

SODIUM CONSERVATION

Physiology

- 85% of sodium filtered in the glomerulus is reabsorbed in the proximal convoluted tubule;
- more is reabsorbed in the loop of Henle and the distal convoluted tubule, the latter being influenced by aldosterone;
- increased concentration of sodium in the distal tubule stimulates secretion of
  —renin by the juxtaglomerular apparatus. Renin releases
  —angiotensin which decreases blood flow through the glomerulus secondary to afferent arteriolar constriction. This
  —reduces GFR, and the amount of sodium filtered is therefore reduced too.
- normally, about
  —30,000 mEq of sodium are filtered by the glomeruli every 24 hours;
  —all but 50 mEq are reabsorbed into the body by the tubules, through passive diffusion across a concentration gradient and by active sodium pumping.

Evaluation of tubular function

- ratio of
  —urine creatinine concentration in milligrams per 100 ml to
  —plasma creatinine concentration in milligrams per 100 ml is a measure of tubular reabsorption of water (creatinine is not reabsorbed); a
- normal kidney working at maximum effort produces a urine to plasma creatinine ratio of about 100.
- this falls to 10 or less in established renal failure. The
- urine/plasma sodium ratio is a more direct measure of tubular function;
- normally this is about 0.1;
- failure of the tubular exchange mechanism may produce urine concentration similar to plasma concentration, and the ratio may be nearly 1.0.

URINE CONCENTRATION

- water is reabsorbed from filtrate as it passes down collecting tubules. This
- concentrates urine and conserves water.
- ability of the kidney to concentrate the urine by reabsorbing water depends on
  —normal collecting tubules, the
  —presence of ADH which controls the collecting tubule's permeability to water, and
  —adequate tubular function to pump sodium out of the tubule into the kidney interstitial tissue, thus increasing tonicity of this peritubular tissue fluid; water is then reabsorbed from the collecting tubules across this osmotic gradient. A
- simple test is to measure urine specific gravity;
- concentrating ability can also be assessed by measuring urine/plasma osmolar ratio, normally greater than 1.3;
- failure of urine concentration makes urine almost isosmotic with plasma. about 1.0.

ONE-HOUR RENAL FUNCTION TEST

- this measures
  —GFR,
  —tubular function and
  —concentrating ability;
- it can be made by taking a single
  —1-hour urine collection and a single
  —serum sample, and calculating the
  —1-hour creatinine clearance for GFR, and the urine/plasma ratios of
  —creatinine (normal, about 100), and
  —sodium (normal, about 0.14) for tubular function, and
  —total osmolarity (normal, greater than 1.3) for concentrating ability.

Prerenal and Renal Failure

CLASSIFICATION OF RENAL FAILURE

- acute renal failure is an inability of the kidneys to maintain the normal internal environment ("milieu intérieur," described by the

French physiologist Claude Bernard);
* oliguria is urine output of less than 20 ml an hour in an adult.
* acute postoperative oliguria and renal failure are almost always due to fluid volume depletion (excessive fluid loss);
* however, the differential diagnosis must include all possible causes of oliguria.
* prerenal oliguria is
  —secondary to reduced blood flow through the kidneys; the
  —kidneys are normal and are trying to correct an abnormal internal environment, e.g., hypotension associated with hemorrhage, fluid loss, heart failure with inadequate cardiac output or dehydration. In
* renal oliguria, the kidneys are abnormal and cannot maintain a normal internal environment; causes include
  —abnormal globin pigment associated with hypotension or hyponatremia,
  —renal ischemia due to hypotension with acute tubular necrosis, or
  —toxic agents, e.g., carbon tetrachloride (carpet cleaner).
* postrenal oliguria is due to urinary tract obstruction which prevents urine reaching the exterior; strictly speaking this is not renal failure, the kidneys are normal.

ETIOLOGY

Predisposing factors

Hypotension
* mean blood pressure (BP) below 40 mm Hg will cause oliguria but will not cause renal failure by itself; however,
* sustained hypotension may make the kidneys vulnerable to other factors which may cause renal failure, so
* arterial pressure should be kept above 60 mm Hg.

Abnormal globin pigment
* abnormal circulating globin pigments may be
  —hemoglobin after transfusion reaction, due to massive intravascular hemolysis; or
  —myoglobin after muscle crush injury, with massive tissue destruction and release of myoglobin;
* these filter into the urine and discolor it; if these
* pigments remain in kidney tubules, they cause renal damage and failure; if

- urine volume is more than 60 ml/hour, renal damage is unlikely, but if
- hypotension and oliguria exist as well, then renal failure is very likely.

Increased renal vascular resistance

- renal vascular resistance may be abnormally increased by
  —crushing injuries or
  —operative stimulation of renal and splanchnic nerves even though cardiac output and total peripheral resistance are normal;
- if this lasts for several days, risk of renal failure is increased.

Precipitating factors

- dehydration or
- hyponatremia, combined with one or more predisposing factors, may precipitate acute renal failure, especially if the abnormal situation persists for several hours.

PATHOGENESIS

- acute postoperative renal failure is usually the result of a combination of two or more abnormal clinical conditions.
- severe hypotension with hypoxia
  —reduces capillary tuft hydrostatic pressure with a consequent fall in GFR and
  —impairs the resorptive capacity of the proximal tubule, where 85% of the sodium in the filtrate is normally reabsorbed. An
- increased content of sodium in the filtrate arriving at the distal tubule stimulates the
  —juxtaglomerular apparatus to secrete renin, which causes release in plasma of
  —angiotensin II. This produces prolonged
  —vasoconstriction of afferent arterioles, thus reducing still further the GFR and tubular function. This is a
- reflex mechanism designed to
  —prevent further loss of sodium and water, but in these circumstances (hypotension and renal ischemia) it merely
  —aggravates an already inadequate renal function, and a
  —vicious circle is established (Fig. 24.1). This
- tubuloglomerular feedback mechanism may reduce GFR to the point where the volume of glomerular filtrate is insufficient to remove

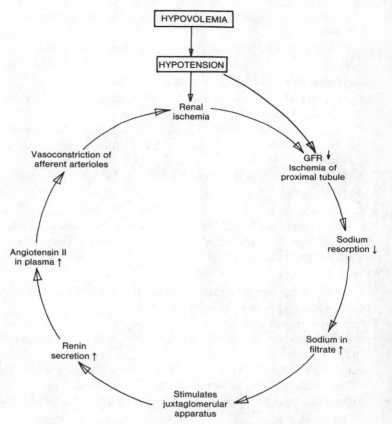

Figure 24.1. Vicious circle of hypovolemia and renal failure.

nitrogenous wastes, with resulting
- oliguria and
- azotemia. If
- renal ischemia is severe, tubular necrosis may occur. In extreme ischemia, massive cortical necrosis results in complete and permanent anuria.
- other complex relationships between renin and angiotensin production, secretion of prostaglandins and neurotransmission are probably involved as well.

DIAGNOSIS

- every patient "at risk" should have his fluid intake and output measured postoperatively until he has regained physiological equilibrium.

Suspicion

- urine volume of
  —less than 30 ml/hour is oliguria, and you should suspect
  —impending or existing acute renal failure of prerenal or renal origin;
- complete anuria never occurs with prerenal renal failure, and rarely with primary (renal) renal failure.

Confirmation

- to confirm your suspicions, perform without delay a routine urinalysis and the 1-hour renal function test and simultaneously
- restore fluid volume with appropriate fluids.
- abnormal results of the 1-hour renal function test confirm that renal failure is
  —impending or that it
  —exists already.
- if oliguria persists after mean arterial blood pressure is restored to more than 80 mm Hg, then acute renal failure with some degree of renal tubular damage already exists.
- with these tests you can differentiate between prerenal and primary (renal) renal failure (Table 24.1).
- raised BUN and serum creatinine concentrations are consequences of acute renal failure, not signs of it. Do not wait for these before starting therapy, or you will be too late.

PREVENTION

- hourly urine output is the cornerstone of objective evaluation of the state of blood volume and cardiorespiratory and renal function in the postoperative patient;
- acute renal failure is one of the most serious postoperative complications; the
- civilian mortality rate of established failure is 60% in the United States in spite of modern progress with dialysis and transplantation;
- during the Korean War, 1 in 200 seriously injured soldiers developed acute renal failure, and 9 of every 10 with acute renal failure died.
- during the Vietnamese War, only 1 in 600 developed renal failure,

Table 24.1
Differentiation between Acute Renal Failure of Prerenal and Renal Origin

Measurement	Pre-Renal Renal Failure	Primary (Renal) Renal Failure
Urine specific gravity	More than 1.015	Less than 1.015
Urine/plasma creatinine ratio	More than 20	Less than 14
Urine sodium concentration in mEq/L	Less than 10	More than 20
Urine osmolality	50 to 100 mOsm greater than plasma	Equal to or less than plasma

indicating an improvement in the prevention of this complication. But still the mortality rate was 90% and had not changed!

- acute renal failure must be anticipated and prevented because treatment is of little avail.
- to prevent acute postoperative failure in a susceptible patient or in a patient who has oliguria and impending renal failure with an abnormal 1-hour renal function test, you must prevent prolonged
  —hypovolemia and hypotension,
  —hypoxia
  —oliguria and renal vasoconstriction;
- correct fluid imbalance by
  —restoration of extracellular fluid volume and
  —circulatory blood volume, to maintain mean arterial blood pressure above 80 mm Hg and GFR above 60 ml/minute;
  —if a prerenal origin is suspected, give 500 to 1,000 ml (depending on the age, size and condition of the patient) of half normal (0.45%) saline over 1 hour. This will rapidly help to correct dehydration;
  —correct hypoxia. These measures may prevent vasoconstriction of renal afferent arterioles.
- restore promptly electrolyte imbalance, especially of extracellular space.

- reduce renin secretion by administration of 25 to 50 gm of mannitol IV to all high-risk patients. Mannitol is more effective before surgery than after it.

TREATMENT

- as soon as diagnosis of impending or existing acute postoperative renal failure is made, start the following treatment:

Maintain ''milieu intérieur''

- renal failure in the postoperative period has a higher mortality rate than does any other kind of renal failure, due to
- disturbance of "milieu intérieur,"
  - —electrolyte
  - —water and
  - —nitrogen imbalance.

Potassium

- potassium is liberated from cells postoperatively due to
  - —accelerated catabolic state and
  - —tissue injury;
- in renal failure, potassium is not excreted and the serum level rises rapidly with
  - —myocardial dysfunction and
  - —ECG changes (tall T wave, small P wave, wide QRS complex) when serum potassium is 7 to 8 mEq, and
  - —cardiac arrest when level is 9 or 10.
- all patients with renal failure must be monitored with ECG, and you must start treatment at first abnormal stage.
- stop administration of K^+ ions contained in
  - —balanced electrolyte solutions, e.g., Ringer's solution, and in
  - —drugs, e.g., aqueous penicillin K^+;
- use ion exchange resins, e.g.,
  - —Kayexalate, 20 gm three to four times a day orally, or by enema, with
  - —sorbitol, 20 ml of 70% solution;
  - —if ECG changes are pronounced, give
- calcium chloride, 10 ml of a 10% solution IV slowly, but not if the patient is digitalized. In this instance, give
- glucose, 500 ml of a 10% solution IV with
- regular insulin, 10 units.
- calcium, glucose and insulin therapy are temporary and only

reduce the serum levels for a while without eliminating potassium from the body. Elimination can only be achieved by ion exchange resin or by

- dialysis
    —hemodialysis (most effective) or
    —peritoneal dialysis.

Water

- repeat frequently the 1-hour renal function test for early diagnosis of acute renal failure. Do not "give fluids and hope the patient urinates!"
- fluids will overhydrate the patient, and this is the next most serious threat to his life. The
- daily water requirement of a totally anuric patient is about 500 ml on a winter day and 1,000 ml or more on a hot, dry summer day;
- if the patient is oliguric, give 500 ml/day (or more, depending on ambient temperature) plus a volume equal to the urine output of the previous 24 hours; the
- constancy of serum sodium concentration is a useful guide to the adequacy of water replacement; the
- patient should lose 0.5 to 1 kg of body weight a day during this period. If he does not, he is overhydrated;
- there is some evidence that if loop diuretics, e.g., furosemide (Lasix), are administered immediately after acute tubular necrosis is suspected, they will increase GFR and will prevent establishment of acute tubular necrosis.

Nitrogen catabolism

- nitrogen catabolism is increased after surgery;
- oliguria prevents adequate excretion of these nitrogenous substances, and uremia (azotemia) develops;
- eliminate all protein from the diet to reduce sources of
    —nitrogen,
    —potassium,
    —phosphates and
    —sulphates.
- to prevent ketosis (metabolic acidosis due to ketone and keto acid products of metabolism of protein and fat) and
- to reduce protein catabolism, give

- glucose
  - —100 to 200 gm daily orally, or
  - —500 to 1,000 ml of 20% or 200 to 400 ml of 50% glucose solution into a large vein (to avoid venous thrombosis). Administer
- vitamins intravenously or intramuscularly, especially
  - —B vitamins and
  - —ascorbic acid (vitamin C).
- dialysis is not usually necessary before 5 to 7 days after the start of oliguria, although
- early and repeated dialysis may prevent death from
  - —hyperkalemia,
  - —water intoxication and
  - —uremia.
- indications for dialysis are serum
  - —BUN more than 120 mg/100 ml,
  - —potassium more than 6.0 mEq/liter, or
  - —creatinine more than 15 mg/100 ml.

Late systemic complications

- the most serious late complications are associated with
  - —hemorrhage,
  - —infection and
  - —drug intoxication.
- massive gastrointestinal bleeding is the major cause of death in patients with acute postoperative renal failure, and is
- due to
  - —coagulation defects associated with renal failure and
  - —stress ulceration of gastric mucosa.
- to prevent or treat this complication
  - —use antacid solutions orally to maintain gastric pH above 6,
  - —avoid gastric irritants, e.g., aspirin, Butazolidin (aspirin also interferes with platelet function and thus aggravates coagulation abnormalities), and
  - —replace clotting factors.
- infection is an important cause of late death in renal failure;
- prevent infection by using strict aseptic techniques for catheterization and similar procedures;
- established infection must be
  - —diagnosed early and

—treated promptly and properly.
- continuation of drugs normally excreted by the kidneys will produce toxic blood levels in a patient with renal failure, e.g.,
  —digitalis and
  —antibiotics;
- resultant drug toxicity may kill the patient, so
- reduce dosages accordingly.

RECOVERY

- if the kidneys are not badly damaged, recovery starts 3 to 5 days
  later.
- if severe tubular necrosis occurs, recovery starts 10 to 21 days later.
- recovery is usually heralded by an
  —increased urine output, but
  —nephrons are not necessarily normal at this time, and
  —increased sodium and water loss may produce
  —hypovolemia and hypotension, with recurrence of acute renal
    failure!
- accurate maintenance of salt and water balance will prevent this
  relapse. A
- normal 1-hour renal function test is the best gauge of renal recovery.

Acute Anuria and Renal Failure of Postrenal Origin

- complete anuria in a postoperative or trauma patient is usually
  indicative of postrenal obstruction.

Etiology

- urethral catheter blocked or misdirected into a false passage;
- urethral or bladder rupture;
- injury to both ureters, usually caused by surgeon at operation!
- bilateral ureteric stones.

Diagnosis

- irrigate catheter and change it if necessary. If the result is negative,
  do a
- urethrogram and/or cystogram as circumstances indicate. If results
  are negative again, do
- cystoscopy and retrograde ureteric catheterization.
- if results are still negative, anuria is probably of renal origin, so
  treat the patient as for primary (renal) renal failure.

Treatment

- institute treatment appropriate to the cause.
    - —surgical repair of injuries,
    - —removal of stones and
    - —nonoperative treatment for primary (renal) renal failure.

Summary

Oliguria

- usually due to inadequate perfusion of kidneys;
- investigate early with routine urinalysis and 1-hour renal function test;
- prevent by
    - —restoration of fluid volumes,
    - —correction of hypoxia and
    - —IV mannitol;
- treat with
    - —restriction of water, electrolyte and protein intake,
    - —hyperalimentation,
    - —ion exchange resin,
    - —calcium chloride or glucose and insulin;
    - —dialysis as a last resort.

Anuria

- usually due to urinary tract obstruction;
- investigate cause and treat it immediately.

chapter 25

Infection and the Body's Response

BODY'S DEFENSES

- outcome of bacterial invasion of the host depends on balance between
  - —host's defenses and
  - —organism's offensive weaponry (virulence), with
- therapeutic armamentarium generally fighting on the host's side.

SKIN

- the most important first line of defense in orthopaedic surgery;
- frequently contaminated, infrequently infected;
- to produce infection, the
  - —tough keratin layer, the
  - —many-layered epithelial layer and the
  - —basement membrane must be breached.
- decontamination occurs by
  - —desquamation of the surface layer and desiccation, and
  - —competition and antibiotic production by resident flora;
  - —lactic acid in sweat and
  - —unsaturated fatty acids in sebaceous secretions are bactericidal.

OTHER TISSUES

- these have individual defense mecahnisms, e.g.,
  - —saliva contains lysozyme and
  - —gastric juice is acidic.

INFLAMMATORY REACTION

- antibacterial activity is a major function of this reaction, through
- polymorphonuclear leukocytes and monocytes (macrophages),
- complement and opsonins and
- antibodies (see Chapter 17)

LYMPHATICS

- regional lymph nodes are the second line of defense;
- incoming lymph enters the
  —cortical sinus,
  —circulates around a reticular network lined by
  —lymphocytes and reticuloendothelial system (RES) cells before leaving the node by efferent vessels from the medullary sinuses.

BLOOD STREAM

- third line of defense;
- blood contains
  —antibacterial substances (complement, opsonins and others),
  —specific, acquired antibodies, and
  —phagocytes (less important here than in local inflammatory exudate).
- reticuloendothelial system, especially cells lining sinuses of the
  —liver,
  —spleen and
  —bone marrow, is the major defense against bacteremia. If the RES fails, then flooding of the bloodstream with pathogenic organisms becomes
- septicemia, and the patient is gravely ill.

IMMUNE RESPONSE

Immunity

- toxic group of organisms produces
  —exotoxins; these are
  —strongly antigenic and provoke
  —humoral antibody response (usually IgG);
- invasive group of organisms does not produce exotoxins and provokes
  —cellular immune response;
- active immunity may be
  —natural, by acquisition of the disease, e.g., a subclinical attack of poliomyelitis virus; or
  —artificial, by vaccination, e.g., Salk vaccine for poliomyelitis, toxoid for tetanus.
- passive immunity may be
  —natural, e.g., the neonate through the mother's milk; or

—passive, by injection of immunoglobulins, e.g., prevention of tetanus;
- passive immunity is short-lived, weeks (adult) or months (infant).
- two immunological systems exist
  —humoral and
  —cell-based. They are mostly
- independent of each other, but in some circumstances they
- work together (synergism) and in others they
- control each other (antagonism);
- both systems are necessary for
- full immunological response.

Immunological cells
- lymphocytes develop from
- reticular stem cells in bone marrow

T lymphocytes
- develop under influence of
- thymus and circulate from the bloodstream through the
- paracortical area (between the cortex and medulla) of lymph nodes or through the
- spleen and thence back to the bloodstream. These lymphocytes
- live for months and are involved in
- cell-mediated immunity.
- sensitized lymphocytes release chemical substances which may
  —kill invading organisms and other
  —foreign cells (graft reaction);
  —prevent a virus from proliferating in a cell already sensitized by viral invasion (interferon);
  —induce and augment an inflammatory reaction, perhaps by chemotaxis on inflammatory cells;
  —increase phagocytic properties of macrophages and
  —immobilize them at the site of invasion, thus localizing the infection;
  —recruit and sensitize more immune cells. Some of these substances may also cause
- delayed hypersensitivity (type IV hypersensitivity, contact dermatitis, tuberculin reaction).

B lymphocytes
- development of B lymphocytes is influenced by
- bursal tissue (so-called after the bursa of Fabricius in birds) in

small intestine (Peyer's patches) and in the appendix and colon. These cells are found infrequently in the bloodstream but stay in

- primary germinal follicles in the cortex of lymph nodes and are the
- first to encounter antigens in incoming lymph draining a more distal area. These are
- short-lived lymphocytes (days) and together with plasma cells (origin unknown) are involved in
- humoral (circulating) antibody production.
- they produce immunoglobulins. These may
  —neutralize exotoxins and help to
  —destroy invading organisms.
- immunoglobins may also cause drug reactions of the following types, where the drug acts as a hapten and combines with host protein to form an antigen:
  —immediate (type I hypersensitivity, IgE, anaphylactic shock),
  —cytotoxic reaction (type II, IgG or IgM, hemolytic anemia),
  —antigen-antibody complexes (type III, IgG, urticaria).

Bacteriology

GENERAL CHARACTERISTICS OF BACTERIUM

Structure

Nucleus
- no limiting membrane;
- rich in DNA;
- basophilic.

Cytoplasm
- ribosomes abundant;
- does not have
  —endoplasmic reticulum,
  —Golgi apparatus,
  —centrosome;
- cytoplasmic membrane is
  —selectively permeable, plays role of
  —osmotic barrier, and controls
  —excretion of specific polysaccharides and proteins (exotoxins).

Cell wall
- protects and maintains shape of organism,
- resists strong intrabacterial osmotic pressure and helps bacterium avoid osmotic lysis,
- determines whether bacterium is Gram-positive or Gram-negative,
- holds somatic antigens.

Capsule
- present in some bacteria;
- determines virulence of some pathogenic bacteria;
- discourages phagocytosis by white cells.

Spores
- some bacteria form spores in adverse conditions;
- can resist
  —relative extremes of temperature, humidity and pressure,
  —ultraviolet irradiation and some
  —chemical agents and antibiotics.

L-forms
- degenerate bacterial variants
  —vary in size and shape,
  —resistant to penicillin;
- named after Joseph Lister (England's answer to Louis Pasteur!).

Pathogenicity
- bacteria are pathogenic when they can
  —multiply in tissues and
  —cause disease, and are
- virulent when they can
  —cause severe disease.
- certain factors enable bacteria to invade and establish themselves in the host's tissues:
- infective dose
  —the more bacteria there are, the better the chances of overcoming the defenses;
- portal of entry
  —tuberculous bacilli are more dangerous in the lung than in the intestine;
- production of chemical substances which may
  —repel (negative chemotaxis) or even

—kill white cells (leukocidin), and other
—exotoxins which may cause many of the manifestations of the
   disease;
- release of surface antigens which can
  —neutralize antibodies (meningococcus);
- discouragement of phagocytosis by unpleasant surface antigens;
- ingestion by white cells which may transport the bacteria elsewhere
   without being able to kill them (e.g., tuberculosis)
- spread of bacterial infection locally by
  —natural passages and spaces, perhaps facilitated by
  —exotoxin production (e.g., hyaluronidase), and
- spread generally by
  —lymphatics and
  —blood stream, encouraged by intermittent contraction of muscles
     which pump fluid up vessels (Hippocrates, 2,500 years ago on
     the Greek island of Cos, advised rest for an inflamed part).

SPECIFIC CHARACTERISTICS

Staphylococci

Morphology

- Gram-positive,
- round, 1 mm diameter, clusters,
- nonmotile, no spores, no capsule.

Pathophysiology

- aerobe and facultative anaerobe, i.e.,
  —prefers aerobic conditions but
  —can survive in anaerobic environment;
- grows on most media;
- strains typed using bacteriophages;
- *Staphylococcus aureus* is invasive and produces
- enzymes
  —coagulase,
  —staphylokinase, lyzes fibrin, and
  —hyaluronidase;
- endotoxins
  —lyze red blood cells and
  —kill white cells. Some strains produce an
- exotoxin which causes food poisoning.
- typical lesion is an abscess.

Streptococci

Morphology

- Gram-positive
- round, little less than 1 μm diameter, chains,
- nonmotile, no spores, some have thin capsules.

Pathophysiology

- aerobe and facultative anaerobe;
- grow best on blood agar;
- three groups exist:
  —alpha, shows a zone of partial hemolysis around the cultured colony,
  —beta, complete hemolysis due to production of a soluble hemolysin,
  —gamma, no hemolysis;
- some beta-hemolytic streptococci may cause serious lesions in man. Lancefield, by serological method,
- subdivided the beta-hemolytic group into 15 subgroups according to the antigen in the bacterial wall. Most human pathogens are in
- Lancefield's group A. These are
- *Streptococcus pyogenes.* Serologically, Griffith
- subdivided group A into more than 50 smaller groups according to the M and T antigens on the surface;
- M antigen inhibits phagocytosis and determines virulence.
- *S. pyogenes* is invasive and produces
- enzymes
  —streptokinase, lyzes fibrin,
  —hyaluronidase and
  —streptodornase, destroys DNA; and
- endotoxins
  —lyze red cells,
  —kill white cells and
  —interfere with heart action. Some strains produce an
- erythrogenic exotoxin (scarlet fever). The
- typical lesion is cellulitis.

Pneumococcus

- *Diplococcus pneumoniae*

Morphology

- Gram-positive
- oval, less than 1 μm diameter, paired,
- nonmotile, no spores, has a capsule.

Pathophysiology

- aerobe and facultative anaerobe;
- grows best on blood agar;
- zone of greenish hemolysis around colony;
- serological typing based on specific soluble substance (SSS) hapten in capsule. This determines the organism's virulence.
- typical lesion is lobar pneumonia.

Gonococcus

- *Neisseria gonorrhoeae*

Morphology

- Gram-negative,
- kidney-shaped, pairs,
- nonmotile, no spores, no capsule.

Pathophysiology

- grows on blood and chocolate agar in the presence of 5% CO_2;
- invasive, produces an
- endotoxin.
- typical disease is
  —gonorrhea contracted by sexual contact; may also cause
  —monarticular arthritis.

Escherichia coli

Morphology

- Gram-negative
- rods,
- motile, no spores, no capsule.

Pathophysiology

- aerobe and facultative anaerobe;
- grows on blood agar and ferments lactose (MacConkey's medium);
- may produce an endotoxin.
- organism is normally present in bowel, and only

- pathogenic when transferred to other tissues;
- produces suppurative lesion.

Proteus vulgaris

Morphology

- Gram-negative
- rods,
- motile, no spores, no capsule.

Pathophysiology

- aerobe and facultative anaerobe;
- grows on blood agar, may swarm over surface in confluent layer; does not ferment lactose;
- smells of fish!
- frequently a normal denizen of the bowel;
- may cause secondary infection of surgical wounds and is
- common cross-infection organism in hospital.

Pseudomonas pyocyanea

Morphology

- Gram-negative
- rod,
- motile, no spores, no capsule.

Pathophysiology

- aerobe and facultative anaerobe;
- blood agar, does not ferment lactose;
- culture and pus is blue-green (clearly seen on nutrient agar and patient's dressings!) because organism produces
  —fluorescein and pyocyanin;
- smells of fruit!
- infrequent inhabitant of bowel;
- common in secondary infection and cross-infection in hospitals; investigation includes serological and bacteriophage typing.
- invasive, especially of blood vessels, and may produce
- septicemia.

Klebsiella

Morphology

- Gram-negative
- rod,
- nonmotile, no spores, has a capsule.

Pathophysiology

- aerobe and facultative anaerobe;
- blood agar;
- causes pneumonia and secondary wound infections.

Clostridia

Morphology

- Gram-positive
- rods, 5 μm long,
- motile, have capsules except *Clostridium welchii*,
- all have spores.

Pathophysiology

- obligatory anaerobes, i.e., cannot grow in the presence of oxygen; so use
- blood agar in McIntosh and Fildes' jar for anerobic atmosphere in laboratory.
- present in soil and urban dust (houses, hospital wards!); *C. welchii* inhabits human bowel;
- spores allow organisms to survive
  —heat and
  —desiccation.
- organisms cause
  —gas gangrene and
  —tetanus
  Gas gangrene organisms
- two groups exist, based on biochemical reactions:
- saccharolytic group ferments sugars and includes the pathogens of gas gangrene
  —*C. welchii*,
  —*C. septicum* and
  —*C. oedematiens*;
- proteolytic group includes
  —*C. sporogenes* and
  —*C. histolyticum*. These break down protein and produce foul gases,
  —hydrogen sulfide and
  —ammonia. This group is responsible for the putrefactive phase of gas gangrene.
- exotoxins and enzymes are numerous and cause systemic

effects of gas gangrene, even though the infection remains localized. These substances include
—lecithinase (alpha toxin) which necrotizes and hemolyses red cells and kills laboratory animals,
—hemolysin,
—collagenase,
—deoxyribonuclease and
—hyaluronidase.

Tetanus
- *C. tetani* is neither saccharolytic nor proteolytic but
- produces a very powerful exotoxin
- tetanospasmin, a neurotoxin; the
- infection is
  —localized, with little or no local reaction, but
  —tetanospasmin travels proximally along
  —peripheral nerves. Here
  —antibodies can neutralize it. But when the toxin reaches the spinal cord and is fixed on the
  —anterior horn cells, antibodies are
  —ineffective.

Mycobacterium tuberculosis

Morphology
- thin rod, 3 μm long,
- nonmotile, no spores,
- waxy content prevents staining by normal methods;
- heated carbol-fuchsin (Ziehl-Neelsen method) stains the organism permanently, and even strong acids and alcohols will not remove the stain. Hence its colloquial name—acid-fast bacillus.

Pathophysiology
- aerobe,
- grows slowly on specialized media, e.g., Löwenstein-Jensen;
- resists drying but not sunlight (ultraviolet).
- clinical disease of tuberculosis in industrial nations caused mainly by
  —human strain, because
  —bovine strain has been largely eliminated from herds and milk is pasteurized (63° C for 30 minutes or 72° C for 20 seconds).

Antibiotics and Other Antibacterial Agents

- half of all the drugs prescribed in North America are antibiotics, and
- many are prescribed without proper indications! So
- drug abuse is not confined to teenagers!!
- prescribe antibiotics for
  —sound and
  —logical reasons;
- antibiotics are most effective as a
  —precision tool to
  —cure an infection caused by an
  —identified organism with
  —known antibiotic sensitivities;
- prophylactic antibiotics may help to
  —prevent postoperative infection if they are given
  —before and during surgery. But they are
  —not a substitute for strict, sterile technique in the operating room.
    Remember your table manners!
- antibiotics and other chemotherapeutic agents are classified in groups
  (families);
- do not prescribe two antibiotics from the same family (you will
  double the disadvantages without doubling the advantages)
- or a bactericidal with a bacteriostatic drug (antagonize each other).

BETA LACTAMINES

- contain a beta-lactamine ring. Some bacteria secrete
- beta lactamase (penicillinase) which inactivates the antibiotic.

  ### Penicillins

  - bactericidal
    —prevent dividing cell from synthesizing cell wall so that
    —bacteria absorb water due to high osmotic pressure, swell and
      explode;
  - probenecid blocks renal excretion of penicillin;
  - toxicity includes
    —allergies (rarely anaphylactic shock) and
    —CNS effects, irritability and convulsions with high doses;
  - synthetic penicillins are made by
    —adding side chains to
    —penicillinic acid, the penicillin nucleus.

Penicillin G

- still the best antibiotic available
  —powerful,
  —relatively broad spectrum,
  —low toxicity and
  —cheap!
- effective against Gram-positive and Gram-negative cocci
  —staphyloccus (nonproducer of penicillinase), streptococcus, pneumococcus,
  —gonococcus; and against
- Gram-positive bacilli in high doses
  —clostridia.
- dosage, 10,000 to 1,000,000 units/kg/day parenterally in divided doses.

Penicillin M

- oxacillin, methicillin (Bristopen and Penistaph are commercial names);
- semisynthetic;
- bactericidal action similar to
  —penicillin G, but also kills
  —staphylococcus that produces penicillinase.
- dosage, 30 to 100 mg/kg/day parenterally in divided doses.

Penicillin A

- ampicillin (Totapen);
- semisynthetic;
- effective against Gram-negative organisms, the enterobacteriaceae,
  —*E. coli*,
  —*Pseudomonas*,
  —*Salmonella*;
- inactive against staphylococcus
- dosage, 50 to 300 mg/kg/day orally or parenterally, in divided doses.

Cloxacillin

- similar to oxacillin but
- oral route gives serum concentrations twice that of oxacillin.
- dosage, 30 to 100 mg/kg/day orally or parenterally, in divided doses.

Dicloxacillin

- absorption from the gastrointestinal tract is better than all other synthetic penicillins;
- active against
  —penicillinase-producing staphylococcus
- dosage, 15 to 30 mg/kg/day orally in divided doses.

Cephalosporins

- cephalothin, cephaloridine and cephalexin are generic names.
- prevent synthesis of bacterial cell wall;
- resistant to penicillinase but
- destroyed by cephalosporinase;
- toxicity
  —allergies, but cross-sensitivity with penicillin is rare;
  —nephrotoxic, so monitor renal function;
- antibacterial spectrum similar to penicillins.
- dosage
  —cephalothin and cephaloridine, 30 to 50 mg/kg/day to a maximum of 4 gm parenterally,
  —cephalexin, 15 to 30 mg/kg/day.

AMINOSIDES

- bactericidal,
  —inhibit bacterial protein production on ribosomes and
  —interfere with cytoplasmic membrane formation;
- toxic to
  —cranial nerve VIII (irreversible) and
  —kidneys (kanamycin and gentamicin).

Streptomycin

- active especially against
  —*Mycobacterium tuberculosis*, but
- bacterial resistance easily develops.
- dosage, 1 gm/day for not more than 90 days, intramuscularly (IM) in a single dose.

Kanamycin and gentamicin

- active form excreted in urine, so
- useful in urinary infections;
- bactericidal against
  —Gram-positive cocci and

—*Enterobacteriaceae* (kanamycin not effective against *Pseudomonas*).
- dosage
  —kanamycin, 1 to 1.5 mg/kg/day IM.
  —gentamicin, 1.5 to 3 mg/kg/day IM, both in divided doses.

OTHER ANTITUBERCULOUS DRUGS

- resistant strains of *M. tuberculosis* develop
  —easily and rapidly to all chemotherapeutic agents; these should
  —never be used alone but should be combined in
  —double or
  —triple therapy, e.g., streptomycin with PAS and isoniazid.
- long-term therapy is essential.

Rifampin

- trade names: Rifadin and Rimactan;
- inhibits bacterial protein synthesis;
- toxicity
  —liver.
- dosage, 10 to 20 mg/kg/day to a maximum of 600 mg/day, orally in one dose.

Isoniazid

- derived from isonicotinic acid;
- diffuses easily into all body fluids and tissues;
- toxicity
  —liver and
  —peripheral neuropathies in poorly nourished patients; give pyridoxine (vitamin B6) at same time to avoid this;
- active against growing *M. tuberculosis.*
- dosage, 300 mg/day orally in one dose.

Aminosalicylic acid

- bacteriostatic;
- prevents organisms from developing resistance to streptomycin and isoniazid;
- toxicity
  —GI tract;
  —contraindicated in renal insufficiency and impaired hepatic function.
- dosage
  —10 to 12 gm/day for adults, orally in a single dose.

Ethambutol
- trade name Myambutol;
- bactericidal,
  —inhibits production of bacterial metabolites,
  —impairs cell metabolism,
  —stops multiplication and
  —kills the cell;
- toxicity
  —decrease in visual acuity;
  —GI tract;
- specific for *Mycobacteria.*
- dosage, 15 mg/kg/day orally in a single dose.

Ethionamide
- trade name Trecator;
- bacteriostatic;
- toxicity
  —GI tract;
  —peripheral neuritis, and may
  —intensify side effects of other antituberculous drugs;
- administer only after adequate treatment with first line drugs (streptomycin, isoniazid and PAS) has failed.
- dosage, 0.5 to 1.0 gm/day for adult, orally in divided doses.

CHLORAMPHENICOL
- bacteriostatic, interferes with bacterial protein and enzyme synthesis;
- toxicity occasionally
  —medullary aplasia with
  —aplastic anemia and
  —agranulocytosis. So
  —monitor regularly RBC and WBC counts during therapy;
- effective against
  —*Salmonella* (typhoid fever especially),
  —*Pseudomonas,*
  —*Brucella* and
  —L-forms.
- dosage, 1 to 4 gm/day orally or parenterally, in divided doses.

TETRACYCLINES
- bacteriostatic, by intefering with bacterial
  —protein and

—enzyme production, and in higher concentrations inhibit
—oxydation reaction, nucleic acid and cell wall synthesis;
- toxicity
  —stain children's teeth brown;
  —diarrhea;
  —nephrotoxicity and
  —catabolic activity causing raised BUN.
- active against
  —*Pseudomonas*,
  —*Brucella*,
  —*Pasteurella pestis* (bubonic plague),
  —*Vibrio cholerae* (cholera) and
  —L-forms.
- dosage, 1 to 2 gm/day orally, 1 gm/day IV, in divided doses.

ERYTHROMYCIN

- a macrolide;
- bacteriostatic against Gram-positive cocci, inhibiting protein synthesis;
- toxicity
  —diarrhea and may interfere with
  —liver function.
- effective especially for
  —L-forms and
  —*Mycoplasma*, but
- resistance may develop.
- dosage, 1 to 4 gm/day orally in divided doses.

AMPHOTERICIN B

- fungistatic or fungicidal
  —interferes with cell membrane;
- toxicity
  —very nephrotoxic,
  —GI disturbance,
  —anemia.
- dosage
  —250 µg/kg/day IV. Can be increased to
  —1.5 mg/kg/day to a
  —maximum total of 4 gm.

ULFONAMIDES

bacteriostatic, compete with PABA (an essential metabolite) for the bacterium's enzymes which catalyze the reaction PABA → folic acid within the cell. Folic acid is a coenzyme in the formation of certain aminoacids and purines and ultimately nucleotide and DNA synthesis;

bacteriostasis

—slows reproduction of bacteria and thereby

—facilitates the work of the white cells.

inhibited by

—pus which contains folic acid and these amino acids and purines. This is

—noncompetitive antagonism;

—competitive antagonism would be excess PABA.

toxicity

—may crystallize in the genitourinary tract and cause renal failure;

—allergies;

—blood dyscrasias;

—neuritis;

active against

—streptococcus,

—gonococcus and

—*E. coli*, especially in urinary tract infections.

dosage, 4 to 6 gm/day orally in divided doses.

chapter 26
Specific Infections

Pyogenic Staphylococcal Infections
SOFT-TISSUE INFECTION

Etiopathology

- *Staphylococcus aureus* (see Chapter 25)
- reaches tissue by
  —blood stream (bacteremia) or by
  —direct inoculation through trauma or surgery.
- organisms multiply and elicit a typical
- acute inflammatory response with
  —much edema,
  —many polymorphonuclear leukocytes followed by
  —macrophages, and
  —large quantities of fibrin, all of which
- localize the infection so that a
- circumscribed abscess is the hallmark of staphylococcal infection.
- if untreated, the abscess bursts onto an epithelial surface and drains, and the
- abscess cavity heals by
  —fibrosis and
  —inward collapse of the cavity walls

Clinical features

- the infected area is
  —painful,
  —red,
  —hot and
  —swollen; these are the
- four cardinal signs of inflammation described by the Roman physician Celsus in the first century AD.

- regional lymph nodes may be enlarged and tender;
- pus is thick, yellow and does not smell.
- fever, raised ESR and leukocytosis.

Complications

- spreading cellulitis;
- bacteremia or septicemia with formation of
- metastatic abscesses.

Treatment

- prompt and appropriate antibiotherapy following the
- culture and sensitivity patterns of the organism, and
- adequate surgical drainage of an abscess (the moon should never see an undrained abscess!) are
- keystones of successful treatment. Drain the abscess in the operating room, not in the ward! Adjuncts are
- rest and elevation of the infected limb and
- supportive therapy, including
  —adequate hydration and nutrition and correction of malnutrition to improve host defenses as well as
  —control of contributing systemic disease, e.g., diabetes mellitus.

ᴀCUTE HEMATOGENOUS OSTEOMYELITIS

Etiopathology

- most common in children;
- *Staphylococcus aureus*, the most common organism,
- reaches bone via the bloodstream during bacteremia from another focus, e.g., nose, infected scratch;
- medullary arterioles in metaphysis are end arteries and turn through 180° beneath the epiphyseal plate to empty into a network of sinusoidal veins. Arterioles do not cross the plate. In the venous sinuses, the blood flow slows; it is
- here that bacteria are able to lodge and proliferate;
- subperiosteal hematoma after a fall or a blow also provides organisms in the bloodstream with suitable "culture medium!"
- organisms proliferate, causing acute inflammatory reaction with
  —localized thrombophlebitis, edema and
  —formation of pus under pressure. This in turn causes
  —more extensive thrombophlebitis and localized arteritis obliterans, more edema and
  —more pus under increased pressure, and thus

—spread of the infection through the metaphysis and into the shaft;

- pressure forces pus through the cortex and beneath the periosteum; this is lifted off bone, subperiosteal abscess forms, and more cortex is deprived of blood supply;
- cancellous and cortical bone in the area of an abscess dies due to
  —toxins realeased by organisms and
  —destruction of blood supply; dead bone forms
  —sequestra (Fig. 26.1).
- abscess cavity in bone has rigid walls which
  —prevent collapse of the cavity and thus
  —impair healing; compare this to the soft-tissue abscess which heals partly by collapse and mechanical closure of the cavity.
- in a child under 1 year old and in an adult after the growth plate closes, infection may spread into adjacent
  —epiphysis, and thence into the
  —joint; the
- metaphyses of the proximal humerus and femoral neck are intracapsular, and metaphyseal pus may erode the cortex and synovium to enter the joint.

Clinical features
- earliest sign is
  —pain and tenderness locally; if untreated,
- clinical features become clearer and include
  —regional lymphadenitis,
  —systemic toxemia with fever, tachycardia, and
  —raised ESR and white cell count. The
- earliest radiological sign is soft-tissue swelling.
- after 10 days, other radiological signs may appear
  —local circumscribed or streaky osteolytic lesions,
  —subperiosteal reaction,
  —breach in cortex,
  —disuse osteoporosis.

Complications
- septicemia and
- pathological fracture early.
- defect in bony continuity after sequestration of full width of shaft or metaphysis when

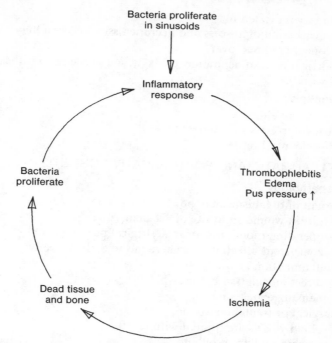

Figure 26.1. Vicious circle in acute hematogenous osteomyelitis.

—involucrum is inadequate due to
—death of periosteum or surgeon performs premature
—sequestrectomy before involucrum has time to form;
• growth-plate disturbance with shortening and axial deformity later.

Treatment
• the earlier, the better!
• broad-spectrum antibiotics until organism is identified and its sensitivities are known by
• culture of aspirated pus or by blood cultures;
• supportive therapy
  —IV fluids and
  —analgesics;
• immobilization of infected limb.

- surgery indicated for
  —evacuation of abscess and necrotic tissue; incision may be left
  —open, or closed over
  —irrigation and aspiration tubes (if you are sure that these will work!).

Prognosis

- lesion will either
- heal completely or progress to
- chronic infection.

POSTTRAUMATIC AND POSTOPERATIVE OSTEITIS

Etiopathology

- origin of organisms may be
  —dirt in wound from site of accident,
  —operating room, instruments, surgical personnel, or
  —concurrent infection elsewhere in the patient's body;
- contamination is usually by
  —direct inoculation but may be
  —hematogenous; in
- surgical or traumatic wound,
  —blood vessels are injured with resultant
  —hematoma formation and
  —bone and tissue necrosis;
  —tissue planes are dissected and
  —dead spaces are formed;
  —implants change vascular patterns. Thus
  —half the invading organism's work is already done for it!
- hematoma and necrotic tissue shield pathogenic organisms from the host's defensive inflammatory response, and infection is established, involving both bone and soft tissue from the beginning.
- open tissue planes enable infection to spread easily through local soft tissues. In
- hematogenous osteomyelitis, pus is under pressure in a closed space and is driven along the
  —medullary canal, through the
  —cortex and under the
  —periosteum; in
- osteitis, pus is not under so much pressure and may
  —not spread so extensively.

- prophylactic antibiotics may modify the infection by
  —attenuating a staphylococcal infection or by
  —allowing other organisms to establish themselves.

Clinical features are

- similar to acute hematogenous osteomyelitis but may be less marked, with
  —pain, increasing instead of diminishing,
  —some redness and edema, and later
  —discharge of seropurulent fluid or frank pus;
- radiography is not usually helpful;
- infection interferes with union of fracture or osteotomy and may cause delayed union or nonunion.

Treatment

- assume infection is deep until proven otherwise (you may fool yourself into thinking the infection is "only superficial," but you will not fool the bacteria!). If infection is deep, then
- surgical drainage as soon as possible
  —remove pus and necrotic tissue,
  —leave internal fixation in place,
  —leave the wound open,
  —immobilize the limb and give
- wide-spectrum antibiotics, but a
- warning: postoperative infection is likely to be due to
  —"hospital organisms"
  —resistant to most antibiotics, so use your
  —knowledge concerning organisms currently in the hospital, and
  —choose antibiotics accordingly; when results of
- culture and sensitivity are known, change to
- appropriate drugs.
- prevention of infection is better than cure, by
  —thorough debridement of open fractures and by
  —strict attention to aseptic techniques in the emergency department, operating room and wards.

CHRONIC BONE INFECTION

Etiopathology and clinical features

- chronic infection is usually secondary to acute osteomyelitis or osteitis which was treated late or was resistant to treatment;
- characterized by

—pain, often a sign of reactivation,

—sinuses which drain continuously or intermittently, often with secondary infection by *Pseudomonas*, *Proteus* or others,

—local soft-tissue scarring and fibrosis, and

—stiff joints proximal and distal to infection; or a

—solitary abscess cavity in a shaft or metaphysis surrounded by a shell of sclerotic bone, a Brodie's abscess.

- radiographs show irregular
  —osteolytic and
  —osteosclerotic areas of varying patterns,
  —cavities,
  —dense subperiosteal new bone and
  —sequestra;
- tomograms may show small sequestra well;
- sinogram shows extent and direction of sinuses and whether they communicate with sequestra.

Complications

- Pathological fracture;
- joint stiffness due to adhesions between muscles and bone, or to periarticular fibrosis, or to direct involvement of the joint;
- growth disturbances;
- epithelioma in sinus tract or
- amyloid disease after many years.

Treatment

- difficult! Includes
- culture and sensitivity studies, then
- appropriate antibiotics, and if
  —abscess forms or
  —sinus reopens and drains or
  —sequestrum causes recurrent infection, then
- surgery to remove
  —all dead and infected soft tissue and bone by the technique of
  —saucerization, leaving the wound open; if dead tissue is left behind in the wound, infection will recur;
  —incision and drainage of abscess is not enough. When the saucerized bed is clean and granulating, a
- small bony defect may be allowed to heal by secondary intention;
- large defect may be

  —filled with autologous cancellous bone and
  —later covered with a split-thickness skin graft if necessary.
- if fracture or osteotomy is not united but is
  —already immobilized by internal fixation, leave this in place, or
    change a small intramedullary (IM) rod for a larger one; if
    bones are not stabilized, then immobilize them with
  —external fixation; plan the
  —cancellous bone graft when infection is under control, because
  —eradication of infection is all but impossible in the presence of
    nonunion. If
- bone is united, then
  —remove internal fixation and
  —treat the infection.
- finally, in chronic infection of bone,
  —cure is
  —only apparent,
  —never certain!

PYOGENIC ARTHRITIS

Etiopathology
- contamination by
  —blood-borne bacteria,
  —spread from epiphyseal infection, or
  —direct inoculation from trauma, surgery or needle;
- synovial response is by
  —increased production of synovial fluid and
  —inflammatory reaction with output of
  —polymorphonuclear leukocytes and monocytes;
- periarticular structures, synovium, capsule and ligaments, as well
  as
- articular cartilage, may be damaged or destroyed by
  —increased intra-articular pressure,
  —direct invasion by the organisms, and
  —enzymes released by organisms and dead or dying white cells.
    This may result in
- invasion of subchondral bone with secondary infection of epiphysis, and
- instability of the joint with subluxation and dislocation (more
  likely in infants and young children).

Clinical features
- pain and muscle spasm with
- hot, red, swollen and immobile joint;
- intra-articular effusion;
- fever, raised ESR and leukocytosis;
- radiographs may show
  —soft-tissue swelling,
  —expanded capsular outline and later
  —osteoporosis;
- aspirated joint fluid shows
  —pus cells and grows
  —bacteria.

Treatment
- wide-spectrum antibiotics, and change them as necessary according to results of
- culture and sensitivities;
- arthrotomy under sterile conditions in the operating room to
  —remove all pus and debris, copious irrigation, then
  —close the wound over
  —irrigation and aspiration tubes because
  —articular cartilage will not survive if the wound is left open;
- immobilize the limb until infection is controlled, then start
- guarded, progressive mobilization of joint to preserve function.

Gas Gangrene

ETIOPATHOLOGY

Superficial wound
- Clostridia may cause
- anaerobic cellulitis with
- serous exudate and gas in fascial planes,
- necrosis, sloughing and
- pain but
- without invasion of muscle.

Deep wound
- presence of
  —dead tissue, especially muscle, where

—oxygen tension is low, is a
—prerequisite for the development of
- gas gangrene (Fig. 26.2).
- saccharolytic bacteria
  —*Clostridium welchii, C. septicum* and *C. oedematiens* (see Chapter 25)
  —ferment sugars, produce
  —odorless gas (crepitation) and
  —powerful exotoxins;
- local inflammatory response is poor and infection
  —spreads rapidly!
- tissue necrosis increases locally due to
  —toxins and
  —local edematous and gaseous compression resulting in

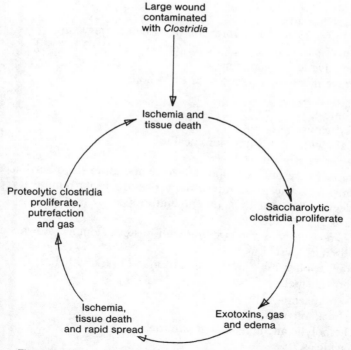

Figure 26.2. Vicious circle of ischemia and clostridial proliferation.

—ischemia; this is
- necrotizing myositis typical of gas gangrene; then
- proteolytic bacteria
  - *Clostridium sporogenes* and *C. histolyticum*
  - break down dead muscle which forms a
  - putrefying, green-black mass with
  - foul-smelling gas (crepitation) causing more tissue death and closing the
  - vicious circle. This is
- gas gangrene, i.e., tissue death with putrefaction.
- systemic toxic reaction is severe, and death follows if condition remains untreated.

CLINICAL FEATURES

- contaminated wound
  - agricultural,
  - war,
  - traffic accident, with
- dead muscle, tissue compression or vascular injury, and
- primary suture of wound are all factors
- conducive to gas gangrene.
- average incubation period is 12 to 24 hours.
- diagnosis is
  - clinical;
- early features are
  - pain with tight, shiny skin locally;
  - fever, confusion, and
  - rapid pulse out of proportion to temperature (in other bacterial infections the pulse rate usually rises 10 beats/minute for each degree Fahrenheit rise in temperature);
- later signs include
  - increasing pain and swelling with blisters, sloughs, brown smelly discharge, crepitus,
  - red, swollen muscles turning green and black with
  - horrid smell;
- severe toxemia with
  - shock, oliguria,
  - hemolytic anemia, hemoglobinuria,
  - acidosis,

—cardiotoxicity and

—death.

DIFFERENTIAL DIAGNOSIS

- Gram-negative bacteria may produce gas without the clinical syndrome of gas gangrene.
- streptococcal myonecrosis has
  —similar clinical features but
  —less severe,
  —inflammatory reaction more marked and
  —no necrotizing myositis.

TREATMENT

Anaerobic cellulitis

- wide surgical decompression and
- antibiotics.

Gas gangrene

- cornerstone is
- surgery
  —remove all necrotic and doubtful tissue,
  —decompress all involved compartments by fasciotomy,
  —irrigate well,
  —leave wound open and
  —immobilize limb.
- if in doubt,
  —amputate to
  —save the patient's life.
- antibiotics are
  —adjunct to surgery; use
  —massive doses of IV penicillins.
- replace blood loss and
- correct electrolyte and fluid imbalance.
- passive immunity is not helpful.

PREVENTION

- better than cure!
- active immunity is not possible; so avoid infection by
- prompt surgical debridement of contaminated wounds,
- leave wound open,
- no constricting

—casts or
—bandages, and give
- antibiotics.

Tetanus

ETIOPATHOLOGY

Clostridium tetani (see Chapter 25)
- spores exist typically in
  —clay soils where population is dense and climate is warm and wet,
  —dust of buildings and clothes,
  —human intestinal tracts, and on
  —skin of outdoor workers.
- entry wound may be insignificant. The
- infection remains localized, but the organism releases
  —neurotropic exotoxins which travel to the spinal cord and
  —interfere with inhibitory impulses at the
  —interneuronal synapse.
- prerequisites for infection include
  —tissue necrosis and
  —low oxygen tension locally.

CLINICAL FEATURES

- incubation period is 2 to 60 days
  —the shorter, the worse the prognosis;
- muscle contractions include
  —risus sardonicus (sardonic smile) due to fascial muscle spasm, often
    the first sign,
  —glottal spasm,
  —increasing spinal lordosis (opisthotonos),
  —arms flexed and
  —legs extended. Muscle contractions are
  —persistent and painful;
- paroxysmal muscle spasms;
- complications may include
  —cardiac arrhythmias,
  —atelectasis and
  —fractures.

TREATMENT

- surgical debridement, and leave wound open;

- passive immunity,
  —3,000 to 6,000 IU gamma globulin in divided doses;
- tracheotomy at earliest sign of
  —pharyngeal or laryngeal spasm;
- sedation
  —quiet, darkened room,
  —valium,
  —sodium pentothal (supervised by an anesthetist);
- antibiotics in massive doses
  —penicillin and
  —streptomycin;
- redress fluid and electrolyte imbalance.
- mortality rate is high.

PROPHYLAXIS

- active immunity is best
  —three IM injections of toxoid over a period of 3 months with a
  —booster 1 year later.
- passive immunity with
  —hyperimmune human gamma globulin,
  —250 IU by IM route.
- surgical debridement of contaminated wound is important, and
  —leave wound open. In this disease
- prevention is much better than cure!

Tuberculosis

ETIOPATHOLOGY

Mycobacterium tuberculosis (see Chapter 25).

- infection contracted by
  —inhalation (human strain) or by
  —ingestion (bovine strain) in contaminated milk where herds are not controlled or milk is not pasteurized.
- initial acute inflammatory response is
  —brief; tubercle bacilli
  —kill polymorphonuclear leukocytes; these are replaced by
- macrophages which
  —phagocytose the bacilli and then change to become
  —epithelioid cells (pale cytoplasm and elongated nuclei), or fuse to form

—Langhans' giant cells;
- lymphocytes and fibroblasts gather around this mass, the center of which
  —necroses and forms a
  —caseous (cheesy) core;
- infective focus now called a
- tuberculous follicle. Similar follicles are seen in some mycoses and in sarcoidosis.
- caseation may continue, with softening and liquefaction, to form a
- tuberculous (cold) abscess. This may
- rupture to exterior and form tuberculous sinus; or it may
- spread locally, by
  —macrophages which carry off the bacilli without killing them; or
- spread further afield along
  —serous cavities, epithelial surfaces,
  —lymphatics (tuberculous lymphadenitis) and
  —bloodstream (miliary and metastatic tuberculosis). Or the focus may
- heal by fibrosis, from surrounding fibroblasts. This may be
  —complete, fibrous nodule, or
  —incomplete, with a fibrous shell around a central caseous core which may slowly calcify and may
  —contain live bacilli for years.

ALLERGY AND IMMUNOLOGY

- primary (initial) infection changes body's response, after 4 to 6 weeks, to a
- second infection by creating an
  —allergic (hypersensitive) reaction to the bacteria's tuberculoprotein (tuberculin), and by
- localization and healing of the second infection,
  —an acquired immunological response which is cell-mediated (lymphocytic), enabling macrophages to kill tubercle bacilli. This immunity to tuberculosis is usually only partial, never as complete as immunity to smallpox.
- BCG is an attenuated bovine strain of the bacillus injected intradermally in nonimmune patients to induce
  —immunity; it also produces
  —hypersensitivity, and this can be shown by the
- Mantoux test, an intradermal injection of PPD (purified protein

derivative of tuberculin) which produces a
—local reaction within 48 hours in hypersensitive individuals; this
• positive reaction is assumed to indicate immunity too, although hypersensitivity and immunity are only partly interdependent.

CLINICAL FEATURES
• infection in industrialized countries is usually pulmonary, with human strain, and causes
—cough and perhaps hemoptysis;
• systemic reaction includes
—fever, raised ESR and monocytosis,
—loss of appetite and weight,
—malaise, and
—pain and limitation of movement when bone or joint is affected.
• Ghon focus occurs in children and is a
—primary area at the edge of the lung, often in midzone, with perhaps
—secondary involvement of hilar nodes (Ghon complex).
• Assmann focus in adults is an
—apical or a subapical lesion with local destruction but
—rarely lymph node involvement. This localization is due perhaps to an
—immune response after previous infection, or
—maturity of adult tissues which are less susceptible to the bacteria.
• bovine strain causes
—enteritis and peritonitis, with little lymphadenitis in adults, and
—extensive mesenteric adenitis with little bowel involvement in children.
• skeletal tuberculosis usually starts 2 or 3 years after the primary focus in the intestine or lung; spreads by the bloodstream. It may start in the
—metaphysis, eroding the growth plate to reach the physis and then the joint, or it may start in the joint as a
—synovitis. Hip and knee are most common joints involved.
• Pott's disease, the most common skeletal focus of tuberculosis, is often
—secondary to urinary tract tuberculosis; the infection usually starts in the
—vertebral body, spreads up and down beneath the longitudinal ligament to

—involve adjacent bodies with the
—destruction of discs,
—anterior collapse and formation of
—kyphosis and
—paravertebral abscess.
- healing of untreated skeletal lesions is usually by
    —fibrous ankylosis and sometimes by
    —ossification with resultant
    —fusion of the joint or adjacent vertebral bodies.

TREATMENT
- triple antibiotic therapy is the cornerstone of treatment (see Chapter 25).
- improvement of the nutritional status of the patient;
- isolation, from the community, of the infectious ("open") tuberculous patient and
- screening of the patient's relatives and close contacts.
- surgey when indicated
    —aspiration or drainage of a persistent abscess;
    —sequestrectomy;
    —synovectomy of a joint with tuberculous synovitis but intact articular cartilage, to preserve mobility of the joint; or
    —arthroplasty or fusion of a painful or an unstable joint damaged beyond redemption.

PREVENTION
- improvement of socioeconomic standards is the single most important factor in prevention of tuberculosis. The incidence of tuberculosis is a good indicator of the socioeconomic conditions of a geographical area;
- vaccination of susceptible (Mantoux-negative) people likely to be exposed to tuberculosis infection, e.g., health workers;
- improvement of conditions in mines and factories where industrial pulmonary disease, e.g., silicosis in coal miners, increases the likelihood of pulmonary tuberculosis;
- mass miniature radiography in screening large populations for early diagnosis.

Acute Anterior Poliomyelitis

VIROLOGY

- polio virus is a
  - —polyhedron with 20 facets (icosahedron),
  - —27 μm (millionths of a millimeter) long;
- central core is RNA, a single chain of about 7,500 nucleotides, which
  - —carries all the genetic information of the virus and can
  - —translate this directly into more viral RNA and protein inside the host cell (polio virus is an obligatory intracellular parasite, like all viruses). RNA is surrounded by
- icosahedral capsid (coat or shell) made of 252 capsomeres (subunits) of protein.
- three types of polio virus infect humans,
  - —types I, II and III, of which
  - —type I is the most common (90%).
- polio virus can exist for weeks outside the body at room temperature, but
- humans are the only reservoir.

PATHOLOGY

- ultimate target cells are motor cells of the spinal cord's anterior horn and cranial motor nerve cells;
- when polio virus has proliferated in intestinal lymphoid tissue and other sites, the
- virus is
  - —absorbed to the target cell wall at a specific receptor site, and the
  - —RNA is released and penetrates the cell to reach the cellular cytoplasm;
- viral RNA then goes into the eclipse phase, during which it
  - —inhibits normal cellular RNA and protein synthesis and
  - —redirects the cell's ribosome system to
  - —replicate viral RNA and protein; then in the
  - —proliferative phase, new complete virus particles are formed within the cellular cytoplasm (100,000 within 6 hours—fast work!) The
- cell dies and bursts, allowing new virus particles to escape and infect other cells.
- acute inflammatory response is invoked, mainly with
  - —lymphocytes and

—macrophages, including microglial cells, which phagocytose cell debris (neuronophagia).

CLINICAL FEATURES

- viruses are
  —ingested in contaminated food or water, and
  —enter Peyer's patches where they multiply before
  —invading the bloodstream (viremia) via the lymphatics to multiply in other extraneural sites; then by the bloodstream again to the
  —central nervous system (beginning of the paralytic phase);
- viruses may be present in stools for several weeks after the initial illness. There are no known carriers. Clinically there are five phases:

Incubation

- incubation period is 3 to 30 days and lasts from ingestion of viruses to the beginning of the paralytic phase.

Prodromal (viremic) phase

- lasts about 3 days, consists of a prodromal syndrome similar to influenza, with
  —fever, runny nose, pharyngitis,
  —generalized muscle and joint pains, and
  —headache; viral invasion of the neuronal cells starts the next phase.

Paralysis

- paralytic phase lasts 2 to 3 days and usually reaches maximum extent within this time. Characteristics are
  —pain and spasm of affected muscles, followed by
  —lower motor neuron paralysis, usually
  —assymetrical, with
  —rapid wasting and
  —negative Babinski;
  —bulbar involvement with untreated respiratory paralysis will kill the patient;
  —sensation is normal, but
  —trophic skin changes occur;
  —fever subsides at the beginning of this phase.
- muscles innervated by a short column of anterior horn cells, e.g., tibialis posterior, are more likely to be completely paralyzed than are those with long-column innervation, e.g. extensor hallucis longus;

- exercise, fatigue, pregnancy, surgery and immunization during an epidemic may increase the paralysis.

Recovery phase

- recovery (convalescent) phase
  —starts about 10 days later and may
  —continue for 2 years. It is rapid at first but is always
  —unpredictable.

Residual phase

- residual (final) phase is that of
  —permanent paralysis with associated
  —deformities, contractures and growth disturbances; this is the phase of
  —reconstructive surgery.

DIFFERENTIAL DIAGNOSIS

- transverse myelitis (Guillain-Barré). Differences are
  —no fever,
  —symmetrical paralysis and
  —hypoesthesia and anesthesia;
- diphtheria
  —paralysis of the
  —palate and of accommodation precedes
  —paraplegia. Diphtheritic polyneuropathy also causes
  —loss of deep sensation and proprioception.
- bacterial meningitis may mimic the meningeal form of polio, but
  —hematological and
  —CSF findings help differentiate these.

TREATMENT

- close monitoring of the respiratory status during the paralytic phase to avoid respiratory failure and death;
- complete bed rest during this phase will reduce the extent of permanent paralysis; position the limbs to avoid joint deformities;
- physiotherapy is given at the beginning of the recovery phase to
  —maintain function of unparalyzed muscles,
  —strengthen recovering muscles and
  —avoid contractures.
- reconstructive surgery generally is not indicated until the patient enters the
  —final phase of

—residual paralysis and deformities. Then surgery may be necessary for

—correction of deformities by soft-tissue release and osteotomy,

—muscle and tendon transfers to reestablish motor power, and

—stabilization of unstable joints by fusion or bone blocks;

• rehabilitation combined with surgery and physiotherapy may

—enable patient to walk, with or without braces, and

—reintegrate into society as an independent and productive person.

PROPHYLAXIS

• virus-neutralizing antibodies (immunoglobulins) prevent virus attaching itself to host cells;

• cell-mediated immunity also is important, through

—sensitized lymphocytes which may secrete interferon and may also kill infected cells and thus their viral contents, and through

—interferon production by infected cells themselves; this antiviral protein may prevent synthesis of viral proteins but does not interfere with normal cellular protein manufacture.

• passive immunity is conferred from mother to newborn; this rapidly disappears when breast feeding stops;

• active immunity may be acquired

—naturally by a subclinical attack of polio; this was common before the use of vaccines became widespread; or

—artificially by vaccination.

Salk vaccine

• virus inactivated by formol, trivalent, i.e. all three types of virus are included;

• does not change intestinal resistance to polio virus infection because

• immunity is due to IgG (circulating immunoglobulins);

• can be combined with other vaccines and toxoids;

• administration by

—two IM injections 4 weeks apart, and a

—third 6 months later and

—booster 1 year after that;

—revaccination may be necessary in face of an epidemic because duration of immunity is uncertain.

Sabin vaccine

• live attenuated virus, trivalent;

• virus infects bowel but does not spread to CNS;

- intestinal infection is uncertain because
  —resident viral flora or
  —enteritis (common in tropics) may prevent this. Several doses of trivalent vaccine may circumvent these difficulties;
- great disadvantage is that vaccine is
  —thermolabile and must
  —remain frozen from manufacturer to patient; this "cold chain" may be difficult to maintain even in North America; imagine the
  —difficulties and risks that may arise in a tropical country!
- immunity is by IgA in intestinal secretions, and also by circulating IgG, and is faster and longer lasting than by inactivated virus;
- contraindications to live viral vaccination include
  —steroid or immunosuppressive therapy,
  —enteritis and
  —pregnancy;
  —neither within 2 weeks of oropharyngeal or dental surgery, nor
  —within 3 weeks of other vaccinations.
- administration is by
  —three oral doses 4 weeks apart, and
  —boosters 1 and 5 years later.

Hospital Infection

GENERAL

- hospital infection is acquired by the patient during hospitalization;
- the organisms are usually
  —resistant to common antibiotics because these have been used worldwide
  —indiscriminately in the past; the resistant population of organisms has
  —emerged by selection and is
  —perpetuated by cross-infection. So the
- vicious circle is fueled by continued
  —injudicious use of antibiotics (Fig. 26.3)

SOURCES AND SPREAD

Staphylococcus aureus

- sources are
  —nose (reservoir of organisms in 25% to 40% of hospital personnel),

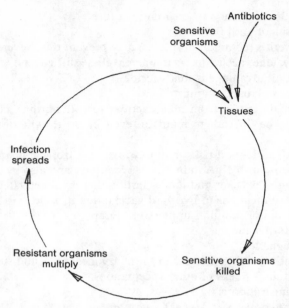

Figure 26.3. Antibiotics drive the vicious circle and increase the population of resistant staphylococci in hospital infection.

—perineum, and any staphylococcal
   —lesions discharging pus;
* transfer to patient (cross-infection) is by
   —hands,
   —other objects (fomites), cups, blankets, or the
   —air;
* patient may infect herself from her own reservoir (auto-infection);
* contamination may occur in the
   —operating room (more likely) or in the
   —surgical wards;
* peroperative contamination may be due to
   —air-borne organisms (test air with sedimentation plate or slit-sampler),
   —personnel (breaks in technique),
   —contaminated instruments,

—the patient's own skin which will harbor the hospital variety within 2 or 3 days of admission, or

—the patient's bloodstream through bacteremia from a distant site;

- infection in the surgical ward due to contaminated
  —air,
  —bed clothes,
  —personnel and other patients who are carriers or have infections; or
  —auto-infection (perhaps secondary to cross-contamination which occurred earlier).
- epidemics caused by
  —certain strains, e.g., type-80 staphylococcus.

Streptococcus pyogenes

- sources are throat and nose;
- transfer is by direct contact.

Enterobacteriaceae

- colon houses
  —*E. coli* always and
  —*Proteus* frequently; so most infections of these organisms are due to
- auto-infection.
- *Pseudomonas pyocyanea* contamination occurs from infected
  —genitourinary tracts and
  —wounds of other patients, and is
- cross-infection by direct contact of
  —ward staff or contaminated
  —instruments (e.g., urinary catheter).

PREVENTION

Operating room

Design

- "clean" operating block isolated from the hospital with
- properly designed
  —patient,
  —personnel,
  —linen and
  —instrument flow to avoid contamination of operating rooms;

- positive pressure ventilation system with filters and controlled
  - —temperature and
  - —humidity.
- "dirty" operating rooms either
  - —isolated from "clean" rooms or at least
  - —reserved only for infected cases.

Personnel

- do not allow the
  - —patient's bed clothes or
  - —personnel with overt straphylococcal infections or
  - —carriers of epidemic staphylococcal strains into the operating suite;
- all personnel entering the area should
  - —remove outer street clothes and wear
  - —gown, cap to cover all hair and overshoes, as well as
  - —mask in the operating rooms themselves;
- careful attention to
  - —sterilization of instruments,
  - —cleanliness of rooms, corridors and equipment, and
  - —aseptic technique throughout the procedure;
- control of
  - —personnel entering and leaving rooms during surgery and control of
  - —spectators.

Surgical wards

- isolate
  - —infected patients,
  - —carriers of epidemic strains, and patients particularly
  - —susceptible to infection; use
- aseptic technique when changing dressings, and
- dispose promptly of contaminated articles and dressings; use
- closed urinary drainage systems;
- keep wards clean and
- disinfect contaminated areas and equipment.

Suggested Further Reading

Gray's Anatomy, edited by Warwick, R., and Williams, P.L., Ed. 35. W.B. Saunders Company, Philadelphia, 1973.

Last, R.J. *Anatomy, Regional and Applied*, Ed. 6. Churchill Livingstone, Edinburgh, 1978.

Walter, J.B., and Israel, M.S. *General Pathology*, Ed. 5. Churchill Livingstone, Edinburgh, 1979.

Textbook of Surgery, edited by Sabiston, D.C., Ed. 11. W.B. Saunders Company, Philadelphia, 1977.

INDEX